The Holistic Treatment of Sleep Disorders

Carolin Marx-Dick

The Holistic Treatment of Sleep Disorders

Complementary Therapy Concept for Physicians and Psychotherapists

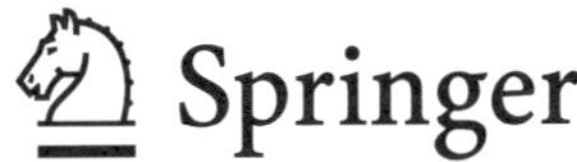

Carolin Marx-Dick
Center for Sleep Health
Psychotherapeutic Practice
Dresden, Germany

ISBN 978-3-662-67175-7   ISBN 978-3-662-67176-4   (eBook)
https://doi.org/10.1007/978-3-662-67176-4

This Springer imprint is published by the registered company Springer-Verlag GmbH, DE, part of Springer Nature.
The registered company address is: Heidelberger Platz 3, 14197 Berlin, Germany

Foreword

Sleep is a basic need of all human beings and thus necessary for life, but above all for a healthy life. Although the sleep center is located right in the middle of the brain, this life-essential center is embedded in a complex machine—the machine of the human body including the human soul.

Dr. Marx-Dick does not consider sleep to be an isolated phenomenon, or a sleep disorder to be an isolated disorder, but she considers our elixir of life—sleep in the context of the whole—namely in the context of the human being, which is uniquely shaped by the physical, mental and spiritual properties.

Only with such a holistic view can an improvement, or even the elimination of the sleep problem be achieved.

To do this, Dr. Marx-Dick describes a variety of mental disorders that can occur simultaneously, as well as in advance, or as a consequence of a sleep disorder.

The readers thus have the opportunity to inform themselves about a whole range of psychological diagnoses and perhaps also to recognize some of them in themselves or in their nearest and dearest and thus to take the right steps in time to prevent and treat them.

Not only other psychological disorders, but also the "normal" physiological processes such as the sleep-wake rhythm and the associated "science of nature rhythms"—chronobiology—are described pictorially and a simple way for the reader.

In addition, it contains many worksheets and information sheets or diaries for psychological therapists and doctors, which are available as download material so that our colleagues also want to work with their clients.

Dr. Marx-Dick had the ambition to make the book as practical as possible and thus offer interested colleagues a quick access to treatment.

The book contains both practical experience of the last 20 years of practical work, as well as theoretical building blocks on the principles of cognitive behavioral therapy, but also on modern approaches such as Mind-Body-Sleep-Dynamic©, which Dr. Marx-Dick uses in her practice.

In addition, the book contains the latest psychological topics such as interpersonal social rhythm therapy, mind-body medicine, sexuality and also lucid dreaming and many other exciting treatment methods.

My colleague Dr. Marx-Dick is a psychologist and sleep therapist by passion who gives her knowledge to her patients with all her heart.

The book is absolutely recommendable and a "must have read"!

March 2022   Prof. Dr. Kneginja Richter

Preface

Working Together to Improve the Care of People with Sleep Disorders

Dear colleagues,
natural sleep is healthy sleep. It provides the perfect conditions for regeneration and the development of vitality and resilience for body and mind. No other state of the body or other conditions are able to do this. Sleep makes us healthy and keeps us healthy, it makes us clever, it rejuvenates us and even makes us physically more attractive.

However, there are many people who suffer from pathological and urgently treatable sleep disorders. Estimates by the German Society for Sleep Research and Sleep Medicine (DGSM) suggest that around 30% of the population in Germany suffer from sleep disorders. There are around 17 million people affected by treatable insomnia, that is, sleep disorders. This is the most common sleep disorder worldwide. A further 10 million people are diagnosed with sleep disorders related to breathing. In addition, there are narcolepsy, nightmares, sleepwalking, night-time movement disorders and many more, which complete the total of over 80 existing sleep disorders.

Those affected seek help in general practitioners', specialists' and psychotherapists' practices and pharmacies. The therapies offered are certainly always very well intentioned, but often do not go beyond the prescription of sleep medication. The German Society for Sleep Research and Sleep Medicine (DGSM) estimates that currently only around 1% of people with insomnia in Germany receive adequate treatment for their condition.

Since 2015, I have been developing targeted methods for the treatment of sleep disorders in my specialized psychotherapeutic practice. This condition is highly dynamic and requires patient-specific treatment concepts. This is also the reason why online and app-based treatment approaches or so-called "sleep schools" cannot achieve comparable treatment success to specific holistic psychotherapy.

I would like to invite you to benefit from my more than 20 years of experience as a scientist and focused psychotherapist and to enable your patients to receive comprehensive treatment.

Originally, a second edition of my first book "Non-organic sleep disorders" (Springer, 2016) was planned. However, when working on the new content, I realized that the framework of a second edition would be blown up, as a lot has happened in sleep research in the past seven years. In addition, I have developed new treatment approaches in my treatments that I do not want to withhold from you. Therefore, you are now holding a new and by far more comprehensive work in your hands. "Sleep disorders—holistic treatment" contains 80% new knowledge and current scientific findings in comparison to its predecessor "Non-organic sleep disorders". The innovative treatment approach started there is supplemented and extended.

I am particularly committed to the holistic view of sleep disorders. Each sleep disorder and its comorbidity has physical correlates. Therefore, I am convinced that only an all-encompassing view can lead to sustainable treatment.

In order to make it easier for you to get started in the treatment of your patients with sleep disorders, I would like to provide you with many information and work sheets, as well as diary templates for your everyday practice, as I use them in my daily work, in addition to the collected knowledge in the book. You will find in this work all instructions for a free download of these materials for use in your treatments. The documents can be found under https://drcarolinmarxdick.de/download_en/.

I am very happy about your feedback on these documents.

Only together can we help all those affected to relieve their suffering, to find a healthy sleep and a fulfilled life. I am happy if I can help you and your patients with this work.

Dr. Carolin Marx-Dick
Psychological Psychotherapist

Contents

1 Healthy Sleep 1
  1.1 Why do We Sleep?—The Evolution Theory 2
  1.2 The Circadian Process 4
  1.3 How do We Sleep? 10
  1.4 The Functions of Sleep 13
  1.5 Hormones that Determine Sleep 21
  References 25

2 Sleep Disorders 29
  2.1 Epidemiology 30
  2.2 The Origin of Sleep Disorders 31
  2.3 Diagnostics and Classification 38
  2.4 Common Comorbidities 57
  2.5 Dealing with People with Sleep Disorders 61
  References 65

**3 Therapy Concept for the Holistic Treatment of Sleep
Disorders** 67
  3.1 Background 68
  3.2 Formal Structure and Framework Conditions
       of Therapy 69
  3.3 Development of the Disorder Model 71
  3.4 Modules of Cognitive Behavioral Therapy 72
  3.5 Nightmare Therapy 131
  3.6 Third Wave of Behavior Therapy 135
  3.7 Mind-Body-Medicine 156
  3.8 Manual Procedures 174
  3.9 Neurotherapy 178
  3.10 Pharmacotherapy: Opportunities and Risks 188
  3.11 Phytotherapeutics 200
  3.12 Dietary Supplements 202
  3.13 Placebo 205
  3.14 Relapse Prevention and Follow-Up 206
  References 207

Case reports 211

Healthy Sleep

Contents

1.1   Why do We Sleep?—The Evolution Theory. 2
   1.1.1   The Evolutionary Development of Human Sleep. 2
   1.1.2   The Evolutionary Protective Functions of Sleep 3
1.2   The Circadian Process 4
   1.2.1   Homeostasis—Balancing of Fatigue and Wakefulness 4
   1.2.2   The 2-Process Model 5
   1.2.3   Light as a Pacemaker 6
   1.2.4   Temperature Course and Heat Regulation 7
   1.2.5   Chronobiology 8
   1.2.6   The Ultradian Rhythm 9
1.3   How do We Sleep? 10
   1.3.1   The Physiology of Sleep. 10
1.4   The Functions of Sleep. 13
   1.4.1   Regeneration. 13
   1.4.2   The Synaptic Homeostasis "tidying up and Making Room for New
           Ones" 14
   1.4.3   Memory Formation. 15
   1.4.4   Emotional regulation 16
   1.4.5   Immune regulation 17
   1.4.6   Metabolism. 19
   1.4.7   Calibration 20
   1.4.8   The Function of Dreams. 20
1.5   Hormones that Determine Sleep. 21
   1.5.1   Adenosine. 21
   1.5.2   Melatonin 22
   1.5.3   Cortisol. 22
   1.5.4   Adrenaline and Noradrenaline 23
   1.5.5   Serotonin. 24
   1.5.6   Dopamine 24
   1.5.7   Orexin. 25
   1.5.8   Other Messengers. 25
References 25

C. Marx-Dick, *The Holistic Treatment of Sleep Disorders*, https://doi.org/10.1007/978-3-662-67176-4_1

▶ The chapter provides an overview of how important a good night's sleep is for health. For a basic understanding, it is essential to know the homeostatic basic process of sleep and wakefulness, the physiology of healthy sleep with sleep architecture, the hormonal cycles as well as the development of the need for sleep over the lifespan of humans. The importance of a good night's sleep is reflected in a variety of its functions, which are impaired by bad nights. For example, sleep deprivation can manifest itself in higher susceptibility to infection due to a weakened immune system or with mental disorders due to dysfunctional emotion regulation. Memory formation and metabolism, and much more, are also regulated during sleep.

Only when we understand healthy sleep can we treat sleep disorders. Healthy sleep comes and goes on its own, does not need to be optimized, generated or forced.

▶ Healthy, natural sleep is our treatment goal.

Without a good night's sleep, the quality of life immediately decreases and the risk of serious physical and mental illness increases in the long term.

1.1 Why do We Sleep?—The Evolution Theory

To understand how and why we sleep, we need to trace the functions that sleep has had for humans and their ancestors at different times in Earth's history and how those functions have changed in dependence on the natural conditions. *We need to understand the evolution of sleep.*

Because of the Earth's rotation, all organisms have been subject to a light-dark, or day-night, rhythm since the beginning of time on Earth. Even the simplest single-celled algae oriented their activity according to the position of the sun. The flowers of various plants also open and close, shoots and leaves are oriented according to the course of the sun's rays, the source of light and temperature. With the beginning of life on Earth, adaptations to the light and temperature conditions of the 24-hour cycle took place as part of evolution. Only those species have survived that were able to adapt and coordinate their metabolism accordingly (Staedt and Stoppe 2001).

> Everything that is against nature does not last in the long run! (Charles Darwin)

But that's not all: Over the course of evolution, nature has adapted the various species to the change between day and night so that they can almost perfectly use the different conditions and thus an enormous variety of species has arisen.

In my treatment practice, I often refer back to the evolutionary development of sleep to illustrate to patients that, for example, a polyphasic sleep (i.e. multiple sleep phases per night or within 24 h) is natural and therefore quite healthy. The aim of therapy is then to bring this natural sleep into harmony with modern social life. For many sufferers, this information is already helpful in alleviating fears and thus improving quality of life.

1.1.1 The Evolutionary Development of Human Sleep

The need for sleep and cognitive performance are inversely proportional to each other: The more cognitive performance an organism has to provide, the greater its need for sleep for regeneration, and the greater its cognitive performance is again. This course was evolutionarily important for the development of brain function: With the increase in brain mass (development of neural networks), cognitive performance could also be increased. For this development process, our ancestors had to expend more energy, that is, find more food. To secure this increasing need for food, it was necessary to remember places with good conditions for food search and hunting. Therefore, more neural structures were needed for better cognitive performance. For this, the expansion of memory was essential. Sleep is one of the most important functions for memory consolidation.

▶ *The further development of neural structures in the brain needed more energy; more energy can only be gained through more food; only "well-rested hunters and gatherers found enough food for this development due to their neurocognitive abilities"* (Staedt and Stoppe 2001).

As a result, the human need for sleep has continuously increased.

1.1.2 The Evolutionary Protective Functions of Sleep

Sleep has a protective function in darkness for diurnal animals like humans. Humans are not "nocturnal animals". They lack the necessary features such as good night vision, a good sense of smell or other orientation options in the dark (e.g. ultrasound in bats). Therefore, one of the main driving forces of evolutionary processes was the protection against dangers. Night-time food search and hunting were very dangerous in the dark, and our ancestors were not able to orient themselves sufficiently in their environment. Therefore, it was "advisable" for Homo sapiens to retire at night and seek shelter to recover from the day's exertions and only "leave the cave" during daylight hours (Allison and van Twyver 1970).

Our human sleep architecture provides that we experience different states of consciousness during sleep. Among other things, we experience a total of up to 2 h of unconsciousness every night, from which only a pain stimulus can wake us up. In addition, these deep sleep phases alternate with phases of lighter sleep and wakefulness, in which even our ancestors were somnolent, that is, not conscious. This means that for nocturnal attackers, man has always been and still is an easy prey. As Allan Rechtschaffen, one of the pioneers of sleep research, so aptly put it:

If sleep did not have a basic life-sustaining function, it would be by far the biggest mistake of evolution. (Rechtschaffen 1978)

It is worth knowing for your patients with sleep disorders that our original night sleep did not take place in one continuous sleep phase. It is now assumed that our ancestors were awake several times during the night and sometimes for longer periods of time in order to look after themselves. Therefore, although nocturnal wakefulness is stressful, it is not necessarily pathological. Moreover, it is remarkable that our body is naturally designed to sleep or rest during the day, for example at noon. Because even the midday nap had evolutionary advantages: The recovery phase at noon enabled early Homo to recover from the morning's exertions and to mobilize sufficient cognitive and physical resources in the afternoon to go in search of food and to defend themselves against threats. This resting phase at noon was therefore essential in order to ensure the survival of the species. Based on this, it makes sense why most people still experience a so-called "midday slump" with reduced body functions today and why many people take a siesta or a midday nap during this time.

The described behaviors of our ancestors are reflected in our current knowledge of sleep and the underlying physiological processes.

The sleep-wake behavior adapted to the light-dark rhythm follows a circadian rhythm, the metronome of which is light and the change in temperature over 24 h.

This rhythm influences almost all human life functions, such as performance, body temperature, blood pressure, heart rate, lung and organ function, hormone concentration, etc., which run periodically at different times of the day.

Thus, the "ineffectiveness" of the human organism in the darkness can be used exceptionally well to prepare body and mind for its functions during daylight (Zulley 2010).

If this process "undisturbed" and adapted to the respective needs and requirements of the sleeper proceeds, the human being remains healthy. Sleep disorders then have no breeding ground. Only the work rhythm of industrialization and the invention of the light bulb made it possible to work also during darkness and at night. Therefore it was necessary to sleep "more effectively": in a long nocturnal sleep phase. From our genetically determined polyphasic sleep pattern (one or more wake phases at night and one or more sleep phases during the day) a monophasic sleep had to become.

▶ The invention of the light bulb (1879) by Thomas Alva Edison was virtually the birth of sleep disorders.

From now on it was possible to be awake at any time of day or night and to do things. The research of the indigenous people confirm this thesis: Before the introduction of electric light, all residents of a group went to bed at about the same time. Through artificial light, the different chronotypes from owl to lark developed and the total sleep time shortened.

Excursus into the Sleep Behavior of Animals

The evolutionary adaptation of the sleep behavior of the various species, regardless of whether they are nocturnal or diurnal, can be very well recognized according to their respective life requirements. For example, many migratory birds that have to fly very long distances in one go can also sleep during the flight. However, this sleep state usually only lasts an average of 30 sec, so that the animals do not crash. These short sleep times add up to several hours over 24 hours, however. Other migratory birds only sleep with one hemisphere of the brain, in order to be able to fly and steer with the other hemisphere while awake. Also the group or flock behavior was adapted to these special conditions by evolution. Thus, the sleeping birds arrange themselves in the middle of the travel group in order not to get lost. After all, common swift can be in the air for up to 10 months without a break.

Many fish sleep while swimming with their eyes open and intact visual reaction ability, in order to be able to recognize potential dangers even during the resting state. The sleep of dolphins is particularly interesting: They only sleep with one hemisphere of the brain, in order to be able to coordinate the surfacing and air-breathing during sleep with the vigilance of the other hemisphere (Kavanau 1997).

If nature had not carried out these environmental adaptation processes as part of evolution, there would be no living beings today that would sleep, because they would not have survived in terms of the food chain or natural selection. However, since sleep has many survival-critical functions, as described below, the lifespan of the respective species would be shortened by a multiple. Tortoises are known to have a life expectancy of up to 100 years. However, if you refuse these animals the winter dormancy, which is equivalent to a sleep, they will only live an average of 30 years.

There is a considerable variance between different organisms in terms of the duration, type and structure of sleep. They show different evolutionary processes of adaptation to their respective environmental and (over) living requirements. A number of studies indicate that the variability of sleep behavior follows a complex genetic architecture. It seems that the existence of a sleep-wake rhythm or a rest-activity periodicity is common to all living beings (Keene and Duboue 2018).

1.2　The Circadian Process

1.2.1　Homeostasis— Balancing of Fatigue and Wakefulness

One of the most important observations of sleep research was that prolonged wakefulness fatigues and subsequent sleep debilitates. From this came the term "sleep pressure".

▶ The longer the wakefulness lasts, the higher the sleep pressure builds up, the more tired we become.

This dynamics is subject to the principle of homeostasis. The term Homeostasis comes from the Greek and means "equality". In the biological-medical context, homeostasis describes a dynamic regulatory process for maintaining physiological balance and constant internal processes in the organism. Homeostasis does not describe a rigid state of balance that is set once and then basically balanced, but it is subject to constant fluctuations and is constantly being re-adjusted—in the sense of a feedback loop. Basically, it is not the case that a longer period of wakefulness also requires a longer period of sleep. Our body is naturally designed to get the sleep it needs. This means that, in order to maintain the balance between fatigue and detraining, our body can "sleep more effectively" in the same amount of time. With two nights of natural sleep, the fatigue of a longer period with too little sleep can usually be compensated.

Alexander Borbély took up this homeostatic process of sleep and wakefulness in 1982. He set the process of fatigue (sleep pressure) against the circadian process, which runs daily parallel to it in the human body. In this process, various hormones such as cortisol and dopamine, body temperature and the sleep-wake rhythm are synchronized in a circadian, that is, approximately 24-hour interval. The decisive factor for this interval are the CLOCK genes in the suprachiasmatic nucleus (SCN), the "internal clock" or the body's "pacemaker". Natural pacemakers such as light, daytime temperature or stable social timekeepers such as clocks, work and meal times can additionally influence the pace of the "internal clock".

1.2.2   The 2-Process Model

In the figure shown here 1.1 you can see Borbély's 2-process model (1982) . The red, rather jagged curve represents the sleep pressure (process S), the yellow, wavy line represents the circadian day curve, process C.

After a refreshing sleep, an organism is so rested that the sleep pressure (process S) is virtually nonexistent at the beginning of the day. With increasing wakefulness, it grows continuously. Because the individual's circadian rhythm (process C) antagonistically suppresses the steadily increasing sleep pressure, the subjectively perceived fatigue does not increase continuously in the morning (Dijk and Edgar 1999; Borbély and Achermann 1999). In order to counter the sleep pressure, the body increasingly sends centrally controlled wake-up signals, represented in process C (also called circadian alerting signal, CAS). These signals cause an increasing release of activating and wake-promoting hormones, so that people remain awake and performant over a longer period of time without feeling the steadily increasing sleep pressure.

Background

After waking up in the morning, the sleep pressure increases continuously throughout the day until it reaches its maximum shortly before falling asleep in the evening. As early as the

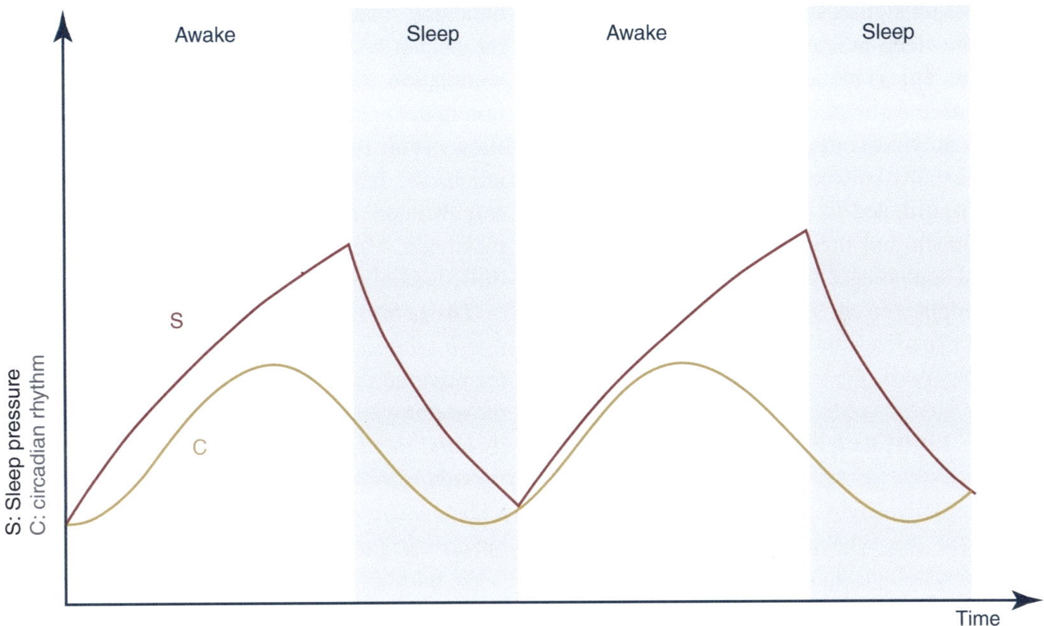

Fig. 1.1   2-Process- Model by Borbély

eighteenth century, the doctor Hufeland spoke of the *"evening fever"* which set in after 12–16 h of *"uninterrupted intense life"* (Hufeland 1797). Today it is known that during this process during the day the fatigue-inducing hormone adenosine accumulates in the body and generates and amplifies the sleep pressure (Cajochen 2009). It acts in the central nervous system as a neuromodulator and blocks the release of activating neurotransmitters such as acetylcholine, noradrenaline and dopamine. Adenosine lowers blood pressure and heart rate, which is necessary at the end of the day to transition from the waking state to sleep. Adenosine also has an inhibitory effect on the wakefulness centers in the hypothalamus and thus induces sleep (Borbély et al. 2016). When sleeping, the enriched adenosine is broken down again.

In the first half of the night, the activation by the circadian system decreases, but the sleep pressure remains pronounced. Therefore, sleep can be well maintained in healthy people at this time. After about four hours of sleep and the passage of several deep sleep phases, the sleep pressure falls sharply together with the adenosine level.

During the day there are breaks in the hormonal wake-up signals that are then felt as fatigue when the sleep pressure is already increased at that time. This is particularly evident in the often experienced "afternoon slump", depending on the chronotypes (early risers or night owls) of a person usually between 13 and 15 o'clock. This is often attributed to the consumption of a too heavy lunch and therefore referred to as postprandial somnolence in professional circles. But even people who eat light meals or nothing at all at noon experience this drop.

1.2.3 Light as a Pacemaker

Evolutionarily, light was an important pacemaker for the synchronization of many endocrine, physiological, but also social processes. Since society has developed much faster in the last 10,000 years than evolution could progress, information for the control of endogenous

processes is genetically anchored in modern humans that date back to the time of our ancestors, the cavemen (Perrez and Baumann 2005).

Daylight is still a very important factor, which is increasingly being overlooked today, for example due to artificial light stimuli during the night shift, due to harmful night-time habits or due to the possibility of staying in the dark during the day. In particular, shift workers suffer from such conditions, and the so-called shift worker syndrome can occur (Angerer and Petru 2010). This leads to a desynchronisation of basic processes in the body and to severe sleep disorders (Rodenbeck 2007).

In the early 1990s, Foster and colleagues (Foster et al. 1991) discovered, in addition to the rods (for light-dark vision) and the cones (for colour vision), a third type of photoreceptor in the retina of mammals: the photosensitive ganglion cells. These are distributed throughout the retina, in contrast to the other two types of photoreceptor. When light stimuli hit these photosensitive ganglion cells in the retina, which contain the photopigment melanopsin, a complex chemical reaction occurs. The impulses are transmitted via the retinohypothalamic tract to the SCN (suprachiasmatic nucleus), the "internal clock" that controls the day-night- rhythm in the human body. There, in the presence of light stimulation, the activation of melatonin secretion in the epiphysis (pineal gland) is suppressed (Lewy et al. 1989). In the absence of light stimulation, the inhibition in the SCN is interrupted and melatonin is secreted from the epiphysis-melatonin. Melatonin secretion is therefore controlled mainly by the SCN.

The secretion of melatonin is naturally inhibited by the light falling into the eye throughout the day and only comes into activation again in the evening hours with increasing darkness. With its rapid increase, it is sleep-inducing and sleep-sustaining. In order to be able to use this natural phenomenon, sleep phases should take place in the dark as far as possible (Kryger et al. 2014).

In addition to synchronizing the circadian rhythm, melatonin can initiate sleep (Lewy et al. 1989). However, pharmacological studies with oral melatonin for sleep initiation showed little efficacy in the treatment of sleep disorders (Macchi and Bruce 2004). During the day, the natural melatonin secretion is rather low in daylight, so the administration of small doses was sufficient to make one sleepy. In the evening or at night, however, the natural melatonin level also increases exponentially. To then achieve potent effects, very high doses of melatonin were needed to even notice any efficacy. In older people, the natural melatonin production is sometimes sluggish, which is why an additional oral administration of melatonin preparations can improve sleep.

In addition to the biological basics, social norms and requirements play a decisive role in the rhythmization of the daily structure. Since there is good artificial light, one is no longer dependent on daylight to be active. This shifts the sleep-wake-rhythm of many people in a sustainable and disadvantageous way.

Interestingly, various hormones, body temperature and the sleep-wake-rhythm synchronize in a roughly 24-hour interval. This also happens without external timekeepers such as light/darkness, time of day, etc. (Cajochen 2009). This illustrates the strong genetic anchoring of the 24-hour rhythm.

All time information is forwarded to the sleep-wake centers of the brain and there summarized by a complex integration of various endogenous, but also social and environmental information to thesleep-wake-rhythm(Reid and Zee 2009).

Excursus: the Color of Light

It is generally known that humans react to various visual, auditory, or olfactory stimuli with emotions and also with vegetative effects. Light not only has an influence on the control of the biorhythm, but also the color of the light can have a significant effect on physiological and psychological processes, such as mood (Rosenthal Jr et al. 1990). This knowledge is already being used to treat depressions.

As a result of intensive research, it is now also known for sleep how great the influence of the different spectra of light on the biorhythm is, and light therapy is increasingly being used to treat sleep disorders. The sensitivity of the photosensitive retinal ganglion cells changes depending on the wavelength of the light. Depending on the time of day, the natural sunlight has different light colors. When the sun is at its highest at noon, the

wavelengths overlap so that the light appears colorless, i.e. white. This is the time of our greatest performance, fatigue or sleep are be thought of at this time. Intensive blue wavelengths are necessary to balance the color spectra to white light, which are also used in many displays (mobile phone, tablet, computer, etc.) today.

If at the end of the day a blue light component hits our retina, the body gets the signal: "It is noon, we are at our most productive, we will not sleep in the next few hours."

Therefore, late screen activity harms our sleep so much (e.g. Thapan et al. 2001).

In Sect. 3.4.6 we will go into detail about how the nature of the light can be used therapeutically.

1.2.4   Temperature Course and Heat Regulation

The circadian rhythm and thus also sleep are fundamentally controlled by the course of the sun. This not only results in fluctuations in the brightness and color of the light, but also in the ambient temperature. The daily temperature changes by an average of about 12 °C in summer and about 5 °C in winter in temperate climate zones. Elsewhere, the fluctuations can be more than 40 °C. The evolutionary response to these daily differences of our body was an adaptation of the body's core temperature with an fluctuation range of about 1 °C. It reaches its maximum in the evening before going to bed and sinks again during the night. In the early morning it is then at its lowest.

The fluctuation of our body temperature explains why many people feel cold at night when they have to get up earlier than their biological clock dictates.

▶   With the drop in body temperature, drowsiness also comes.

This temperature low point then starts the first sleep cycle, so that we quickly find ourselves in the Non-REM and finally in the REM sleep. During REM sleep, it is hardly possible for humans to regulate their body temperature. This can lead to night sweats or phases of freezing. In Non-REM sleep, however, this happens as in the waking state. For a healthy and restful sleep, it is important and necessary that our body can go through this variability of body and ambient temperature. Heating and air conditioning make this natural regulation more difficult.

The physiological change of thebody temperatureover a 24-hour cycle has been intensively researched. Over the course of a day, the body temperature follows a sinusoidal curve that reaches its low point at 2:00 a.m. and its maximum in the afternoon (Zulley 1976). In animal experiments it has been shown that prolongedsleep deprivationleads to a metabolic disorder that ends fatally in rats via a dysregulation of body temperature (Everson 1995). In humans, sleep deprivation over 5–10 days did not result in lasting psychological or physical damage. This was followed by a strong fatigue that made it impossible to keep the subjects awake for several minutes, they immediately fell asleep again (Vaitl 2012). It is not known that people have died from prolonged sleep deprivation, as there is a central protection mechanism that causes the person to fall asleep beforehand.

1.2.5 Chronobiology

An individual's biorhythm results in their chronotype. The chronotype is determined by the body's internal clock and the hormones associated with it, as well as performance, rest, and exhaustion phases, body temperature, and sleep and wakefulness phases. Depending on the time of day, the circadian rhythms vary in individual intensity.

▶ The different chronotypes are wakeful or sleepy, performant or in a performance trough, at different times.

The corresponding wake-up and bedtimes as well as the course of the day should be aligned with the respective chronotype of the person in order to maintain well-being and long-term health. The Center for Chronobiology at Ludwig Maximilian University of Munich has done groundbreaking research in this area. With a sample of over 150,000 subjects, a total of seven essential chronotypes could be distinguished from each other (Roenneberg et al. 2019), as shown in Table 1.1.

It becomes apparent that only about 30% of the population can cope with the typical office hours of 9 a.m. to 5 p.m. in accordance with their chronotype with optimal and healthy performance. Earlier types should therefore be allowed to start earlier and later types correspondingly later. Flexible working hours and flexitime benefit employees and employers

Table 1.1 Chronotypes and their properties (all times are approximate and can vary individually)

Chronotype	Sleep times	Performance high[*]	Break[*]	Happy Hour[*]
extreme early type approx. 1% of the population	9 pm to 5 am	6 am to 11 am; 1 pm to 3 pm	11 am to 1 pm	4 pm to 6 pm
moderate early type approx. 15% of the population	10 p.m. to 6 a.m.	7 a.m. to 12 p.m.; 2 p.m. to 4 p.m.	12 p.m. to 2 p.m.	5 p.m. to 7 p.m.
light early type approx. 20% of the population	11 p.m. to 7 a.m.	8 a.m. to 1 p.m.; 3 p.m. to 5 p.m.	1 p.m. to 3 p.m.	6 p.m. to 8 p.m.
Normal type approx. 30% of the population	0 to 8 o'clock	9 to 2 o'clock; 4 to 6 o'clock	2 to 4 o'clock	7 to 9 o'clock
slight late type approx. 25% of the population	1 to 9 o'clock	10 to 3 o'clock, 5 to 7 o'clock	3 to 5 o'clock	8 to 10 o'clock
moderate late type approx. 8% of the population	2 to 10 pm	11 am to 4 pm; 6 pm to 8 pm	4 pm to 6 pm	9 pm to 11 pm
extreme late type approx. 1% of the population	4/5 to 12/13 pm	1 pm to 5 pm; 7 pm to 9 pm	5 pm to 7 pm	10 pm to 12 am

* These times are based on experience

alike, as the overall performance is significantly higher, fewer sick days are taken and people enjoy their work more.

▶ Whether owl or lark—the productivity of these people is the same.

Break Times

It is important to set break times according to one's chronotype and the circadian hormone course. After about 4–5 h of productivity, a time window for recovery must be created. This does not mean that during these recovery times the feet necessarily have to be raised. It is important here to do other activities than the actual work. People with physically passive office work should use this time to move more. This can also include physically more active activities within the scope of work tasks, such as picking up or dropping off mail, filing or simply working standing up. The lunch break should also be designed accordingly, for example with a walk after eating. The most important thing is that during this time the actual workstation is left for as long as possible. For people who do physically active work, such as scaffolders, cleaning and maintenance services, gardeners, etc., the opposite applies. They should actually rest physically during the rest periods. This can also include work tasks, such as writing invoices, purchasing goods or bookkeeping.

▶ Break is everything that is different from work.

Excursus: Social Jetlag

Based on the data of the Center for Chronobiology at the Ludwig Maximilian University of Munich, it was possible to assess how the duration of sleep and the sleep period change in the different seasons and over the lifespan.

The study results show that more than 60% of the working population experience a so-called "social jetlag" (Roenneberg et al. 2012).

They switch between workdays and weekends, or on days off in different "time zones".

The workdays and nights are determined by the alarm clock, the days off by the internal clock. So it can happen that on workdays the affected people sleep more than two hours less than on weekends. Here it should be noted that sleep can only be "advanced" or "made up" to

a small extent. The "social jetlag" is a common cause of sleep disorders.

1.2.6   The Ultradian Rhythm

The ultradian process arises from complex hormonal interactions that control REM, non-REM sleep and wakefulness, build up fatigue, and finally initiate sleep by activating or inhibiting hormone secretion. Thus, dopaminergic, serotonergic and adrenergic activity is high during wakefulness, decreases during non-REM sleep, and is almost completely suppressed during REM sleep. In contrast, cholinergic activity is always high during wakefulness and REM sleep. For many of these hormones, feedback loops are assumed that control the regular secretion independently of the circadian system (Bourguignon and Storch 2017).

The sleep-wake rhythm is exclusively ultradian in newborns. In the first weeks to months after birth, several sleep-wake cycles occur during the day for newborns. The circadian rhythm with only one sleep and wake phase during the day develops just later (Rivkees 2003). While the sleep-wake phases change to the circadian rhythm, the ultradian rhythm is not lost, but both integrate harmoniously. So there are short periods of "activity spurts" alternated with longer periods of wakefulness and sleep.

▶ In everyday life, the ultradian 4-hour rhythm can also be observed in the distribution of meals.

The circadian system is coupled to the "internal clock" and, together with many other processes, is synchronized by the biorhythm. Thus, it reacts rather slowly to changes. If we want or need to resynchronize our biorhythm, e.g. when starting a new job that starts much earlier, when children start school after kindergarten, etc., it takes weeks of consistent adherence to the new times.

Sleep pressure and the ultradian system, on the other hand, depend on daily specialties in life and vary depending on bedtime, activity, or intake of caffeine or meals. The key to a healthy and restful sleep is the synchronization of sleep pressure and biorhythm. That is why it is so important for sleep-disordered people to maintain regular sleep times and to align their daily routine accordingly.

The alternation of REM and non-REM phases also follows a recurring rhythm. Since the alternation of these phases is much faster than the circadian rhythm, it is referred to as ultradian (Borbély and Achermann 1999).

1.3 How do We Sleep?

1.3.1 The Physiology of Sleep

Sleep Architecture

Healthy sleep is subject to intact sleep architecture and proceeds in four sleep stages (AASM, American Academy of Sleep Medicine 2005): three non-rapid eye movement (NREM, without rapid eye movements) and one rapid eye movement phase (REM, with rapid eye movements). Rechtschaffen and Kales (1968) originally proposed a 5-stage classification, according to which, in addition to REM sleep, four NREM phases were distinguished. Due to the great similarity and the difficult delimitation of phases

3 and 4 in the hypnogram (sleep profile), they were finally combined into N3, deep sleep, also known as slow-wave sleep (SWS). Figure 1.2 shows a schematic representation of the sleep architecture of a healthy night, called a hypnogram in professional circles. The time course is plotted on the x-axis and the depth of sleep is plotted on the y-axis in descending order. The yellow line represents the course of sleep, the light gray shaded bars represent the REM sleep proportions.

A sleep cycle consists of NREM and REM sleep and lasts between 80 and 110 min in adults, who experience it 4 to 7 times per night. Each sleep cycle begins with light sleep (N1). This is followed very quickly by deeper sleep (N2) and deep sleep (N3). REM sleep completes a sleep cycle. This means: At the end of each sleep cycle, after about 90 min, sleep is shallower and lighter. People with sleep disorders then report experiencing wakefulness between sleep cycles (after 1.5 h, 3 h, or 4.5 h). Good sleepers quickly fall back into a deeper sleep after a sleep cycle. Deep sleep occurs more frequently in the first half of the night. However, deep sleep does not occur in every cycle. Sleep is overall lighter and more fragmented in the morning hours, so it is "normal" to wake up

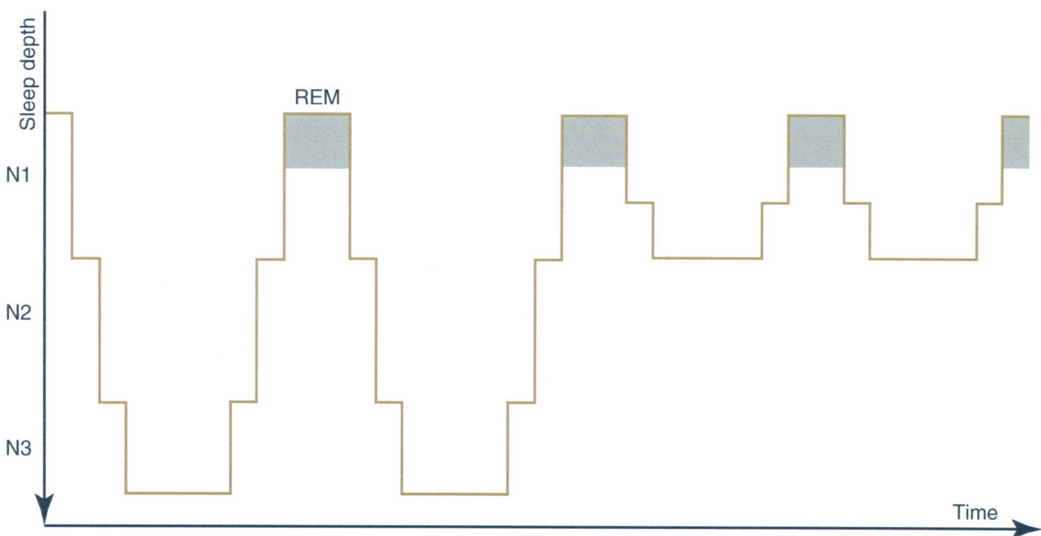

Fig. 1.2 Schematic representation of a hypnogram (the sleep architecture) of a natural night

more often, as long as you fall asleep quickly again.

Brain Activity During Sleep

Figure 1.3 shows the different brain waves (waves of the electroencephalogram; EEG waves) of the different sleep stages as well as different sleep phenomena.

In order to sleep well, an attentive state of wakefulness should turn into a relaxed state of wakefulness. This is preceded by alpha activity in the sleep stage N1. The vertex spikes visible in the figure indicate the onset of sleep on a psychophysiological level.

In the more robust sleep N2, brain activity becomes slow-wave, which means that the individual brain cells increasingly work in unison. The K-complexes shown in the figure indicate the perception and processing of external stimuli in the state of wakefulness. In connection with sleep, it is assumed that they initiate wakefulness reactions (arousals). They often go hand in

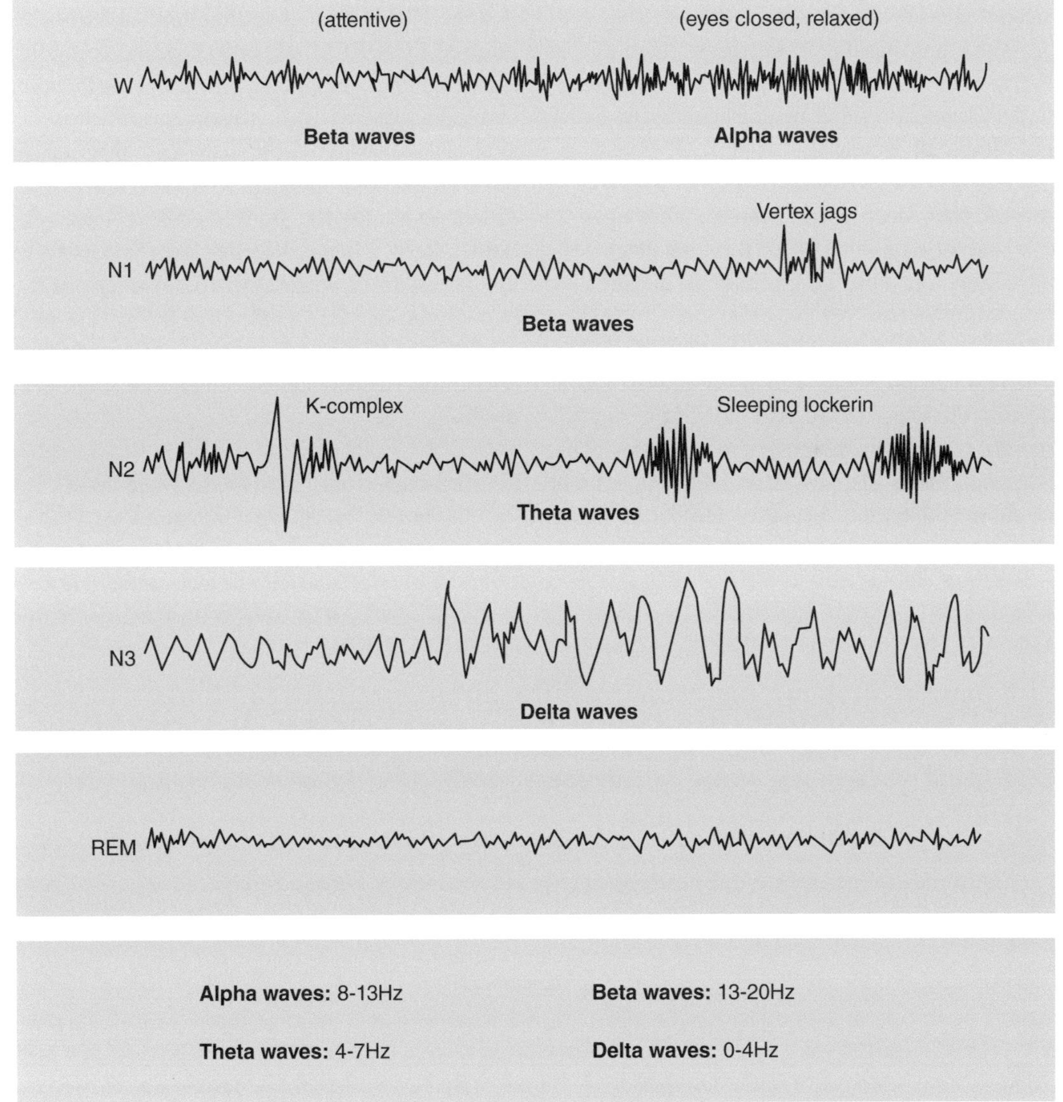

Fig. 1.3 The brain waves (EEG) during the different sleep stages (with the kind permission of Daizu GmbH, Berlin)

hand with sleep spindles. The function of sleep spindles has not yet been exhaustively investigated. However, connections have been found to early childhood brain development, memory processes and the suppression of acoustic stimuli in particular.

In the deep sleep stage N3, slow-wave sleep takes place. It shows that all brain areas are now communicating with each other in unison. Delta activity is only found in healthy people during deep sleep and in very experienced deep meditators.

The typical characteristics of the individual sleep stages are shown in Table 1.2.

When transitioning from sleep phase N1 to N2 and to N3, muscle tone, heart rate, pulse, body temperature, and responsiveness to external stimuli all decrease.

▶ A deep sleep phase, which makes up a total of about 25% of the total sleep time, can only be aroused by a pain stimulus.

The first half of the night is mostly composed of deep sleep, while the second half of the night is mostly composed of lighter sleep phases. This does not mean that the first half of the night is more important, because many important processes for maintaining homeostasis also take place during lighter sleep.

The sleep stage N1 is described as the transition from wakefulness to sleep, the stage N2 as stable sleep and the stage N3 as deep sleep (Stuck et al. 2018). When falling asleep, the healthy sleeper wanders through the NREM 1–2 phases very quickly. These phases together take up to 60% of the total sleep time. Afterwards, the healthy sleeper spends the first sleep cycle, according to his sleep needs, up to one hour in deep sleep. After this first sleep cycle, the depth of sleep loosens up to the stage N2, N1 and the REM sleep. The time until then is also referred to as REM sleep latency and is a polysomnographic parameter for the classification and diagnosis of sleep disorders (Shrivastava et al. 2014). The REM sleep can take up to 25% of the total sleep time in a healthy adult (Stuck et al. 2018). Between the cycles with lighter sleep it is possible that the sleepers wake up. The state of wakefulness is also part of the hypnogram and can take up to 5% of the total sleep time. If this wakefulness is shorter than 3 min, the sleepers cannot remember it the next morning.

▶ It is therefore "normal" to wake up at night and fall asleep again quickly.

Table 1.2 Characteristics of the sleep stages in adults according to AASM (2005)

Stage	EEG	EOG	EMG
Awake	Predominant alpha and beta activity	Eye blinks, rapid eye movements, occasional slow, sometimes rolling eye movements at the transition to N1	High muscle tone, movement artifacts
N1	Theta activity, (vertex spikes)	Slow, sometimes rolling eye movements	Decrease in muscle tone (< W)
N2	Theta activity, K-complexes, sleep spindles	No eye movements, EEG artifacts, occasionally slow, sometimes rolling eye movements during transition from N1	Decrease in muscle tone (< N1)
N3	Delta waves < 2 Hz (*slow waves*): > 20%	No eye movements, EEG artifacts	Decrease in muscle tone (< N2)
REM	Theta activity (also slow alpha activity), sawtooth waves	Conjugate, rapid eye movements, REM	Lowest average tone (≤ N3), partly phasic activation

Then the sleeper falls back into a deeper sleep. This cycle is repeated 2- to 4-times during the night.

The REM sleep has fascinated science for many decades. The exact functions of the REM sleep are still unknown today. It is often equated with the dream sleep, as dreams are predominantly dreamed in these phases. However, in recent studies, dreams have also been reported by sleepers who had no REM sleep (Siclari et al. 2013). It seems to play an important role in memory formation, emotion regulation and problem-solving skills. In addition, the REM sleep is very sensitive to the effects of medication (Shrivastava et al. 2014).

1.4   The Functions of Sleep

Sleep research is similar to deep-sea research in one essential respect: There are more aspects that we do not know yet than are known to us. It is certain that sleep has a variety of functions in the organism, which have not yet been exhaustively investigated. Horne (1988) and Koella (1988) summarized the state of research at the time by seeing the only proven function of sleep as the so-called fatigue-relief-effect. Pollmächer and Lauer (1992) supported this thesis with the statement: "At the present time, not a single one of the possible functions can be clearly demonstrated experimentally." Over time, various hypotheses have been put forward and theoretically underpinned. In the last 20 years, groundbreaking and fascinating findings have been made. However, for everyday clinical practice, it is enough to ask our patients after one or more "bad nights" which symptoms and deficits they feel. Based on the resulting daytime symptomatology of sleep disorders, we can derive how much sleep contributes to the maintenance of our performance and our health. Here you will find an insight into the essential functions of sleep, which are particularly useful for your therapy.

1.4.1   Regeneration

For a long time it was believed that sleep served only the recovery of the organs, since apparently all body functions are reduced: heart rate, pulse, blood pressure, respiration, body temperature, etc. With the improvement of the examination possibilities of the human body, research in this field also increased greatly. Today we know that sleep has far more functions. A basic and well-known property of sleep is the reduction of sleep pressure in order to be active and both physically and cognitively fit the next day (Borbély 1982).

After intense physical activity, the duration of deep sleep (slow wave sleep, SWS), which usually takes place more in the first half of the night, increases significantly (Baekeland and Lasky 1966). Thus, physical regeneration is the first function that is carried out with the highest priority even after prolonged sleep deprivation. During deep sleep, our growth hormone somatotrophin (growth hormone, GH) is secreted from the pituitary gland to a much greater extent (Adamson et al. 1974). These sleep phases are particularly important for growth and physical and mental development in children and adolescents. But even adults need somatotrophin (GH) for the regeneration and maintenance of the vitality of body structures. GH follows the circadian periodicity, its concentration thus changes in a 24-hour cycle. Since cortisol (our stress or performance hormone) is not secreted or only secreted in small concentrations during deep sleep and cortisol inhibits the secretion of GH, deep sleep is therefore absolutely necessary for health-promoting regeneration. GH is also significantly involved in the consolidation of declarative memory (Van Cauter and Copinschi 2000).

Interestingly, GH was the first hormone that could be directly linked to sleep (Takahashi et al. 1968; Sassin et al. 1969).

The human peripheral nervous system tolerates sleep deprivation surprisingly well and often regenerates after one or two nights of restful sleep. In the central nervous system (CNS), however, insufficient sleep leads to clear neurocognitive deficits and emotional instability, up to psychotic symptoms (Koella 1988).

Excursus: Rebound Effect

In this regard, paradoxically and particularly interesting is that in the first night after sleep deprivation, deep sleep is "demanded" mainly at the expense of REM sleep. Only in the second night—after intensive sleep deprivation—more REM sleep phases occur. This is referred to as the "rebound effect" and could also be seen as a "catch-up sleep". In total, about three quarters of the deep sleep is "recovered", but only about one third of the REM sleep time.

These rebound effects therefore take place in two phases:

- *the core sleep, which is mainly responsible for the maintenance and regeneration of basic structures and is absolutely essential for survival, and*
- *the adaptive sleep, which allows the organism to constantly adapt to its environment and events taking place in it* (Horne 1988).

In addition, there is a high correlation between wakefulness and subsequent deep sleep duration. The REM sleep time is more oriented towards the circadian periodicity (Dijk and Czeisler 1995).

For the basic recovery of the body, resting in the waking state is sufficient. However, it should be noted that awake, resting test subjects need about one third more energy than sleeping (Van Cauter and Copinschi 2000; Jung et al. 2011). In sleep, energy is also saved in this way. Researchers from Harvard Medical School discovered in animal experiments that during the deep sleep phases, the energy carrier adenosine triphosphate (ATP) accumulates in the brain (Jung et al. 2011). It became clear that brain regions particularly stressed during the day are flooded with ATP after falling asleep (Dworak et al. 2010). However, if the rats were prevented from sleeping, there was no increased ATP concentration.

Conclusion: *For simple recovery of the body, resting in the awake state is sufficient. However, if the sleep pressure is extremely high, this is no longer enough: Before the human organism fails, that is, the human dies, the body forces sleep. This means that we certainly do not die from not sleeping. Nevertheless, fatigue can be dangerous, for example, the microsleep at the steering wheel.*

Body and psyche get exactly the kind of sleep they need to make regeneration as optimal as possible. First, our body balances what was demanded the day before: If we have physically exerted ourselves a lot, the body demands more deep sleep. The processing of emotional challenges takes place mainly in light and REM sleep. So if you want to sleep really well, for example on vacation, you should exhaust yourself sufficiently with physical and mental activity beforehand.

1.4.2　The Synaptic Homeostasis "tidying up and Making Room for New Ones"

In my opinion, synaptic homeostasis is a great achievement of nature and the most fascinating function of sleep. During deep sleep, we humans are completely unconscious and lose the ability to respond to external stimuli completely. Only pain stimuli (haptic or acoustic) can end this state intentionally. There must therefore be a very important function that justifies this survival risk every night.

> ▶　There is no doubt that one of the most important functions of sleep is to restore the balance of nerve cells in the central nervous system. Only in this way it is possible to maintain the plasticity of the brain and to perform corresponding neurocognitive functions.

During the day, countless stimuli flow to a person, which are received consciously or unconsciously. It is important to know that our consciousness "only" processes 40 bits (approx. 4–5 individual stimuli) per second. Our unconscious, on the other hand, registers 11 million bits, that is, approx. 1.1 million individual stimuli per second (from Kopp 2015). Even the unconscious stimuli form nerve pathways and memory nodes. In this way, countless nerve connections are created that are unnecessary and hinder our cognitive processing capacity. From the information received during the day, memory is finally formed, even redundant information (often acoustic: street noise; or visual: moving vehicles) is then stored.

In 2005, Tononi and Cirelli first observed in an experiment with rats that during deep sleep the so-called "synaptic downscaling" (breakdown of synaptic activity) takes place. During the waking phase, countless stimuli flow to the organism and thus to the CNS. In this way, new synaptic connections are formed between the nerve cells through long-term potentiation. If the excitement of these neurons continued, new connections would be established without interruption. During deep sleep, this activity is interrupted by the synchronization of several neuronal groups with long-wave potentials (delta waves) visible in the EEG (measurement of electrical activity in the brain). The connection strength between the synapses decreases and only the strong connections are retained. This is necessary for the selection between important and unimportant information, to protect against overload of the CNS and to establish the necessary plasticity for new synaptic activity (Tononi and Cirelli 2021).

Conclusion: We take most sensory impressions during the day rather unconsciously. However, since our brain processes all information, it is necessary to distinguish between important and unimportant. In order to preserve processing capacity and plasticity, it must therefore be determined which information is to be prepared for storage in memory and what can be forgotten. The unconsciousness during deep sleep is therefore essential for the plasticity of the brain.

1.4.3 Memory Formation

Memory formation, especially the formation of long-term memory, takes place to a large extent during sleep. The basic mechanism for this function is also the "switching off" of the perception of external stimuli during deep sleep. This process of cognitive processing is another explanation for why there is a complete loss of consciousness during sleep (Marshall and Born 2007). Since the brain uses the same neural networks to process external stimuli and to form a long-term memory, the capacity is limited. Through the circadian rhythm, the brain can process sensory impressions during the day and establish corresponding neural links (Walker and Strickgold 2004). At night, memorable and important-seeming information is transferred to long-term memory through reactivation and feedback. In deep sleep, the release of performance and stress hormones, such as cortisol, adrenaline, noradrenaline, is partly completely suppressed. This mechanism is very important for memory formation. Without this inhibition, long-term storage and elaboration of new information is impaired. Thus, sleep is essential for memory formation (Marshall and Born 2007).

Basically, declarative and procedural memory are distinguished. Declarative memory has factual knowledge, such as dates, vocabulary, that were "learned" consciously. The consolidation of declarative memory content is based on feedback between the hippocampus and the neocortex. The hippocampus is the intermediate memory of our brain and thus the switch between short- and long-term memory. New neurons can be formed there throughout life, which is essential for memory processes. Through very complex internal circuits, the new neurons are integrated into the existing structures of the hippocampus. It is assumed that the information to be stored first circulates in the hippocampal network (Winocur et al. 2010). This reactivates old memory content in the hippocampus. Thus, a shift or representation of the information to the neocortex is stimulated. This way, further links can be formed and the memory can be built up and consolidated. The slow-wave brain activity of deep sleep synchronizes the hippocampus and neocortex. Thus, in the first night quarter with large deep sleep shares, corresponding synaptic connections are first marked, which are consolidated in the last night quarter in REM sleep (Born et al. 2006). Sleep can be used specifically to learn more effectively, for example in exam preparation. If the learner sleeps shortly after reading, working through, etc., that is, encoding, the consolidation of the previously perceived content is more effective than without sleep (Gais et al. 2006). Also, daytime sleep phases without deep sleep components are helpful.

> ▶ *The consumption of alcohol severely disrupts this mechanism because alcohol acts as a cell poison and inhibits deep sleep. Therefore, it is not advisable to help oneself to an alcoholic drink at the end of an intense learning or further education day in order to switch off and relax.*

This means: both deep and REM sleep are necessary for memory formation. At the same time, this mechanism explains why massive memory deficits are often a key component of all sleep disorders. It is good to know at this point that this memory mechanism is already restored the next good night. However, the memory deficits that have arisen by then cannot be restored.

Procedural memory mainly takes in sensory impressions and stores movement sequences, such as riding a bike. These pieces of information contain a very large number of unconscious components. While it was long assumed that declarative memory is built up during deep sleep and procedural memory during REM sleep. We now know that sensory impressions and movement sequences are first activated and elaborated during deep sleep, and then further processed procedurally during REM sleep. These processes are often reflected in sometimes bizarre dreams in which the movement sequences to be stored are manifested in cortical trial actions. But that's not all: Brand et al. (2010) were able to show in an experiment that subjects who had practiced the execution of various neurocognitive tests (e.g. Tower of Hanoi) before going to sleep the next day performed better on similar and complicated tasks than subjects without prior training. Furthermore, it is assumed that in REM sleep, associations of already stored information are activated and thus an elaboration with various neuronal links of new memory content takes place (Strickgold and Walker 2007). This means that even very long-standing experiences, problem-solving processes, experiences

and feelings can be made accessible through this reactivation. Current problem-solving and processing processes are included. In addition, REM sleep promotes the ability to metacognitions, that is, to think about oneself and one's own thinking processes as well as introspections. An inward-looking perception of one's own thoughts and feelings is only made possible in this way (Wagner et al. 2004). These processes alone make it possible to acquire implicit knowledge through logical and complex reasoning (Fischer et al. 2006).

This may explain why retrieving certain memories is easier than others. The recall of procedural, non-declarative memory content requires fundamentally less processing capacity and is usually also possible after sleep deprivation. Even after a bad night, we can ride a bike or ski and, above all, operate the coffee machine. The retrieval of facts, on the other hand, requires concentration, which is restricted but locally available after bad nights.

Conclusion: *Memory formation and thus learning tend to take place at night. The human being can store all facts better if he had a sufficient sleep both before and after the learning phase. The recall of memory content also works better after a good night. This does not necessarily require learning facts by heart. A relaxed reading of the things, so a priming, brings an enormous gain in memory performance.*

1.4.4 Emotional regulation

The relationship between sleep, emotions and social behavior is very complex. The underlying mechanisms are not fully known yet (Beattie et al. 2015). It is certain, however, that REM sleep, together with non-declarative memory formation, plays a decisive role in the formation of emotional memory (Walker and Van der Helm 2009). The spontaneous primary evaluations of the day's experiences are intensively reconciled and re-evaluated during sleep.

In the hippocampus, the intermediate memory of our brain, the experiences of the day are reconciled in feedback loops with already processed emotional experiences in memory. Contrary to the long-held assumption that only dreams have the function of emotional processing, it is now known that emotional regulation takes place primarily in the deep sleep phases. This so-called "replay" is to a large extent unconscious, that is, it is not initially reflected in the dream content of REM sleep. Subsequently, the unconsciously and consciously activated information is linked together in REM sleep in the second half of the night and probably also in dreams (Wagner et al. 2001). In this way, the day-to-day situations are linked with already coped emotions. At this point, the human being benefits from previous experiences that were felt in similar situations or how he proceeded afterwards.

This is why the widely held grandmotherly advice: "Sleep on it. Tomorrow the world will look different" gets its meaning. Of course, the world does not change overnight. But sleep changes the evaluation of emotional events, which is why many situations look less stressful or dangerous in "daylight" than the day before.

By reactivating short- and long-term memory in the hippocampus, only the core of emotional experiences is transferred, the essentials have already been filtered out for further processing. The information is enriched with current topics on the way into and out of the hippocampal structures. In this way, the memory content changes and can be stored emotionally re-evaluated.

The hippocampus is also a switch to and in between the structures of the limbic system. In addition to emotion-regulating processes, the limbic system is also said to be involved in the control of motivation, vegetative regulation (in particular the hormone axes of the sympathetic nervous system), nutrition, digestion, libido and much more. Therefore, it is not surprising that the various sleep disorders have close comorbidities with depression, stress reaction, burnout and adjustment disorders, anxiety, eating and metabolism disorders.

Minkel et al. (2011) were able to show in a study that sleep-deprived people showed significantly fewer emotional facial expressions than people who had slept before watching emotional film scenes. Even greater differences were found in funny films (Cooper et al. 2008). In addition, sleep-deprived people have difficulty attributing the right emotion to certain facial expressions (Franzen et al. 2008).

Neuroimaging studies found in people who reported poor sleep quality, a pathological activation of the amygdala, as is also found in depression and anxiety disorders (Prather et al. 2013). Chuah et al. (2010) showed in sleep-deprived people a significantly higher connectivity between the prefrontal cortex and the amygdala. Minkel et al. (2012) carried out magnetic resonance imaging (MRI) studies on emotion regulation and asked the subjects to "get a grip" on their emotions after presenting certain exciting stimuli. In people who had not slept well, a clear psychopathological activation of the amygdala was again observed during this process. Inhibition of behavior is also more difficult for sleep-deprived people. Therefore, typical symptoms are mood swings with pronounced weepiness, euphoric phases or frequent irritability. In addition, emotional intelligence decreases, emotional reactions are overall less pronounced, and thus social interactions are more complicated (Beattie et al. 2015).

Emotions play an important role in memory retrieval. So people with depression can more easily remember painful things and have a corresponding negative view of the future. The same applies to manic or anxious people, because memory and future vision are emotion-congruent.

Conclusion: Good sleep quality is essential for a healthy psyche. Therefore, sleep disorders occur in most cases comorbid with mental disorders.

1.4.5 Immune regulation

A very important effect of sleep is the building and maintaining of the immune system (Bryant et al. 2004). Sleep regulates hormones that influence the immune system. The secretion of cortisol, norepinephrine and adrenaline is inhibited during sleep, while the secretion of growth hormone and prolactin is promoted (Lange and Born 2011).

Unlike in the periphery of the body, the CNS does not have a lymph drainage system that can remove toxins. Therefore, it is very interesting to know that during sleep the cellular structure of the brain changes, whereby the neurons contract and thus gaps between the cells arise, as scientists discovered in experiments with mice. Into these gaps, cerebrospinal fluid can flow at night and wash away waste products (Xie et al. 2013). The cerebrospinal fluid outflow rate is twice as high at night as during the day. Among other things, prions and plaques, which play a major role in the development of dementia and Alzheimer's disease, are transported to a greater extent. This means that sufficient sleep can protect against the onset of severe neurodegenerative diseases (Iliff et al. 2013). This process is controlled, among other things, by a blockade of norepinephrine.

During sleep, the number of leukocytes and lymphocytes increases. If an infection is present, the number of cells can increase several times during the night's sleep. The need for sleep of acutely slightly ill people (e.g. infection with influenza viruses, corona, rhinitis, pharyngitis) increases to a high degree. During sleep, interleukins and other messenger substances are released more frequently, which on the one hand trigger sleep and on the other hand fight the infection. This is also where the term "sleeping healthy" comes from. In addition, sleep strengthens the "memory" of immune reactions, so that viruses and bacteria can be recognized more quickly in the future and thus eliminated more specifically. Supporting this, it was found in a study on immune response after hepatitis A vaccination that significantly more antibodies were formed in people who had a normal night's sleep after vaccination than in subjects who were supposed to stay awake for about 36 h (Efe 2012). Therefore, people should not drink alcohol after vaccination and allow as much sleep as possible. Then the best possible antibody response takes place. Irwin et al. found (1999) that sleep

deprivation leads to a reduced activity of lymphocytes. They have the function of recognizing and eliminating pathogens in the organism. Already after three hours of sleep deprivation, the function of these T-helper cells and thus of the entire immune system is impaired. It was also found that sleep deprivation increases the cortisol concentration in the blood and in turn decreases the spleen weight. The spleen is basically the place for the formation, maturation and storage of lymphocytes. Thus, the total number of lymphocytes also decreases. After sufficient recovery sleep, the lymphocyte count grew again (Zager et al. 2007). Furthermore, lymphocytes capture and eliminate mutated cells from which tumors may arise. Therefore, the risk of cancer is increased in patients suffering from sleep disorders, people who sleep too little, and especially in people who work in shifts. For this reason, the WHO included night work as a major risk factor for the development of cancer.

> *Short-term sleep deprivation does not cause lasting damage to the immune system and a few good nights regenerate it quickly. However, in the case of long-term sleep deprivation, it can take months for the immune system to be rebuilt.*

Sleep promotes wound healing. In particular, during deep sleep, more growth hormones are released. These are involved in cell renewal and cell exchange, that is, the regeneration of tissue. For example, it was observed that deep injuries of bears heal much better after winter sleep than during the summer active phase. Also in rats it was found that burns heal much better if the rodents were allowed to sleep than in case of sleep deprivation (Gumustekin et al. 2004).

Targeted studies of various diseases showed a high correlation between disturbed sleep or permanently shortened sleep duration and somatic diseases such as diabetes mellitus (Rafaelsen et al. 2010), obesity and hypertension (Gangwisch et al. 2006), heart failure (Ayas et al. 2003) and early onset of dementia (Spira et al. 2014). Further studies describe so-called endotoxin effects during sleep (Haak et al. 2001). Endotoxins are released during the breakdown of certain bacteria and can cause inflammation and fever in the human body. They first cause a lighter, short-wave sleep. After the body's immune response to the endotoxins, deep sleep occurs more frequently in order to fight them specifically.

Conclusion: Sleep is also significantly involved in maintaining our body's health.

1.4.6 Metabolism

The alternation between wakefulness and sleep and thus the adaptation to the circadian periodicity is essential for health, performance and resilience. By switching all physiological and neurological processes, all cells are prepared for the tasks ahead during the day. Various genes are activated and deactivated, intestinal cells are adjusted to the different digestive functions, the final digestion takes place mainly at night, the cells of the hormone glands are regenerated, and the CNS is prepared for a performant wakefulness by the synchronization of the neurotransmitters. For these processes, the organism needs energy. Therefore, it is not surprising that we need only about 30% less energy in the sleep state than in the wake state.

If the sleep duration is too short, the risk of developing a metabolic disease, such as overweight, obesity or diabetes, increases by a multiple. The blood sugar-regulating hormone insulin is involved to a large extent. New research has shown a circadian course of insulin secretion, as it can not only regulate blood sugar levels for energy production, but also act as a clock for the synchronization of the internal clock (Okubo et al. 2014). The circadian rhythm can be thrown off track by irregular meals and especially night-time eating in shift work and jet lag. Conversely, regular food intake can be used to stabilize the internal clock and to treat non-organic sleep disorders.

A hypoglycaemic episode during the night or large variations in blood sugar levels have a big influence on sleep quality. If the body is hypoglycaemic at night, it starts a stress-awakening reaction in order to allow the person to take in food. This process is also set in motion in the opposite direction in the case of chronically elevated muscle tone and the resulting sleep disorders. The nocturnal arousals and awakening processes, which are also caused by external wake-up stimuli such as noise, sleep interruptions by children or bed partners, put the body under enormous stress. Every wake-up reaction causes an adrenaline release in the nervous system. This in turn leads to an increase in blood sugar levels. Evolutionarily, this process was essential for survival, as our ancestors had to build up acute stress reactions quickly in the event of night-time risks. However, due to the chronic stress of our population, this vicious circle leads to serious illnesses.

Even a short-term lack of sleep can cause the cells to be unable to take up enough sugar from the blood due to a lack of insulin (Rao et al. 2015). If people sleep for less than five hours a night on a permanent basis, insulin resistance is a possible consequence and leads to type 2 diabetes.

▶ Diabetes patients should therefore pay more attention to getting enough and restful sleep, as they will need less insulin and be more stable in their disease management.

Healthy people have a higher metabolism than people with sleep disorders (Bonnet and Arand 2003). As a result, people with sleep disorders are significantly more likely to be overweight than healthy people (Knutson and Van Cauter 2008). People who sleep an average of five hours have a 50% higher risk of being overweight than people who sleep between seven and nine hours. However, it is not the effective sleep time of the patients that is decisive, but the time at which the affected people go to bed: people who go to bed very late are significantly more likely to be overweight than people who go to bed earlier (Markwald et al. 2013).

However, sleep does not take over the complete hormonal control of energy metabolism, but rather influences the feeling of hunger or satiety. Sleep disorders throw the synthesis and release of the hormones ghrelin and orexin out of balance. Ghrelin is an acronym for *Growth Hormone Release Inducing*, i.e. responsible for initiating the release of growth hormone, which primarily takes place during deep sleep. It is also part of the regulation of food intake. When hungry and sleep-deprived, ghrelin levels in the blood rise, and after food intake they level off again (Yildiz et al. 2004).

The hormone orexin stabilizes wakefulness and stimulates hunger, so it is appetite-enhancing. Therefore, if you have a late dinner or a nighttime snack, you get into a vicious circle of wakefulness and increased food intake. This is how the close connection between sleep disorders and obesity and their consequences arises.

In addition, orexin increases body temperature, promotes wakefulness and attention. Orexin inhibitors, on the other hand, stabilize sleep and thus create fewer wakefulness periods during the night. An orexin inhibitor is therefore also appetite-regulating with its sleep-stabilizing effect. Therefore, orexin inhibitors are currently the subject of many research efforts as a means of medical therapy for sleep disorders.

This very complex hormone system also controls digestion and sleep. Digestion also works overtime at night.

Basically, you can divide the digestive process into three overlapping phases:

- The cephalic phase begins with the perception of the smell as well as the sight and taste of the food. The entire digestive tract is prepared for the upcoming food. So if we eat carelessly, too quickly and "the wrong thing", this process can not run smoothly.
- This is followed by the gastric phase, the comminution and mixing of the food in the stomach.
- Finally, the intestinal phase follows, in which the food is broken down in the small intestine. Now the cellular uptake of nutrients, the distribution in the body and the transport of non-digestible and "dangerous" substances take place. This phase is already part of the final digestion, which can last 18 h or more.

For this, the body needs rest and no overstrain by excessive stress or the intake of new food. During sleep, the final digestion can take place undisturbed. Therefore, about 4 h should pass before going to bed to avoid disturbing this process. At the end of digestion and preferably at the end of the night, the remaining food mass accumulates in the large intestine, where only water is removed. Good digestion can be recognized, among other things, by the fact that a regular bowel movement takes place in the morning, either immediately after getting up, morning gymnastics or breakfast.

Conclusion: Metabolism in the body and sleep influence each other. Therefore, certain principles of nutrition should be observed for a restful sleep. In return, enough restful sleep is necessary for a more regulated metabolism.

1.4.7   Calibration

If you draw a conclusion from all the functions described, you can say that sleep essentially serves the calibration of the human body. It integrates all the functions of sleep. The healthy, sufficient sleep should synchronize all processes in the body (metabolism, processing of physical and chemical stimuli) for a smooth operation. During the waking phases, very different demands are placed on the body, depending on how active or passive the individual is, which and how much food it takes in, etc. This means that the cardiovascular system as well as the hormonal, neuronal and gastrointestinal systems work at different speeds with different intensities. This disturbs the balance of the body and is balanced again by a balanced and rhythmic night's sleep (Dijk and Lockley 2002) and supports the basic homeostasis theory.

1.4.8   The Function of Dreams

A dream is defined as "the memory of mental activity during sleep" (Stuck et al. 2018). The dream content is experienced as a whole with sensory perceptions, cognition and emotions.

The function of dreams has not been clarified fundamentally to this day. In science, this is hypothetically spoken of with regard to the processes and functions in the dream content. The methodological basis of dream research is still the main obstacle to finding answers to many questions. Dreams cannot be measured or made visible from the outside. The researchers are always dependent on the dream memories of the subjects.

▶ From today's point of view of science, it is certain that all people dream. Dream phases can occur in all non-REM and also in the REM phase. However, it is certain that all people dream in the REM sleep.

One of the unanswered questions is: Why do some people remember their dreams and others not? This is precisely the focus of dream research at the moment. So there will be answers soon.

Overall, dream studies have found a balanced ratio between positive and negative dream experiences. Unless the people are blind from birth, dreams always contain visual images. The auditory impressions concentrate more on language, less on noise. The body perception rather shows kinesthetic, i.e. movement sensations, but rarely pain, heat, cold, etc. Taste, smell and touch are rarely dreamed.

As described above, during dreaming, memory contents are consolidated and elaborated. In particular, the consolidation of motor sequences is attributed to the dream. Emotion regulation also takes place in part during dreaming. Evolutionarily, it is assumed that the survival-necessary fear was consolidated in the dream in connection with various situations experienced during the day. Subjects who were prevented from REM sleep were more moody, irritable, and their social behavior was less empathetic (1966), than when they were allowed to dream.

Excursus: The "Mastery Hypothesis"
This hypothesis about the content of dreams assumes that dreams are the unconscious attempts to find solutions to problems. In dreams, people reflect on their tasks, problems, and concerns. In particular, themes that cannot be solved by conscious thinking (2020). It is also said that in dreams problems are dealt with more creatively. The periodic table of elements is said to have finally appeared to Dimitri Mendeleev in a dream after decades of research.

In contrast, it is assumed that we need the dream to forget unnecessary information. Dreams arise through the willful activation of the neocortex (cerebral cortex). Thus, even irrelevant information is activated and can be "deleted". Crick and Mitchison reported 1983 in the highly respected journal *Nature* that there is a "reverse learning mechanism" during REM sleep. In sleep activated, unconscious memory contents are weakened rather than strengthened in the dream.

Conclusion: *In summary, it can be said that dreams are involved in all functions of sleep.*

1.5 Hormones that Determine Sleep

1.5.1 Adenosine

Adenosine accumulates throughout the period of wakefulness and generates sleep pressure. It has a fatiguing effect, which is why it is also referred to as a "somnogenic" or "hypnogenic" substance. During sleep, it is slowly broken down over the course of sleep. It suppresses various activating arousal processes in the central nervous system and initiates non-REM sleep. In the first half of the night it is only broken down to a moderate extent in order to stabilize sleep. Even after only 3–4 h of sleep, one still feels significant fatigue. In the second half of the night, however, the increased breakdown takes place, which is why one does not feel tired after 5–6 h of sleep and the sleep deficit only becomes apparent during the day (Stuck et al. 2018). The interplay of circadian rhythm and wakefulness-promoting hormones ensures that the fatigue of adenosine is suppressed during the day and only experienced before falling asleep. However, people with sleep disorders also feel this fatigue during phases of low performance during the day. The night sleep is not sufficient to sufficiently reduce the sleep pressure, i.e. the adenosine.

A popular way to stay awake and receptive during the day is coffee, black or green tea, for many people.

▶ The caffeine in the drinks (also called teein in tea) blocks the adenosine receptors, which temporarily inhibits the perception of fatigue. Cocoa (dark chocolate) also contains caffeine.

1.5.2 Melatonin

Melatonin is known to the population as our sleep hormone. In a narrower sense, this is not quite right, because melatonin is a sleep-preparing hormone. If the melatonin concentration increases sharply, it is tiring, sleep-initiating and -maintaining. Melatonin is produced mainly in the pineal gland, which is located in the brain directly above the optic nerve. Information about light and darkness is transmitted directly from the optic nerve to the pineal gland. In bright light, melatonin production is suppressed (Czeisler et al. 1986). The entire nervous system therefore receives the information that it is light, thus wakefulness, and the cells and glands secrete activating neurotransmitters and hormones. With the onset of darkness, the pineal gland receives the signal that now the night begins and initiates the release of melatonin. This is secreted into the bloodstream and can thus signal throughout the body that now the night is coming and that the activating performance processes of the day must be switched to the regenerating sleep processes. Melatonin spreads throughout the body via the circulation and triggers complex reactions that calm, tire and promote sleep.

For example, melatonin regulates the body temperature in the evening, which reaches its minimum temperature early in the morning (Cagnacci et al. 1997). The thyroid gland switches off the dopaminergic activity and the immune system is stimulated. In the morning, with the onset of light, the melatonin level drops again.

Strong artificial light in the evening can also inhibit melatonin production. For this reason, it is essential to avoid long periods of screen time and bright light exposure before bedtime (Rheinberg and Ashkenazi 2008). On the other hand, longer periods of darkness during the day, for example in winter, and long-term stays in moderately lit rooms can also stimulate melatonin production and cause unwanted fatigue and lethargy. In such cases, light therapy is a good option for seasonal depression and milder sleep disorders (Rosenthal et al. 1990).

The raw material for melatonin production is tryptophan. Many foods contain this essential amino acid. Tryptophan, for example, is found in nuts, legumes, fish and cereal flakes. Various minerals, fats and vitamins are also involved in the conversion of tryptophan to melatonin. Therefore, a sleep-promoting diet is an important part of the therapy of a sleep disorder.

1.5.3 Cortisol

Cortisol is commonly referred to as our "stress hormone." In fact, it is the hormone that makes us performant in the first place. It has an activating and performance-enhancing effect. It is secreted more in stress situations, and chronic stress can lead to serious illnesses. Cortisol also has important functions in the sleep-wake regulation. The secretion of cortisol is subject to circadian periodicity, that is, a regular 24-hour rhythm. In Fig. 1.4 the natural course of cortisol of a healthy adult of the most common chronotypes (light early and normal type) is shown.

It is evident that a high secretion takes place in the morning and early afternoon. In these periods, activity and performance increase. On the other hand, cortisol also causes the well-known "midday slump." The reason for this is a short-term drop in cortisol levels, which leads to a decrease in performance and the fatigue caused by the enriched adenosine becomes noticeable. In general, a healthy cortisol level decreases in the evening and reaches its lowest point in the first half of sleep. The highest

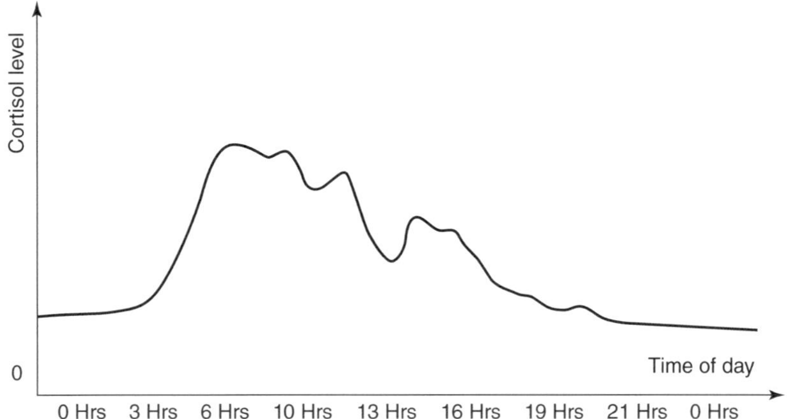

Fig. 1.4 Cortisol profile of a healthy adult of the mild early and normal types.

cortisol secretion can be observed in the morning, shortly after waking up. It is called the "cortisol awakening response." The cortisol awakening response provides a morning high of energy and motivation. During the evening, the healthy cortisol level then decreases again with slight fluctuations.

The physiological secretion of cortisol reaches its minimum in the evening and at night. The work of Rodenbeck and Hajak (2001) is particularly impressive in this regard. The working group found a close correlation between the concentration of cortisol secreted in the period from 5:00 pm to 8:00 pm and the quality of the subsequent night's sleep. Healthy subjects with an increased cortisol level at this time of day slept significantly worse than people with a normal cortisol level. In people with chronic sleep disorders, the cortisol level was generally increased.

Alertness develops throughout the morning and reaches its peak in the midday hours (Zulley 1979). This is consistent with the 2-process-model of sleep regulation by Borbély (1982), which states that the activating hormones of the circadian rhythm are fully developed after a midday lull to counteract the accumulating sleep pressure (Dijk and Edgar 1999). This means that the early afternoon is once again a good time for many people to solve cognitively demanding tasks.

▶ The natural course of cortisol can be influenced by the subjective experience and behavior.

In stressful situations, anger or conflict, the body reacts with increased cortisol secretion. Cortisol creates readiness for action in these moments and puts the person in a state of readiness for fight or flight. Over millions of years, this reaction was essential for our ancestors' survival. Our body is prepared for these occasional moments of stress and can cope with them well. However, with chronic stress and constant tension, cortisol is secreted permanently and also at night. The readiness for flight and fight remains active and the constant vigilance impairs sleep. If the tension is not released and the cortisol profile remains high, chronic insomnia can develop. As a result, light sleep phases increase while the deep sleep percentage decreases. Sleep becomes less restful and increasingly fragmented overall.

1.5.4   Adrenaline and Noradrenaline

Similar to cortisol, adrenaline is known as a stress hormone. The "adrenaline rush" is often experienced during dangerous situations or during sports. Norepinephrine is less well known, although it is the actual main agent in the acute stress system. With sudden stress events, there is an increased production of norepinephrine. This triggers a number of physiological reactions, such as increased heart rate and blood pressure, accelerated breathing, muscle tension, sweating and increased attention. It activates the fight-or-flight reflex (fight-or-flight mode), which prepares all resources for a fight or a quick retreat. In prehistoric times, this reaction was essential for our ancestors' survival. The connection with sleep is quickly apparent. When there is a threat, the entire organism remains "alert", and consequently does not enter a (deep) sleep. Pharmacological studies show that the direct administration of norepinephrine or corresponding agonists increases wakefulness overall (Berridge et al. 2005).

Therefore, these two hormones can also be the reason why it is difficult to fall asleep. If the usual sleep point is missed, the body enters a stress state that, through this mechanism, increases readiness and alertness. This activity is then difficult to shut down. For this reason, it is advisable to go to sleep at the same time every night and only to cross this time in exceptional cases.

1.5.5 Serotonin

Serotonin is also known as the "happiness hormone" in layman's terms. However, its functions are much more diverse. This hormone is mood-enhancing during the day and responsible for initiating and regulating deep sleep at night. REM sleep, on the other hand, is inhibited by serotonin.

Serotonergic neurons are particularly located in the raphe nuclei and project to various areas of the brain. Neuronal connections between the raphe nuclei and the thalamus suggest that serotonin promotes the formation of sleep spindles during sleep (Ursin 2002). This allows the corresponding developmental and cognitive processing during sleep as well as the transition from lighter to deeper sleep phases. Sleep spindles typically occur in non-REM phase 2 and inhibit stimuli from the environment to support falling asleep and staying asleep (Lecci et al. 2017).

In depression, there is a deficit in serotonin production, which is why sleep disorders are closely linked to affective disorders, among other things. Serotonin is the precursor of the hormone melatonin, so a deficiency can restrict melatonin production and thus the initiation and maintenance of sleep. Selective serotonin reuptake inhibitors (SSRIs) prevent the breakdown of serotonin, so that more of the hormone is active and available. SSRIs have a good efficacy as antidepressants. Therefore, certain preparations also have a sleep-inducing effect and lead to an improvement in sleep. Serotonin is mainly produced from the amino acid tryptophan and some vitamins and minerals. Therefore, a balanced diet can have a very positive effect on serotonin levels.

1.5.6 Dopamine

Dopamine also belongs to our "happy hormones". It promotes drive and motivation. So far, it is less well known that dopamine also follows a circadian rhythm and plays an important role in controlling wakefulness. The "inner clock" and dopamine are in close interaction. The production of dopamine is controlled by the so-called CLOCK genes in the suprachiasmatic nucleus (SCN), which follows the circadian rhythm (McClung et al. 2005). At the same time, dopamine is an important component of the retina (retina) and is involved in the adaptation of brightness and the conversion of the photopigment melanopsin (Van Hook et al. 2012). With the conversion of melanopsin, signals are sent to the SCN. There, the release of melatonin is regulated and thus the sleep-wake rhythm is controlled.

In REM sleep, the dopamine concentration controls muscle tone. The experimental reduction in dopamine concentration led to conspicuous muscle movements during REM sleep, which is normally associated with muscle atony. Both dopamine deficiency and the absence of muscle atony are typical features of REM sleep behavior disorder (Kharraz-Tavakol Pahlewan 2005). More than half of the patients with Parkinson's disease, the symptomatology of which is due to the degeneration of dopaminergic cells, report sleep disorders. These are largely due to dysfunction of the dopaminergic system (Li et al. 2017).

Blum and colleagues (2014) were able to show that different dopamine concentrations follow ultradian rhythms (shorter than the 24-hour circadian rhythms, Sect. 1.2.6) and, on the other hand, act regulatory on the ultradian process. Through changing dopamine concentrations, ultradian rhythms can become shorter or longer (Bourguignon and Storch 2017). This regular increase and decrease of dopamine in about 4-hour periods is reflected in everyday life with activity spurts and changing motivation. Compared to the circadian rhythm, these ultradian phases are much more flexible and adapt to changes in everyday life more quickly. If dopamine production is interrupted, there is a significant loss of spontaneous drive and motivation (Zhou and Palmiter 1995). Thus, the release of dopamine seems to be fundamentally responsible for action impulses and willingness to perform, which are correlated with a restful or non-restful sleep.

1.5.7 Orexin

The name orexin comes from the Greek and means "desire" or "appetite". In addition to regulating food intake and digestion, orexin also affects the sleep-wake rhythm by stabilizing the waking state. In our evolution, it provided our ancestors with sufficient motivation to search for food by stimulating appetite and hunger, maintaining wakefulness and simultaneously increasing attention to food search. In addition, it increases body temperature, which mobilizes physiological activity on the one hand and prevents transition to sleep on the other. The release of orexin is additionally increased when carbohydrates are taken. Therefore, one should not eat carbohydrate-rich food late at night. Proteins, on the other hand, have little effect on the release of orexin.

Orexin is closely related to the awakening disorder narcolepsy. A faulty orexin neurotransmission in the hypothalamus causes a deficiency of the hormone. Narcolepsy is accompanied by cataplectic attacks (sudden loss of muscle tone) and chronic drowsiness (Saper et al. 2010). In narcoleptics with an orexin deficiency, the hormone cannot prevent unwanted transitions from wakefulness to sleep.

Orexin antagonists are currently being researched as possible sleep aids.

1.5.8 Other Messengers

Gamma-Aminobutyric Acid (GABA)

Gamma-Aminobutyric Acid, GABA for short, is the most important inhibitory neurotransmitter. GABA supports the initiation of sleep by reducing the activity of the important arousal system ARAS (ascending reticular activating system) in the brainstem. GABA binds to two different receptors, with $GABA_A$ receptors in particular mediating sleep-promoting, anxiety-reducing and muscle-relaxing processes.

Histamine

Histamine is known for triggering allergic reactions. In the central nervous system, histamine is an important hormone of the arousal network. It is mainly activated during the waking state. Blocking histamine receptors with antagonist substances has a drowsy and sleep-stimulating effect. During non-REM and REM sleep, histamine is almost inactive, histamine-producing neurons only fire during the waking state (Franco-Pérez et al. 2012). This means that histamine also promotes wakefulness. Antihistamines are therefore used as hypnotics and also in allergies. The drowsy effect is an unpleasant side effect in allergy sufferers.

References

Adamson JW, Dale DC, Elin RJ (1974) Hematopoiesis in the grey collie dog. Studies of the regulation of erythropoiesis. J Clin Invest 54:965

Allison T, van Twyver H (1970) The evolution of sleep. Nat Hist 79:56–65

American Academy of Sleep Medicine. AASM (2005) International classification of sleep disorders.

Diagnostic and coding manual (ICSD-2) Westchester, IL. http://www.aasmnet.org

Angerer P, Petru R (2010) Schichtarbeit in der modernen Industriegesellschaft und gesundheitliche Folgen. Somnologie 14:88–97

Ayas NT, White DP, Manson JE et al (2003) A prospective study of sleep duration and coronary heart disease in women. Arch Intern Med 163:205–209

Baekeland F, Lasky R (1966) Exercise and sleep patterns in college athletes. Percept Mot Skills 23:1203–1207

Beattie L, Kyle SD, Espie CA, Biello SM (2015) Social interactions, emotion and sleep: a systematic review and research agenda. Sleep Med Rev 24C:83–100

Berridge CW, Stellick RL, Schmeichel BE (2005) Wake-promoting actions of medial basal forebrain β_2 receptor stimulation. Behav Neurosci 119(3):743–751

Bonnet MH, Arand DL (2003) Insomnia, metabolic rate and sleep restoration. J Intern Med 254:23–31

Borbély AA (1982) A two process model of sleep regulation. Hum Neurobiol 1(3):195–204

Borbély AA, Achermann P (1999) Sleep homeostasis and models of sleep regulation. J Biol Rhythm 14:557–568

Borbély AA, Daan S, Wirz-Justice A, Deboer T (2016) The two-process model of sleep regulation: a reappraisal. J Sleep Res 25(2):131–143

Born J, Rasch B, Gais S (2006) Sleep to remember. Neuroscientist 12:410

Bourguignon C, Storch KF (2017) Control of rest: activity by a dopaminergic ultradian oscillator and the circadian clock. Front Neurol 8:614

Brand S, Opwis K, Hatzinger M, Holsboer-Trachsler E (2010) REM sleep is related to the transfer of implicit procedural knowledge following metacognitive learning. Somnologie 14:213–220

Bryant PA, Trinder J, Curtis N (2004) Sick and tired: does sleep have a vital role in the immune system? Nat Rev Immunol 4:457–467

Cagnacci A, Kräuchi K, Wirz-Justice A, Volpe A (1997) Homeostatic versus circadian effects of melatonin on core body temperature in humans. J Biol Rhythm 12:509–517

Cajochen C (2009) Schlafregulation. Somnologie 13:64–71. Springer

Chuah LYM, Dolcos F, Chen AK et al (2010) Sleep deprivation and interference by emotional distracters. Sleep 33:1305–1313

Cooper RM, Rowe AC, Penton-Voak IS (2008) The role of trait anxiety in recognition of emotional facial expressions. J Anxiety Disord 22:1120–1127

Crick F, Mitchison G (1983) The function of dream sleep. Nature 304(5922):111–114

Czeisler CA, Allan JS, Strogatz SH et al (1986) Bright light resets the human circadian pacemaker independent of the timing of the sleep-wake cycle. Science 233(4764):667–671

Dement W, Greenberg S, Klein R (1966) The effect of partial REM sleep deprivation and delayed recovery. J Psychiatr Res 4(3):141–152

Dijk DJ, Edgar DM (1999) Circadian and homeostatic control of wakefulness and sleep. In: Turek FW, Zee PC (Hrsg) Regulation of sleep and circadian rhythms. Marcel Dekker, New York-Basel, S 111–148

Dijk DJ, Czeisler CA (1995) Contribution of the circadian pacemaker and the sleep homeostat to sleep propensity, sleep structure, electroencephalographic slow waves, and sleep spindle activity in humans. J Neurosci 15:3526–3538

Dijk DJ, Lockley SW (2002) Integration of human sleep-wake regulation and circadian rhythmicity. J Appl Physiol 92:852–862

Dworak M, McCarley RW, Kim T et al (2010) Sleep and brain energy levels: ATP changes during sleep. J Neurosci 30(26):9007–9016

Efe D (2012) Einfluss des Schlafes auf den Impferfolg nach Hepatitis-A-Impfung. Dissertation, Universität zu Lübeck, Medizinische Fakultät

Everson CA (1995) Functional consequences of sustained sleep deprivation in the rat. Behav Brain Res 69(1–2):43–54

Fischer S, Drosoupolos S, Tsen J, Born J (2006) Implicit learning-explicit knowing: a role for sleep in memory system interaction. J Cogn Neurosci 18:311–319

Foster RG, Provencio I, Hudson D, Fiske S, De Grip W, Menaker M (1991) Circadian photoreception in the retinally degenerate mouse. rd/rd. J Comp Physiol A 169(1):39–50

Franco-Pérez J et al (2012) Major neurotransmitters involved in the regulation of sleep-wake cycle. Rev Investig Clin 64(2):182–191

Franzen PL, Siegle GJ, Buysse DJ (2008) Relationship between affect, vigilance, and sleepiness following sleep deprivation. J Sleep Res 17:11–34

Gais S, Lucas B, Born J (2006) Sleep after learning aids memory recall. Learn Mem 13:259–262

Gangwisch JE, Heymsfield SB, Boden-Albala B et al (2006) Short sleep duration as a risk factor for hypertension: analyses of the first National Health and Nutrition Examination Survey. Hypertension 47:833–839

Gazzillo F, Silberschatz G, Fimiani R, De Luca E, Bush M (2020) Dreaming and adaptation: the perspective of control-mastery theory. Psychoanal Psychol 37(3):185–198

Glühbirne (1879) Patent „US223898A: Electric Lamp. Angemeldet am 4. November 1879, veröffentlicht am 27. Januar 1880, Erfinder: Thomas Alva Edison.“

Gumustekin K, Seven B, Karabulut N et al (2004) Effects of sleep deprivation, nicotine, and selenium on wound healing in rats. Int J Neurosci 114(11):1433–1442

Haack M, Schuld A, Kraus T, Pollmächer T (2001) Effects of sleep on endotoxin-induced host responses in healthy men. Psychosom Med 63(4):568–578

Horne J (1988) Why we sleep. Oxford University Press, Oxford

Hufeland CW (1797) Die Kunst, das menschliche Leben zu verlängern. Akademische Buchhandlung, Jena

Iliff JJ, Lee H, Yu M et al (2013) Brain-wide pathway for waste clearence captured by contrast-enhanced MRI. J Clin Invest 123(3):1299–1309

Irwin M, Thompson J, Miller C, Gillin JC, Zieglert M (1999) Effects of sleep and sleep deprivation on catecholamine and interleukin-2 levels in humans: clinical implications. J Clin Endocrinol Metabol 84(6):1979–1985

Sassin JF, Parker DC, Mace JW, Gotlin RW, Johnsonand LC, Rossman LG (1969) Human growth hormone release: relation to slow-wave sleep and sleep-waking cycles. Science 165(3892):513–515

Jung CM, Melanson EL, Frydendall EJ et al (2011) Energy expenditure during sleep, sleep deprivation and sleep following sleep deprivation in adult humans. J Physiol 589:235–244

Kavanau JL (1997) Origin and evolution of sleep: roles of vision and endothermy. University of California, Department of Biology, Los Angeles, California, 90095-1606, USA

Keene AC, Duboue ER (2018) The origins and evolution of sleep. J Exp Biol 221(Pt 11):jeb159533

Kharraz-Tavakol Pahlewan B (2005) Assoziation von D2-Rezeptor-und Dopamin-Transporter-Störungen mit erhöhter Muskelaktivität während des REM-Schlafes. Doctoral dissertation, LMU

Knutson KL, Van Cauter E (2008) Associations between sleep loss and increased risk of obesity and diabetes. Ann N Y Acad Sci 1129:287–304

Koella WP (1988) Die Physiologie des Schlafs. Fischer, Stuttgart

Kryger MH, Avidan AY, Berry RB (Hrsg) (2014) Atlas of clinical sleep medicine, 2nd edn. Elsevier Sounders, Philadelphia

Lange T, Born J (2011) The immune recovery function of sleep – tracked by neutrophil counts. Brain Behav Immun 25(1):14–15

Lecci S, Fernandez LMJ, Weber FD, Cardis R, Chatton J-Y, Born J, Lüthi A (2017) Coordinated infraslow neural and cardiac oscillations mark fragility and offline periods in mammalian sleep. Science. Advances 3

Lewy AJ, Bauer VK, Ahmed S, Thomas KH, Cutler NL, Singer CM, Moffit MT, Sack RL (1989) The human phase response curve. PRC. to melatonin is about 12 hours out of phase with the prc to light. Chronobiol Int 15(1):71–83

Li S, Wang Y, Wang F et al (2017) A new perspective for Parkinson's disease: circadian rhythm. Neurosci Bull 33:62–72

Macchi MM, Bruce JN (2004) Human pineal physiology and functional significance of melatonin. Front Neuroendocrinol 25(3–4):177–195

Markwald RR, Melanson EL, Smith MR et al (2013) Impact of insufficient sleep on total daily energy expenditure, food intake, and weight gain. Proc Natl Acad Sci USA 110(14):5695–5700

Marshall L, Born J (2007) The contribution of sleep to hippocampus-dependent memory consolidation. Trends Cogn Sci 11(10):442–450

McClung CA, Sidiropoulou K, Vitaterna M, Takahashi JS, White FJ, Cooper DC et al (2005) Regulation of dopaminergic transmission and cocaine reward by the Clock gene. Proc Natl Acad Sci U S A 2005(102):9377–9381

Minkel J, Htaik O, Banks S, Dinges D (2011) Emotional expressiveness in sleep-deprivated healthy adults. Behav Sleep Med 9:5–14

Minkel JD, McNealy KN, Gianaros PJ et al (2012) Sleep quality and neural circuit function supporting emotion regulation. Biol Mood Anxiety Dis 2:1–9

Okubo N, Matsuzaka M, Takahashi I, Sawada K, Sato S, Akimoto N, Umeda T, Nakaji S, Hirosaki University Graduate School of Medicine (2014) Relationship between self-reported sleep quality and metabolic syndrome in general population. BMC Public Health volume 14, Article number: 562

Perrez M, Baumann U (Hrsg) (2005) Lehrbuch Klinische Psychologie – Psychotherapie. 3., vollständig überarbeitete Aufl. Huber, Bern

Pollmächer T, Lauer C (1992) Physiologie von Schlaf und Schlafregulation. In: Berger M (Hrsg) Handbuch des normalen und gestörten Schlafs. Springer, Berlin Heidelberg New York, S 1–44

Prather AA, Bogdan R, Hariri AR (2013) Impact of sleep quality on amygdala reactivity, negative affect, and percieved stress. Psychosom Med 75:350–358

Rafaelsen L, Donahue RP, Stranges S et al (2010) Short sleep duration is associated with the development of impaired fasting glucose: the western New York health study. Ann Epidemiol 20(12):883–889

Rao MN, Neylan TC, Grunfeld C, Mulligan K, Schambelan M, Schwarz JM (2015) Subchronic sleep restriction causes tissuespecific insulin resistance. J Clin Endocrinol Metab 100(4):1664–1671

Rechtschaffen A, Kahles A (1968) A manual of standardized terminology, techniques and scoring system for sleep stages of human subjects. University of California, Brain Information Service/Brain Research Institute, Los Angeles, CA

Rechtschaffen A (1978) The single-mindedness and isolation of dreams. Sleep (1):97–109

Reid KJ, Zee PC (2009) Circadian rhythm disorders. Semin Neurol 29:393–405

Rheinberg A, Ashkenazi L (2008) Internal desynchronization of circadian rhythms and tolerance to shiftwork. Chronobiol Int 25:625–643

Rivkees SA (2003) Developing circadian rhythmicity in infants. Pediatrics 112:373–381

Rodenbeck A, Hajak G (2001) Neuroendocrine dysregulation in primary insomnia. Rev Neurol 157(11 Pt 2):57–61

Rodenbeck A (2007) Zirkadiane Rhythmusschlafstörungen. In: Peter H, Penzel T, Peter JH (Hrsg) Enzyklopädie der Schlafmedizin. Springer, Berlin

Roenneberg T, Allebrandt KV, Merrow M, Vetter C (2012) Social Jetlag and Obesity. Curr Biol 22(10):P939–P943

Roenneberg T, Pilz LK, Zerbini G, Winnebeck EC (2019) Chronotype and Social Jetlag: A (Self-) Critical Review. Biology (Basel) 8(3):54

Rosenthal NE Jr, Levendorsky AA, Johnston SH et al (1990) Phase-shifting effects of bright morning light as treatment for delayed sleep phase syndrome. Sleep 13(4):354–361

Saper CB, Fuller PM, Pedersen NP, Lu J, Scammell TE (2010) Sleep state switching. J Neuron 68:1023–1042

Shrivastava D, Jung S, Saasat M et al (2014) How to interpret the results of a sleep study. J Community Hosp Intern Med Perspect 4(5):24983

Siclari F, LaRocque JJ, Postle BR, Tononi G (2013) Assessing sleep consciousness within subjects using serial awaking paradigm. Front Psychol 4(542):1–8

Spira AP, Chen-Edinboro LP, Wu MN, Yaffe K (2014) Impact of sleep on the risk of cognitive decline and dementia. Curr Opin Psychiatry 27(6):478–483

Staedt J, Stoppe G (2001) Evolution und Funktion des Schlafes. Fortschr Neurol Psychiatrie 69:51–57

Strickgold R, Walker M (2007) Sleep-dependent memory consolidation and reconsolidation. Sleep Med 8:331–343

Stickold R (2016) Physiologie: Schlaf drüber! Spektrum der Wissenschaft; Magazin 05.04.2016. https://www.spektrum.de/magazin/physiologie-was-beim-schlafen-im-gehirn-passiert/1402373

Stuck BA, Maurer JT, Schlarb AA, Schredl M, Weeß HG (2018) Praxis der Schlafmedizin – Diagnostik, Differenzialdiagnostik und Therapie bei Erwachsenen und Kindern. 3. Aufl., vollständig ak. und erw. Aufl. Springer, Berlin Heidelberg New York

Takahashi Y, Kipnis DM, Daughaday WH (1968) Growth hormone secretion during sleep. J Clinical Investigation 47(9):2079–2090

Thapan K, Arendt J, Skene DJ (2001) An action spectrum for melatonin suppression: evidence for a novel non-rod, non-cone photoreceptor system in humans. J Physiol 535(Pt 1):261–267

Tononi G, Cirelli C (2005) Sleep function and synaptic homeostasis. Sleep Med Rev 10(1):49–62

Tononi G, Cirelli C (2021) The why and how of sleep-dependent synaptic down-selection. Semin Cell Dev Biol. S1084-9521. 21.00031-8

Ursin R (2002) Serotonin and sleep. Sleep Med Rev 6(1):57–69

Vaitl D (2012) Veränderte Bewusstseinszustände. Schattauer, Stuttgart

Van Cauter E, Copinschi G (2000) Interrelations between growth hormone and sleep. Growth Horm 10(Suppl B):57–62

Van Hook MJ, Wong KY, Berson DM (2012) Dopaminergic modulation of ganglion-cell photoreceptors in rat. Eur J Neurosci 35:507–518

Von Kopp D (2015) Focussing. Springer, Berlin

Wagner U, Gais S, Born J (2001) Emotional memory formation is enhanced across sleep intervals with high amounts of rapid eye movement sleep. Learn Mem 8:112–119

Wagner U, Gais S, Haider H et al (2004) Sleep inspires insight. Nature 427(6972):352–355

Walker MP, Strickgold R (2004) Sleep-dependent learning and memory consolidation. Neuron 44:121–133

Walker MP, Van der Helm E (2009) Overnight therapy? The role of sleep in emotional brain processing. Psychol Bull 135:731–748

Winocur G, Moscovitch M, Rosenbaum RS, Sekeres M (2010) An investigation of the effects of hippocampal lesions in rats on pre- and postoperatively acquired spatial memory in a complex environment. Hippocampus 20:1350–1365

Xie L, Kang H, Xo Q et al (2013) Sleep drives metabolite clearance from the adult brain. Science 342:373–377

Yildiz BO, Suchard MA, Wong ML, McCann SM, Licinio J (2004) Alterations in the dynamics of circulating ghrelin, adiponectin, and leptin in human obesity. Proc Natl Acad Sci USA. 101, Nr. 28

Zager A, Andersen ML, Ruiz FS et al (2007) Effects of acute and chronic sleep loss on immune modulation of rats. Am J Phys Regul Integr Comp Phys 293(1):R504–R509

Zhou QY, Palmiter RD (1995) Dopamine-deficient mice are severely hypoactive, adipsic, and aphagic. Cell 83:1197–1209

Zulley J (2010) Mein Buch vom guten Schlaf: Endlich wieder richtig schlafen. Goldmann, München

Zulley J (1976) Schlaf und Temperatur unter freilaufenden Bedingungen. 30. Kongr Dtsch Ges Psychol, Berlin. S 398–399

Zulley J (1979) Der Einfluß von Zeitgebern auf den Schlaf des Menschen. R. G. Fischer, Frankfurt am Main

Sleep Disorders

Contents

2.1 Epidemiology 30
  2.1.1 Risk Factors 30
2.2 The Origin of Sleep Disorders 31
  2.2.1 Mind-Body-Sleep-Dynamics©. 31
  2.2.2 Causes of Sleep Disorders 35
2.3 Diagnostics and Classification 38
  2.3.1 Diagnosis 38
  2.3.2 Classification 39
  2.3.3 The Diagnostic Process 49
2.4 Common Comorbidities 57
  2.4.1 Affective Disorders. 57
  2.4.2 Anxiety Disorders. 58
  2.4.3 Stress and Adjustment Disorders 58
  2.4.4 Obsessive-compulsive Disorders 59
  2.4.5 Addiction Disorders 59
  2.4.6 Eating Disorders. 60
  2.4.7 Pain Disorders. 60
2.5 Dealing with People with Sleep Disorders 61
  2.5.1 Difficult Therapy Situations 61
  2.5.2 Common Personality Aspects in People with Sleep Disorders 64

▶ After the most important basics of healthy sleep were explained in Chap. 1, Chap. 2 is about sleep disorders. First, an insight into the epidemiology is given. Then the development of sleep disorders is discussed. In this part you will find the model of Mind-Body-Sleep-Dynamics©. It is a multidimensional model of the development and maintenance of sleep disorders that can both increase your understanding of sleep disorders and serve the patient as an explanatory model of their illness. Furthermore, the many different possible causes of sleep disorders are described. A detailed part is dedicated to the classification and diagnosis as well as the comorbidities. You will find practicable instructions, guidelines and questionnaires for the diagnosis of sleep disorders, which are also available to you as working material for your practice as a download. At the end of the chapter, recommendations are given on how to deal with people with sleep disorders.

© The Author(s), under exclusive license to Springer-Verlag GmbH, DE, part of Springer Nature 2023
C. Marx-Dick, *The Holistic Treatment of Sleep Disorders*, https://doi.org/10.1007/978-3-662-67176-4_2

2.1 Epidemiology

80% of employees in Germany sleep poorly (Storm et al. 2017). Fortunately, not everyone of these employees has a sleep disorder requiring treatment. Only when insufficient sleep duration or poor sleep quality persists over a long period of time and thus leads to clinically significant suffering and fatigue during the day, can one speak of a sleep disorder.

> ▶ Many people simply do not take enough time to sleep on weekdays and try to compensate for the lack of sleep at the weekend.

Others hurry through the day and also do not come to rest in the evening. Psychological overstimulation and lack of physical exercise promote sleep disorders to a large extent. In order to prevent pathological sleep disorders from the outset under these unfavorable conditions, sleep hygiene measures can contribute to relief. However, this is by no means sufficient in the case of persistent and complex symptom pictures.

Poor sleep is still too rarely recognized as a clinical disorder, as few colleagues know the disorder well. Unfortunately, it is still not part of the mandatory training for doctors or psychotherapists. Only half of the patients with sleep disorders are recognized, and in turn only half of the patients with this diagnosis receive treatment, usually with hypnotics, neuroleptics and antidepressants. Psychotherapy is only rarely used. The exception are patients with sleep-related breathing disorders, such as sleep apnea syndrome. The knowledge and care situation is also significantly better in neurological sleep-wake disorders.

Almost every second general practitioner patient reports about sleep disorders. According to current estimates, about a quarter of the German population suffers from longer-lasting insomnia, the most common sleep disorder. The frequency data of international studies for insomnia fluctuate between 4% and 26% (Ohayon 2011), with less than 20% of those affected by insomnia being correctly diagnosed. Sleep disorders increase in the population with age. At the same time, women are affected in all age groups more often than men. From the age of 50, almost twice as many women are diagnosed with sleep disorders as men. In total, a point prevalence rate of approximately 5.7% could be uncovered for insomnia in Germany. Of these 5.7%, in turn, only about a third of those affected seek out a doctor or other treatment (Schlack et al. 2013). So many sleep disorders remain untreated. There is a high comorbidity with other mental and physical disorders with a prevalence rate of 75% (Roth 2007). So insomnia and sleep disorders almost always occur with affective disorders, dementia and schizophrenia (Riemann et al. 2017). According to the BARMER health report (Grobe et al. 2019), people with sleep disorders show more than twice as many other clinically relevant mental and behavioral disorders than non-affected people. So up to four times more depression, anxiety disorders, adjustment disorders and eating disorders were recorded in patients with sleep disorders. Five times as often, in addition, obsessive-compulsive disorder or personality disorder was diagnosed. Over 90% of those surveyed showed another neurological disorder in addition to the sleep disorder. In more than 80% of the patients, in addition, mental or behavioral disorders were diagnosed.

> ▶ Sleep disorders are very serious diseases. They represent an enormous risk factor for the development of other physical and somatic diseases, in addition to the basic symptoms such as insomnia, poor sleep quality and daytime fatigue.

2.1.1 Risk Factors

Various risk factors promote the development of sleep disorders. These include the type of origin, the place of residence and the population density (e.g. large cities with more noise and light), the employment conditions (temporary work, shift work, fixed-term contracts) as well as other diseases and mental disorders. Clinical predictors are substance disorders, affective disorders, neurotic, stress and adjustment disorders, hyperkinetic disorders, extrapyramidal diseases and movement disorders, headaches, chronic pain, chronic respiratory diseases as well as diseases of the spine and back.

▶ The highest incidence rates are for women aged 50 to 54 and men aged 60 to 64. The lowest incidence rates are for men and women aged 30 to 34.

2.2 The Origin of Sleep Disorders

Depending on the type and dynamics of the sleep disorder, the origin is very individual. However, it is often the case that many sufferers can link the beginning of their sleep disorder to an event or a particularly stressful time. The body signals with the sleep disorder over-stimulation or overload. This seems particularly paradoxical in insomnia: despite being busy during the day and sufficient fatigue, it is not possible to fall asleep in the evening. Sleep disorders—regardless of their type—are often accompanied by typical symptoms of an adjustment disorder in the form of depressive mood, anxiety, worry, loss of pleasure, loss of motivation, social withdrawal, restlessness and tension. Due to the constant fatigue and exhaustion, these acute reactions often lead to depressive episodes that can persist or recur .

▶ Psychological over-stimulation and lack of physical activity are typical conditions of today's time and the main cause of most sleep disorders.

Due to the over-stimulation, patients are not able to "shut down" in the evening, the lack of movement leads to physical tension and pain and an insufficient physical fatigue. It is precisely this insufficient physical work-out that leads to a massive deterioration of sleep quality. Another typical starting point of sleep disorders

is chronic stress. This can be of professional or private nature. Due to the constant stress, the cortisol level is permanently increased. This can lead to very severe sleep disorders.

2.2.1 Mind-Body-Sleep-Dynamics©

Sleep is an essential pillar of human health. We already feel the effects of too little sleep after one bad night. After several nights of insufficient sleep or sleep quality, this has a lasting effect on our overall well-being:

- We are less able to concentrate, remember and think.
- We feel emotionally unstable, more anxious, more irritable and less resilient.
- We no longer show our full performance, postpone appointments, tasks or report sick.
- We feel dizzy, have headaches, feel a queasy feeling in our stomach and feel generally weak.
- We can only perceive the beautiful things and duties that make up our life in our private, professional and social environment to a limited extent.

These examples show the multi-layered and complex nature of a sleep disorder. At the same time, they also indicate possible comorbidities and systemic problems.

In addition, there are many mental and physical illnesses, medications and life circumstances that can lead to sleep disorders.

All of these factors affect each other, so that when a sleep disorder occurs, one always has to assume a multi-dimensional model of conditions. In everyday clinical practice, it is often difficult to grasp this complex dynamics. However, in order to treat a sleep disorder in a holistic and sustainable way, it is necessary to recognize these factors. The model of Mind-Body-Sleep-Dynamics© was developed over 20 years of practical experience in dealing with people with sleep disorders (Marx-Dick 2020). It can represent the often complex symptomatology of a sleep disorder.

▶ Using structured questionnaires and evaluation forms, the overall symptomatology is recorded in the diagnostic process and then specific therapy modules can be selected. This approach makes it possible to treat most sleep disorders causally and not just symptomatically.

This ensures sustainable treatment success and actively and responsibly involves the patient in his or her recovery process.

The Model of Mind-body-sleep Dynamics©

The model of mind-body-sleep dynamics© is shown in Fig. 2.1.

It basically consists of 4 levels:

Mind level 1: Cognition: neurocognitive deficits, thoughts, worries and rumination etc.

Mind level 2: Emotion: joy, fear, anger, curiosity, disgust, sadness, love, surprise, shame, guilt, contempt and numerous mixed feelings etc.

Mind-body level: Behavior: habits, (compulsive) rituals, overload, avoidance and sparing etc.

Body level: Body: pain, nausea, dizziness, pulmonary, gastrointestinal or neurological symptoms etc.

Each level contains a dynamics of mutually conditioning factors that lead to disturbed sleep. Each cycle on a level follows a 5-step process. After insufficient sleep duration or quality, day-time symptoms inevitably occur, which can be expressed, for example, in worries, anxious mood, avoidance of effort and headaches (1. day-time symptoms). This feeling leads to reduced performance and capacity (2.). In everyday life, the patient may then experience himself as inadequate and develop further fears, for example of a serious physical illness or the boss's dismissal due to frequent absences (3.

experience in everyday life). As a result of the thus stimulated problem and worry chain, the patient becomes tense (4. effects on sleep). This can increase in the course of the day until it is so massive in the evening that restful sleep is no longer conceivable (5. Sleep disturbance).

The experience of the overall symptomatology takes place in the patient's system. This means that all of the patient's living conditions must always be included in the diagnostic and therapeutic process. These include: family, partnership, friends, professional life, financial situation, housing and location, hobbies, childhood and further development, age, previous illnesses and all other circumstances that play a role in a person's life. All factors of the 4 levels interact with each other and can activate and inhibit each other. These activation and inhibition processes are very important for therapy, as often several aspects of the disorder can be addressed with a targeted intervention.

In the targeted analysis of the individual factors of sleep disorder, those that are responsible for the development and maintenance of the occurring symptoms are uncovered. This is also where the symptoms of all comorbidities find their place. As a result of this holistic approach, all symptoms are recognized and can be taken into account in therapy planning.

In this complex system "of a person's life", the symptoms and the disease dynamics of sleep disorder are specifically recorded on the 4 levels and then transferred into corresponding therapy modules.

Acute sleep disorders are usually an immediate reaction to a specific life event or life phase that can be both joyful and stressful. If the stressor is eliminated quickly or after the positive excitement, that is, after the elimination of the cause of the sleep disorder, the symptomatology can sometimes come to an end quickly. However, if the causes remain longer, it leads to chronicization and the overall symptomatology culminates in a complex vicious circle. The holistic model of Mind-Body-Sleep-Dynamics© (MBSD) shows this multidimensional pathogenesis of sleep disorders.

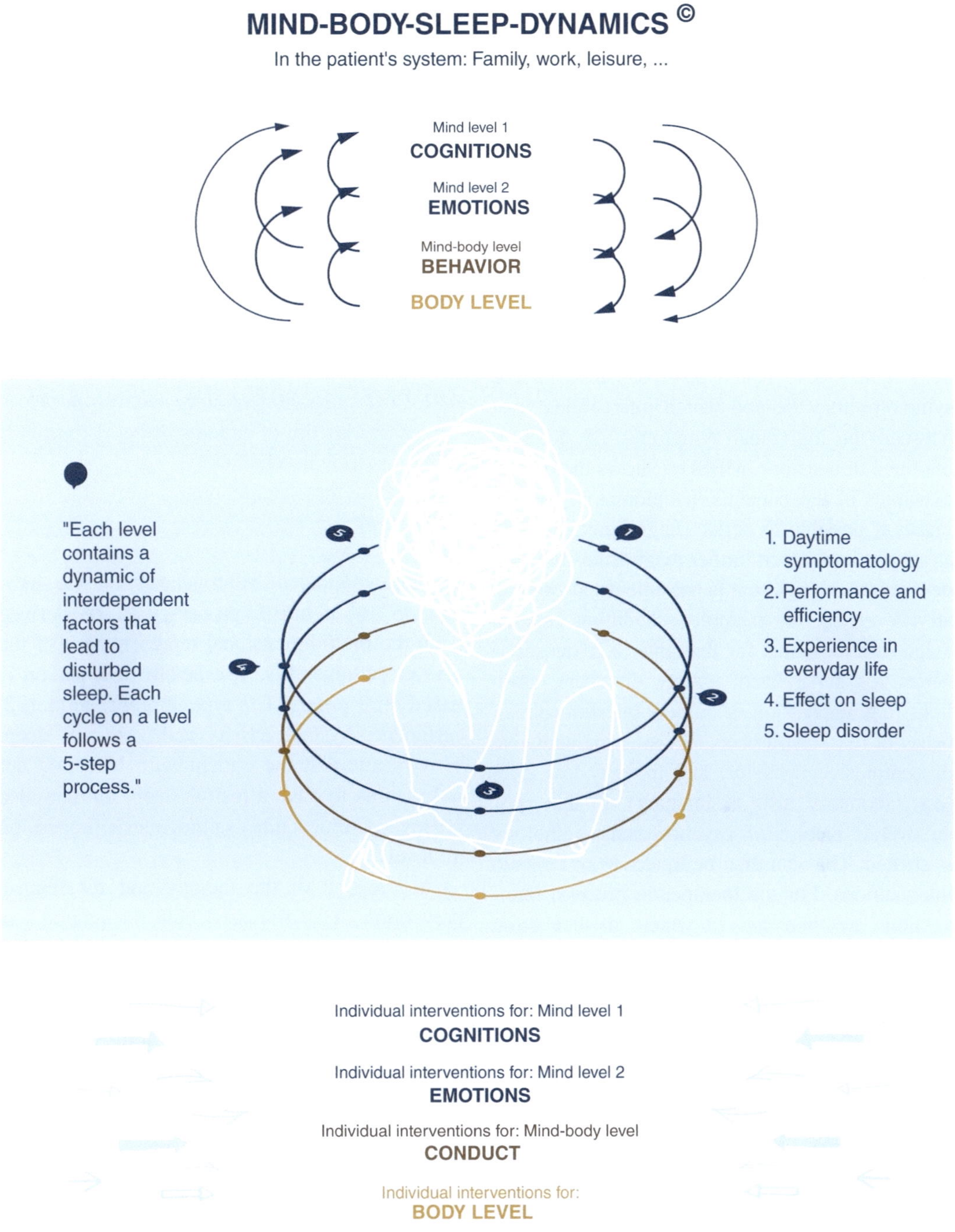

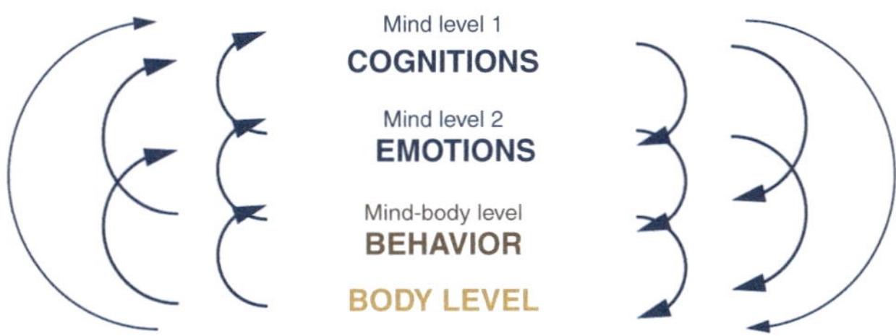

Fig. 2.1 Model of mind-body-sleep dynamics© (Marx-Dick 2020)

Working with the Model of Mind-Body-Sleep-Dynamics©

MBSD© is a bio-psycho-dynamic condition model that can be worked out together with the patients. For this purpose, the individual areas of mind (emotion and cognition), mind-body (behavior) and body (physical) are first considered separately and only later combined to form the overall picture. This makes it possible to represent which symptoms are present as a whole, including all comorbidities, both somatic and mental in nature. From this, initial findings can be obtained as to where possible causes of the symptoms may lie and which interactions exist between the individual symptoms. By combining the 4 dimensions, MBSD© shows the overall dynamics of the patient's symptomatology. This makes it possible to derive diagnoses or to gain an insight into which further diagnostics may still be required. Here too, it is possible to proceed on all 4 levels by, for example, scheduling targeted diagnostic measures for thoughts (e.g. questionnaires for generalized anxiety disorder), emotions (e.g. depression or anxiety questionnaires), behavior (e.g. instruments for assessing addictive or compulsive behavior) and the physical level (e.g. laboratory tests or imaging). In this way, an overall picture of psycho-somato-pathology is created. This can then be treated with targeted interventions. For the therapeutic process, interventions are then derived which, in their sum, can do justice to the overall symptomatology. Here, MBSD© can be a good therapy companion, as the therapy process can be supplemented, adjusted and checked on an ongoing basis.

> In practice, the following sequence has proven to be favorable:
>
> 1. Thorough medical history and, if necessary, targeted diagnostics
> 2. Explanation of the current symptomatology, feedback of the diagnosis(es) and rough idea of the treatment plan
> 3. Rapid relief of the massive suffering pressure in the first therapy sessions (e.g. with bed rest restrictions and change of daily routine)
> 4. Accompanying psychoeducation: the patient becomes an expert on his illness
> 5. Working out concrete therapeutic topics that (possible) causes of sleep disorders can be (e.g. by means of lifestyle change, acceptance-commitment therapy or cognitive behavioral therapy)
> 6. Presentation and practice of interventions that should be integrated into everyday life later
> 7. Implementation of interventions in the everyday life of patients, support for the transition into habits
> 8. Follow-up care and relapse prevention

The interventions of salutogenesis, i.e. the "production" of a health process, can be derived from the multidimensional representation of the overall pathogenesis. The health of a person is based on 3 pillars: 1. a type-appropriate diet, 2. sufficient physical activity and 3. restful sleep. This means that the patient with MBSD© not only learns to have a restful sleep, but can also positively influence his salutogenesis process on all levels.

At the end of the therapy and for relapse prevention, it is discussed how the patient can integrate the respective interventions of the disease treatment into his everyday life and which measures are necessary to change the lifestyle in a health-promoting way in the long term. This strengthens self-efficacy and enables sustainable treatment success.

There are disease dynamics that require only 3–5 sessions of therapy in this way to lead to treatment success. But there are also pathologies that require long-term therapy.

> ▶ It is important in all cases that patients be enabled to move from a self-responsible disease treatment (disease management) to a self-efficacious motivated health management.

In this way, those affected can take immediate action on new or recurring symptoms and the disease does not recur.

2.2.2   Causes of Sleep Disorders

Psychological Causes

Dysfunctional Cognitions

Worry and rumination are among the most commonly reported symptoms of sleep disorders. It has long been scientifically proven that worry and rumination increase muscle tone (Borkovec et al. 1991). This leads to physical tension. However, a relaxed awake state is necessary for falling asleep. This mechanism is also important at night. If the patient wakes up from one of the following light sleep phases or a short wakefulness phase due to sleep architecture, the usual rumination thoughts often start automatically and unconsciously in many patients. This leads to a rapid increase in body tension and makes it impossible to fall asleep again quickly.

Due to neurocognitive deficits, patients experience themselves as less capable, they are more easily distracted, have reduced receptivity and can solve problems less well. As a result, patients experience themselves as insufficient, which in turn fuels negative worries and rumination. Many patients are also tormented throughout the day by the thought of not being able to fall asleep or sleep through the night again. In this way, stress is also created in the body, which has a lasting negative effect on sleep.

Dysfunctional Emotions

Feelings always have the right! They secure our survival and are therefore very important. Since we have our feelings evolutionarily still from the time when our ancestors lived as cavemen, some brain structures and reflexes are "overcautious" or too sensitive to support us functionally in the modern world. Emotional reactions can also have a negative effect on sleep. Anger and rage make us ready for battle, so they activate our sympathetic nervous system and the entire body physiology. Any kind of fear wakes up the flight reflex, which also leads to a sympathetic reaction. The relaxation necessary for falling asleep is inhibited. Emotions such as being freshly in love or looking forward to the vacation, the wedding etc. can make falling asleep much more difficult. Positive life events can also be a stress for the psyche.

Patients who have been suffering from sleep disorders for a long time already fear going to bed. This expectation anxiety about a sleepless night or longer nocturnal wakefulness can already set in after morning waking and persist throughout the day. Such feelings increase muscle tone and cause restlessness and tension. This also hinders the relaxed state of wakefulness, which is essential to find sleep. Sadness and depressed mood, as is typical for a depressive episode, can lead to a loss of motivation. The depressive symptomatology is closely related to insomnia due to a pronounced avoidance behavior or hypersomnia after a massive load (e.g. burn-out) or by significantly increased fatigue.

▶ Any kind of intense feelings can lead to sleepless nights. If these are temporary states that only exist for a certain period of time, this is no problem, and a healthy person can cope with them well. However, caution is advised if these structures become chronic.

Dysfunctional Behavior

Sleep is a completely natural process that works automatically and on its own for most people for a long time. Therefore, many people are not aware when they behave in a sleep-disturbing way. By having an unstructured day without regularity in meals, performance and rest phases, as well as bedtime and wake-up times, the circadian rhythm can be thrown off balance and sleep disorders can occur.

Dysfunctional behaviors, such as turning on the light at night, eating, or getting angry about not being able to sleep again, can further intensify the evening or nighttime wakefulness. Using the bedroom for sports, housework, home office, etc. disturbs sleep. The consumption of substances or late internet research, news consumption, phone calls, arguments, etc. also have a negative effect on sleep. This list could be continued almost endlessly. Basically, all behaviors that are harmful to health in general, such as lack of exercise, stress, and actions that disturb the circadian rhythm, disturb the restful night's sleep.

Somatic Causes

When looking for the causes of sleep disorders, somatic triggers should also be considered. Diseases that cause hormonal changes can cause sleep disorders. A thyroid dysfunction, female cycle problems, or other hormonal changes can be the cause here.

Many diseases cause pain, mobility restrictions, cognitive deficits, etc. This usually results in an illness-related need for rest, which in turn can lead to a lack of exercise, movement, and exhaustion. If the body and mind are not sufficiently tired, there is no need for deep regenerative sleep. An illness itself and the healing process can put a tremendous strain on the body and mind, which is why the sick person needs significantly more sleep than usual. Insomnia, hypersomnia, and circadian rhythm disorders can then occur more frequently.

If a person is in pain, they cannot or can only sleep very poorly. Pain can only wake us up from stage 3, deep sleep. Consequently, pain can pull sufferers out of any phase of sleep or prevent them from falling asleep in the first place. Analogous to sleep disorders, pain can also become chronic. Insomnia, in turn, can intensify the experience of pain. These impairments then condition each other and maintain each other. Therefore, everything should be kept in mind that can cause pain, such as musculoskeletal diseases, injuries, rheumatism, postoperative events, etc.

▶ Nausea, dizziness and headaches can also interfere with sleep. Therefore, sleep disorders occur more frequently in cancer, inflammatory and metabolic diseases, cardiovascular diseases and respiratory diseases.

In the transition from the waking state to deep sleep, the entire body physiology calms down: heart rate, pulse and blood pressure drop, breathing volume and body temperature decrease. For these processes, the body needs flexibility to adapt these functions. If there are diseases, such as hypertension, which make it impossible for the body to perform these regulatory processes, no healthy sleep can occur.

Autoimmune diseases are usually closely related to the cortisol balance. The resulting imbalance can have an unfavorable effect on the cortisol course and thus also on sleep. The administration of cortisone-containing medications, especially intravenously or orally, can also lead to severe sleep disorders.

Many neurological diseases such as multiple sclerosis, seizure disorders, tumors, strokes and especially degenerative diseases can lead to sleep disorders. Patients with Parkinson's disease are particularly affected by this. The resulting dopamine deficiency also disturbs sleep, since dopamine is a neurotransmitter of the sleep-wake regulation and also subject to the circadian rhythm. Dementia also usually comes with a sleep disorder. Through the loss of sense of time, day structures and routines are softened. This lack of structure can lead to a floating day-night and sleep-wake rhythm and thus to sleep disorders. Diseases of the diencephalon can lead to inexplicable daytime sleepiness and hypersomnia. Obesity and thus also type 2 diabetes are closely related to the sleep apnea syndrome.

Substances

Most people affected notice very quickly that they can fall asleep more easily and maintain it better if they drink a "beer" or a "glass of red wine" in the evening. There is nothing wrong with doing this occasionally and especially for enjoyment. However, using alcohol deliberately as a sleep aid is tantamount to abuse and increases the risk of addiction very significantly, because alcohol is a substance that is physically addictive. This means that with regular use, tolerance develops: either the alcohol no longer works at all or the affected person needs much more to achieve the same effect. Alcohol does have a relaxing effect and thus allows a faster transition from the waking state to sleep, but it largely suppresses deep sleep, thus destroying Sleep architecture and thus limiting the recovery function of sleep. Similar is the case with substances such as marijuana, other drugs and to some extent also with sleep aids. At first they seem to contribute to relaxation and shorten the time it takes to fall asleep. However, in the medium and especially in the long term, this use is of no use, as tolerance develops and above all a psychological dependence occurs.

When studying the package inserts of many medications, sleep disorders occur very frequently. This is not surprising, as sleep is highly complex and involved in many physical and psychological processes.

▶ It is extremely important to ask in the first conversations which medications are taken in which dose at what time of day.

Substances of any kind and a variety of medications for the most diverse diseases can interfere with the healthy natural regulatory processes of the body. Therefore, they should be considered in the search for the cause of sleep disorders.

Everyday Life and Lifestyle

Paradoxically, but true, some people simply do not take enough time to sleep. Affected people often find no conclusion in the evening because they have to do housework, do Internet research or answer news and e-mails. For many people, the time before going to bed is the only "time for themselves". Taking time to sleep does not just mean allocating enough bedtime. It is also important to plan time to "slow down", arrive and find peace.

Sleep disorders have a major impact on every aspect of life, making it impossible to deal with the topic of sleep in a relaxed manner anymore. The thoughts of those affected often revolve around it, and many everyday behaviors are geared towards hopefully being able to sleep well at night. For example, many people with sleep disorders no longer drink any coffee or black or green tea at all because they are afraid of not being able to fall asleep at night due to the caffeine. They sleep separately from their partner, do not take morning appointments, do not go out in the evening anymore, and they plan a disproportionate amount of time for the bed in order to get the corresponding amount of sleep and recovery. They rarely or seldom go on vacation, and they don't like to stay overnight away from home because they can't do their usual nighttime rituals there. By behaving in this way, they impair their overall quality of life and often also burden relatives and friends.

It is also striking that there is a nearly pathological search for information on all articles, programs, websites, newspapers and books that can be found on the topic of sleep and sleep disorders. The constant thought of sleep is a strong maintaining factor of the disorder, quite contrary to the sleep-promoting process: »The way away from sleep is the way towards sleep« (Crönlein 2010).

Disturbing influences from the outside can have a massive impact on sleep. Possible causes are noise, light, heat, stuffy air, a bad mattress or also itching and urination.

Children are popular sleep thieves. The first two years are usually the most stressful, as children have a very fragmented sleep. Some children fall asleep relatively quickly, but there are also children who wake up more often at night, want to drink something or just need closeness. Once this first period is over, childhood diseases and nightmares follow. Then comes the adolescence, with worries that rob the parents of their sleep. Fortunately, there are wonderful moments and restful nights in between, which make the time with children very valuable.

▶ Almost 20% of employees work in shifts. For "sensitive sleepers", the different working, resting and sleeping times are a huge challenge.

Life with shift work is usually accompanied by a shift in sleep-wake rhythms. Thus, the circadian rhythm is softened and it can lead to massive sleep disturbances and health problems. It is particularly critical if those affected only work in night shifts, such as security guards. Even if a regular sleep rhythm during the day would be possible, this can cause strong shifts in the hormone and neurotransmitter balance, because humans are diurnal and not "nocturnal animals".

Sleep is a very sensitive construct. Disturbances or overstrain in everyday life are often first reflected in sleep. Since a refreshing sleep is urgently needed in order to be able to perform and stay fit during the day, it has to work. As long as that is the case, few people waste thoughts on sleep. Only when sleep is no longer refreshing, a clear suffering pressure sets in.

2.3 Diagnostics and Classification

When the media or the general population talk about sleep disorders, they usually mean insomnia. This is a psychologically caused sleep deficit. However, there are over 80 different sleep disorders. Therefore, a thorough diagnosis is an important foundation for the treatment and alleviation of symptoms in the group of sleep disorders.

In the ICD-10 (International Statistical Classification of Diseases and Related Health Problems ICD-10-WHO Version 2019), organic sleep disorders were still distinguished from non-organic sleep disorders. By this categorization, the treating physicians and the therapy measures were already fixed. However, this separation turned out to be unfavorable due to the increasingly holistic view of all diseases (mind-body-medicine). Therefore, a separate category for all sleep disorders was introduced in the ICD 11 (WHO 2022). This change allows for better interdisciplinary exchange and the possibility of holistic treatment of all sleep disorders.

2.3.1 Diagnosis

Basically, in most cases the diagnosis of a sleep disorder is not difficult. The underlying symptoms can be queried by means of self- and external anamnesis. Targeted standardized questionnaires also provide diagnostic tools with which specific information on sleep quality, sleep duration and above all daytime sleepiness can be collected. Nevertheless, one should not be deceived by this superficial diagnosis by means of ICD-10 and -11 diagnostic criteria. Under the superficial subjectively felt and reported symptoms of the sleep disorder usually lies a complex dynamics. The overall pathology with subclinical syndromes and comorbidities is partly very difficult to grasp and yet relevant. Therefore, it is important in the diagnostic phase at the beginning of a treatment not to fall into a tunnel vision and only have the symptoms of the different sleep disorders in mind. It is important to gain a structured overview.

Psychotherapy offers wonderful screening instruments and general psychopathology questionnaires, which ensure that a doctor or therapist is not tempted by clinical gut feeling. A one-sided diagnosis and therapy would be the result. Experience has shown that too one-sided treatment does not lead to sustainable success.

A thorough medical history and a physical examination should also be carried out to discuss how physical health factors play a role in the dynamics of sleep disorders. Particular attention should be paid to hormonal, neurological, cardiovascular, gastrointestinal, pain and auto-immune diseases. In addition, special attention should be paid to the medications used, as these can often cause sleep disturbances as a side effect. Physical fitness and eating habits also play an essential role.

> ▶ The central question in the medical history and diagnosis of sleep disorders is: "How is your daily fitness?"

It sounds banal, but not all sleep disorders automatically lead to reduced daily fitness or daytime symptoms or fatigue during the day. Conversely, it is not automatically the case that a sleep disorder exists if people do not feel rested and powerful during the day. Therefore, four different constellations are possible (Table 2.1).

Table 2.1 Matrix for diagnosing various sleep disorders

	With subjectively poor sleep quality	Sleep is perceived as deep and sound
With daytime sleepiness	Insomnia, sleep-wake rhythm disorder etc.	Sleep apnea syndrome etc.
No or only sporadic daytime sleepiness	Paradoxical insomnia	Probably no sleep disorder, the suffering is located elsewhere.

Every now and then, people come to my practice and report an unpleasant fatigue during the day around noon and in the evening. This "midday slump" is genetically determined and demanded by the healthy circadian rhythm. In addition, it is "normal" and even healthy to feel tired and exhausted after a busy day in the evening. If the night's sleep makes you feel well-rested the next morning and reasonably energetic during the day, there is no pathology in this regard.

2.3.2 Classification

The American Academy of Sleep Medicine (AASM) regularly develops and updates the "International Classification of Sleep Disorders" (ICSD) to reflect the latest research.

The current version of the ICSD-3 (AASM 2014) differentiates between 88 forms of disturbed sleep, which are divided into six main categories.

1. Insomnia (sleep deprivation due to difficulties falling asleep and staying asleep)
2. Sleep-related breathing disorders (e.g., obstructive sleep apnea syndrome)
3. Hypersomnias of central nervous origin (e.g., narcolepsy or as a result of drug abuse)
4. Circadian rhythm disorders
5. Parasomnias (e.g., sleepwalking or nightmares)
6. Sleep-related movement disorders (e.g., "restless legs syndrome" or teeth grinding [bruxism])

For the everyday treatment in medical and psychotherapeutic practices, ICD-10 and, since 2022, ICD-11 are the best basis. Due to the structure and the regulations of ICD-10, sleep disorders could so far often only be counted as a symptom of another mental disorder and not be explicitly coded as a diagnosis or comorbidity. ICD-10 stipulates that the non-organic sleep disorder should only be given as an additional diagnosis if "the sleep disorder is one of the main complaints and is considered as an independent condition" (Dilling and Mombour 2013). So far, only the primary sleep disorders (non-organic insomnia, non-organic hypersomnia) have been taken into account in the diagnosis and also in the (psycho-)therapy. This caused great misunderstandings, as many doctors and colleagues did not know the non-organic sleep disorders (especially insomnia, hypersomnia and nightmares) as an independent diagnosis and always assumed a depressive underlying disease. As a result, many sufferers felt not taken seriously, because they had no depressive symptoms. If comorbid symptoms occurred, the sleep disorders were not included in the diagnosis and treatment in return. Therefore, the sleep disorder was hardly taken into account in the therapy process. If necessary, sleeping pills were prescribed in the inpatient or partial inpatient setting. Targeted psychotherapy took and takes place in the rarest of cases.

It is all the more gratifying that the diagnosis has been adapted in ICD-11 and now there is a separate category for all sleep disorders.

▶ In ICD-11, the subdivision into organic and non-organic sleep disorders is dispensed with: Intensive research in recent years has shown that all sleep disorders can have somatic and psychological components.

Sleep disorders are taken out of the individual chapters V (mental and behavioral disorders, F-diagnoses), VI (diseases of the nervous system, G-diagnoses), IV (endocrine, nutritional and metabolic diseases, E-diagnoses) and XVI (certain conditions originating in the perinatal period, P-diagnoses) and summarized in the new chapter 07 *with the title* "Sleep-wake disorders".

Even if ICD-11 will not be mandatory until 2027, the diagnosis is already explained here using the new coding system, as it has many advantages over the classification with ICD-10.

Table 2.2 shows the classification of sleep disorders according to ICD-11, ICD-10 and the categories of ICSD

Insomnia (7A00–7A0Z)

The term insomnia comes from Latin and means "sleeplessness". However, the diagnosis of insomnia is not equated with not sleeping, but rather refers to a condition that can be equated with a lack of sleep. This can include difficulty falling asleep or staying asleep, as well as waking up much too early, as shown in Fig. 2.2.

There is chronic (ZA00), acute (ZA01) and unspecified insomnia (ZA0Z).

Patients complain of poor sleep quality, which adversely affects their social and occupational performance (WHO 1946). Sleep onset disorders are characterized by an extended sleep latency (time to fall asleep) that exceeds the "normal" amount. There are no uniform time limits for a "normal" amount in the literature. In practice, an approximate 30 min is assumed. The key factor in this component is the patient's distress, which can already begin with a sleep latency of 20 min. Sleep maintenance disorders are characterized by multiple awakenings during the night and a delayed ability to fall back asleep. Re-sleep times of 2 h or more are reported. If a person cannot fall back asleep after a night or early morning awakening, it is called an early morning awakening or sleep maintenance disorder. Again, there are no uniform time limits for how long the sleep latency or the night awakening

may last or how early the person may wake up in order to be considered insomnia. The patient's distress and social norms must be taken into account. For example, if a person wakes up at 8:00 a.m. even though he or she wanted to sleep until 11:00 a.m., it cannot be considered a sleep disorder according to social norms. Nevertheless, there may be a great deal of distress. In addition, sleep does not have a refreshing effect and performance in everyday life is impaired (Dilling and Mombour 2013).

These symptoms must occur at least 3 times a week for diagnosis, this corresponds to the acute insomnia. If the symptoms last longer than 3 months, it is called chronic insomnia. The course of chronic insomnia often lasts for many years and even decades. It usually shows an episodic course with recurrent phases of sleep disorders, which last for several weeks or months and then pass into a milder symptomatology.

▶   According to estimates, every fourth adult in industrialized countries suffers from sleep and wakefulness disorders, which lead to a reduced total sleep time, a lower sleep quality and thus a lack of feeling of recovery the next morning.

This is accompanied by a pronounced daytime symptomatology with fatigue, depressive mood, irritability, general discomfort, pain, nausea, exhaustion and cognitive impairment with concentration and memory deficits, etc.

In addition, more than 80% of employees sleep too little, partly because they do not take enough time to sleep. This is referred to as "sleep deprivation syndrome" in ICSD-3. In ICD-11, this is coded under "sleep-wake disorders, not otherwise specified".

▶   Insomnia can be diagnosed with a thorough anamnesis, sleep diaries and specific questionnaires. Patients usually do not need to go to a sleep laboratory.

Table 2.2 Classification of sleep disorders according to ICD-11, ICD-10 and ICSD

ICD-11-Code	Title ICD-11	ICD-10-Code	Title ICD-10	ICSD category
7A00–7A0Z, Insomnia				
7A0Z	Insomnia, unspecified	F51.0	Nonorganic insomnia	1
7A0Z	Insomnia, unspecified	G47.0	Sleep onset and sleep maintenance disorders	1
7A20–7A2Z, hypersomnia				
7A20.Z	Narcolepsy, unspecified	G47.4	Narcolepsy and cataplexy	3
7A21	Idiopathic hypersomnia	G47.1	Pathologically increased need for sleep (hypersomnia)	3
7A26	Insufficient sleep syndrome	F51.1	Non-organic hypersomnia	3
7A40–7A4Z, Sleep-related breathing disorders				
7A4Z	Sleep-related breathing disorders, not otherwise specified	G47.3	Sleep apnea syndrome	2
7A40.1	Primary central sleep apnea in infancy	P28.3	Primary sleep apnea of newborn	2
7A42.0	Sleep-related hypoventilation or hypoxemia disorders	E66.2	Excessive obesity with alveolar hypoventilation	2
7A60–7A6Z, Circadian sleep-wake disorders				
7A6Z	Sleep-wake disorders of the circadian rhythm, not otherwise specified	G47.2, F51.2	(nonorganic) disorders of the sleep-wake rhythm	4
7A80–7A8Z Sleep-related movement disorders				
7A80	Restless-Legs-Syndrom	G25.81	Restless-Legs-Syndrom	6
7B00–7B0Z, Parasomnien				
7B00.1	sleep walking	F51.3	sleep walking	5
7B00.2	Pavor Nocturnus	F51.4	Pavor Nocturnus	5
7B01.2	Nightmares	F51.5	Nightmares	5
7B2Z, Sleep-wake disorders, unspecified, other sleep-wake disorders.				
7B2Z	Sleep-wake disorders, not otherwise specified	F51.8	Other specified sleep disorders	1
7B2Z	Sleep-wake disorders, not otherwise specified	F51.9	Sleep disorder, not otherwise specified	4
7B2Z	Sleep-wake disorders, not otherwise specified	G47	Sleep disorders, (subcategory)	1
7B2Z	Sleep-wake disorders, not otherwise specified	G47.9	Bruxism, (sleep disorders, not otherwise specified)	6

Fig. 2.2 Forms of insomnia

If the overall symptomatology cannot be related to each other and thus is not clearly explicable, a polysomnography should be scheduled. This is the case, for example, if

- the patient sleeps sufficiently with a subjectively good sleep quality, but still feels fresh and fit,
- massive sleep disorders exist, which do not improve even with therapy,
- persistent daytime sleepiness exists without any recognizable cause,
- a subjective *insomnia* is reported with good daytime fitness without fatigue (sleep perception disorder).

Subtype Paradoxical Insomnia (Sleep Perception Disorder)

In a paradoxical insomnia, or a sleep perception disorder, the patients report that they have hardly or not slept at all for several days or even weeks. They describe nocturnal brooding and daydream images with partial perception of external stimuli (church tower clock, tram, nocturnal awakening of the partner), which give the patients the feeling of being constantly awake. In addition, there is hypersensitivity to external stimuli during the sleep period, which further burdens the patients. The bed partners, on the other hand, often report that they have experienced the patients asleep.

The patients feel burdened by the extremely long perceived waking times and frequent nocturnal awakenings with long periods of wakefulness. Since the daytime fitness appears to be hardly or not restricted in relation to the subjectively experienced insomnia, the suffering of the patients lies in the tormenting subjectively experienced as endless wakefulness. The patients are often surprised that despite severe sleep deprivation, they hardly feel any fatigue or restrictions during the day. At the same time, they are plagued by fears, as sleep deprivation can lead to serious physical and mental illnesses and a shortened life expectancy.

▶ Objective data from a polysomnography, however, show that the patients'

sleep is sufficiently long and of good quality, which in turn explains the good daytime fitness.

Paradoxical insomnia occurs just as often in comorbid depression or post-traumatic stress disorder as in actual sleep deprivation. In the general population, an incidence of approximately 5% is currently assumed. The sleep perception disorder therefore seems to occur much more frequently than initially assumed. The therapy is very demanding due to the lack of awareness of the disease.

The specific classification of the subtypes is not foreseen in the ICD. The ICSD-3 offers precise classification options here (Table 2.3).

Differential Diagnosis

It is important to differentiate between sleep-related breathing disorders and insomnia, as some clinical pictures appear phenotypically identical. Depressive symptoms, such as lack of drive, dysphoria, loss of appetite, as well as pronounced daytime sleepiness can also occur in insomnia. The decisive diagnostic question here is: Is the patient sleeping or is the nocturnal wakefulness the cause of the daytime symptoms? People with sleep-related breathing disorders usually have no sleep or wakefulness disorders.

For most forms of insomnia, a psychotherapist specializing in sleep disorders should be the first point of contact.

Hypersomnia (7A20–7A2Z)

In contrast to insomnia, hypersomnia is characterized by a significantly extended sleep duration or increased sleepiness up to excessive sleepiness. Hypersomnias are characterized by daytime sleepiness that is not due to another sleep-wake disorder (e.g. disturbed night sleep, wrongly aligned circadian rhythm or breathing disorder). People with excessive sleepiness may have deficits in concentration and attention, reduced vigilance, distractibility, reduced motivation, energy, dysphoria, fatigue, irritability, restlessness and coordination disorders. A hypersomnia is also said to be present when

Table 2.3 Overview of the different classification forms of insomnia

Classification of insomnia according to ICSD-3	Measure
Short-term insomnia—insomnia as an adjustment disorder • Temporarily • As a result of a clearly defined event • Full remission if stressor is turned off	→ Psychotherapy
Psychophysiological insomnia • Increased level of arousal • Dysfunctional cognitions about sleep	→ Psychotherapy
Paradoxical Insomnia—Sleep Perception Disorder • Characterized by partly massive underestimation of the effective sleep time • Hardly to no performance loss during the day • Hardly to no daytime symptomatology	→ Psychotherapy
Idiopathic Insomnia • Similar to psychophysiological insomnia • Disease onset in early childhood • Cause possibly genetic/neurological	→ Referral to the family doctor or neurologist
Insomnia in the context of mental illness • Sleep disorders together with depressions, anxiety disorders, mania, schizophrenia, eating disorders, dementia • In the context of addiction	→ Psychotherapy

the person has great difficulty transitioning from sleep to wakefulness.

The non-organic hypersomnia is classified in the ICD-11 as *Idiopathic hypersomnia* (7A21) or *insufficient sleep syndrome* (7A26). These syndromes often occur in connection with depressive disorders.

Subtype Narcolepsy

Narcolepsy (7A20) also belongs to hypersomnias. This disorder is known by the apparent, sudden falling asleep of those affected. However, they actually experience cataplexies, that is an emotionally triggered loss of tone of the striped muscles while remaining conscious. In ICSD-3, narcolepsy type 1 with cataplexy and narcolepsy type 2 without cataplexy are distinguished. Both forms have a partly enormous increased daytime sleepiness, which is associated with considerable suffering of the affected.

The following also belong to this diagnosis category:

- Kleine-Levin-Syndrom (7A22)
- Hypersomnia due to a disease (7A23)
- Hypersomnia due to a medication or substance (7A24)
- Hypersomnia in connection with a mental disorder (7A25)
- Hypersomnolence disorders, not otherwise specified (7A2Z)

If there is suspicion of hypersomnia, interdisciplinary cooperation should take place. First, a thorough anamnesis, a polysomnography in the sleep laboratory and a subsequent case conference with a neurologist and a psychotherapist are desirable. With the confirmed diagnosis, medical therapy can be carried out by the neurologist. In addition, a relieving psychotherapy can alleviate the suffering of the affected.

Sleep-related Respiratory Disorders (7A40–7A4Z)

The term sleep-related breathing disorders refers to the widespread sleep apnea syndrome (SAS, 7A40). Those affected experience nocturnal breathing pauses, which lead to a reduced oxygen saturation in the entire body and also in the brain. The cause is a closure of the airways (e.g. due to overweight or relaxation of the tissue in the throat area). The patients suffer from an enormous amount of daytime sleepiness, as their sleep is not restful. Usually, the partners are disturbed by very loud snoring. They often notice the breathing pauses first.

▶ The patients report an excessive amount of daytime sleepiness, up to the involuntary nodding off in some dangerous or embarrassing situations. The main complaints are very similar to those of depression, so a precise differential diagnosis must be made here.

The disorders are divided into central sleep apnea, obstructive sleep apnea and sleep-related hypoventilation disorders (reduced ventilation of the lungs) or hypoxemia disorders (reduction of oxygen content in the blood).

Central sleep apnea is characterized by a reduction or interruption of airflow due to absent or reduced effort to breathe. In obstructive apnea, there are temporary breathing pauses due to closures of the upper airways. Both central apnea (apnea) and hypopnea (severely reduced breathing) can occur cyclically or intermittently. Both apnea forms lead to a reduction in blood oxygen saturation and are usually terminated by arousals (micro-awakening reactions).

The diagnosis criteria for sleep apnea syndrome (SAS) are met if more than 15 respiratory events (apneas, hypopneas) occur per hour. Mild forms of SAS can be diagnosed if fewer than 15 but more than five respiratory events occur per hour and other symptoms are present, such as

- excessive sleepiness,
- nocturnal dyspnea or apnea (observed by bed partner),
- habitual snoring,
- hypertension, affective disorders, cognitive dysfunction, heart disease, increased stroke risk or type 2 diabetes mellitus.

In children, SAS is already diagnosed if there are more than one obstructive event per hour and there are signs of respiratory disorders.

In the differential diagnosis of depressive disorder, the corresponding risk factors of SAS should be considered:

Risk Factors of SAS
- Increased age
- Male gender
- Obesity
- Smoking and alcohol consumption
- Intake of relaxants and sleeping pills

Some symptoms of SAS and depression are identical:

- Lethargy and depressed mood
- Partly massive loss of motivation
- Severe fatigue during the day
- Neurocognitive deficits, especially memory and concentration disorders
- Loss of libido and appetite

Typical SAS symptoms that should be asked during the anamnesis are:

- No recovery despite sufficient sleep duration or significantly longer sleep duration
- Snoring
- Sudden awakening with partly tachycardia and shortness of breath
- Dry mouth upon waking
- Severe headaches in the morning

▶ An SAS must always be diagnosed with a polysomnography. Therefore, if there is suspicion of an SAS, the patient must always be referred to a pulmonary sleep laboratory.

The therapy with a CPAP device ("Continuous Positive Airway Pressure") quickly brings relief. In this case, the airways of the affected persons are blown free with air which is blown into the nose (and possibly mouth) under increased pressure. A pulmonologist in the sleep laboratory is the right contact person here.

Circadian Sleep-wake Disorders (7A60–7A6Z)

The category of circadian sleep-wake disorders in the ICD-11 was referred to as non-organic sleep-wake rhythm disorder in the ICD-10. Here, the sleep and wake phases of the affected person are shifted in time so that they collide with the social rhythm and thus lead to suffering. In turn, the delayed sleep phase disorder can be distinguished from the advanced sleep phase disorder. Many adolescents, for example, suffer from the delayed sleep phase syndrome during puberty. Even if they have to get up at 6 a.m. to go to school, they do not find themselves in bed before 11 p.m. due to hormonal reasons. In older people, an advanced sleep phase syndrome is often found. Since the current generation of older people has been getting up very early all their lives, many of them retain this sleep behavior. Since even healthy older people can no longer sleep for more than 5 h a night, they are tired during the day and want to go to bed early. Therefore, it is not uncommon for seniors to go to bed at 9 p.m. and wake up completely again between 2 and 3 a.m.

Sleep can also be highly fragmented and sleep or wakefulness can occur at any time of day or night.

▶ Patients show both specific symptoms of insomnia and hypersomnia.

This often affects people who work in shifts or who often have to travel through different time zones for work and then experience jet lag. Retired people, people with chronic illnesses, job seekers and other people who lack a daily structure due to commitments can suffer from circadian sleep-wake disorders.

A visit to the sleep laboratory is not necessary at first. Psychotherapists can help with targeted cognitive behavioral therapy to synchronize the sleep-wake rhythm and adapt it to the living conditions (occupation, family, chronotype, etc.).

Subtype Shift Worker Syndrome

About 20% of the working population in industrialized countries works in shifts, about 40% of these employees suffer from sleep disorders. So the shift worker syndrome is not a rare symptom. Due to constantly changing active and inactive times, which often run contrary to the course of the day (light and temperature) as well as other external timekeepers, such as social contacts and meals, many people experience a shift in their sleep-wake rhythm, which then leads to sleep disorders. This can lead to insomnia symptoms as well as an undesired circadian shift in the sleep-wake rhythm.

If the symptoms occur for at least one month and can be directly related to shift work, this subtype can be classified. However, helping people on shift work is very difficult because our natural sleep-wake rhythm is linked to light and darkness, meals and social rhythms. Even the best psychotherapy cannot work miracles here.

Sleep-related Movement Disorders (7A80–7A8Z)

Sleep-related movement disorders include involuntary, simple and stereotyped movements that disturb sleep. Various muscles can be involved. They often occur in the transition from the waking state to sleep or exactly when the person wants to rest. They not only involve actual muscle movements, but also sometimes very unpleasant to painful sensations.

Subtype Restless Legs Syndrome

Among the sleep-related movement disorders is the restless legs syndrome (syndrome of restless legs, RLS) described. RLS patients report very unpleasant restlessness and sensations in the legs and also in the arms when they want to come to rest in the evening or sleep. It is characterized by:

- periodic leg movements in sleep (PLMS)
- sleep-related leg cramps
- sleep-related rhythmic movement disorders
- strong and partly very painful sensations (tingling, burning, pulling, etc.)

▶ Restless Legs cause insomnia in many effected people, which significantly increases the suffering.

A neurological sleep laboratory is the right contact here. In addition, a psychotherapy should be scheduled to support, as the RLS can be exacerbated by stress in general and emotional stress.

While in the ICD-10, nocturnal teeth grinding (bruxism) was counted among the nocturnal movement disorders, it is now found in the ICD-11 under the diseases of the mouth, salivary glands and jaws (K00-K14). Bruxism is the result of excessive chronic tension, usually caused by stress in everyday life. The affected people suffer from headaches and teeth as well as physical tension with sometimes un-recoverable sleep. First, the patient should consult a dentist to assess the current dental and jaw status as well as to exclude organic causes. Subsequently, the cause of bruxism should be clarified by psychotherapy and appropriate psychotherapeutic measures should be initiated.

Parasomnias (7B00–7B0Z)

Parasomnias are behaviors or physiological phenomena that occur during sleep onset, sleep, or awakening from sleep. Parasomnias can occur during both non-REM and REM sleep and during the transition between sleep stages, as well as during sleep onset or awakening. This can lead to very complex movements, behaviors, and dreams. The ICD-11 distinguishes between parasomnias in REM and non-REM sleep.

Arousal Disorder in Non-REM sleep (7B00)

Arrousal disorders in Non-REM sleep are characterized by sleep-related phenomena such as confusion, behavior with sometimes violent movements or extreme autonomic arousal. They occur in deep non-REM sleep (N3).

Sleep drunkenness (7B00.0)

Sleep drunkenness includes symptoms such as disorientation, unresponsiveness, impaired or slow speech, and amnesia. It often occurs upon awakening from deep sleep. Sleep drunkenness is a relatively harmless wake-up phenomenon. Only when the experience leads to significant suffering or impairment in important areas of functioning should a thorough diagnosis and therapy be scheduled.

Sleepwalking (7B00.1)

In *sleepwalking* (somnambulism), those affected show stereotypical movements up to very complex automated behaviors during sleep (e.g. going to the toilet, making coffee). They are not clearly conscious, but have partial attention. Such episodes can last from a few seconds to a few minutes, rarely longer. Only a few sleepwalkers leave the bed while they are asleep. The walking phases occur each time during the transition from Non-REM 2 to Non-REM 3, that is, during the middle and deep sleep, and back again. Those affected are in a changed state of consciousness at this time. The eyes are open and it is possible that these people appear responsive and react adequately. However, they can also be unresponsive and act unusually. After waking up, most affected people cannot remember their nocturnal outing.

The cause of sleepwalking is thought to be an insufficient inhibition in the thalamus. This inhibition is responsible for shielding external stimuli from the sleeper and for not converting imaginative dream images into actual muscle movements or speech. Children are more often affected than adults, as their central nervous system and thalamus are not yet fully developed.

If sleepwalking occurs only occasionally, sleep duration and quality are not impaired. If sleepwalking is pathological, those affected complain after the nights in which they sleepwalked about increased fatigue, exhaustion, poor concentration and poorer memory. In addition, those affected often suffer from the fear of doing something dangerous or embarrassing during sleepwalking. To avoid accidents and injuries, the sleeping environment should be well secured. In principle, sleepwalking is rather a non-pathological phenomenon. If sleepwalking, however, leads to significant suffering, daytime sleepiness and other restrictions, therapy should be scheduled.

▶ Differential diagnosis is very important to exclude REM sleep behavior disorder.

Pavor Nocturnus (7B00.2)

Pavor nocturnus ("sleep terror") is characterized by a sudden awakening from non-REM sleep stage 3, that is, deep sleep. It therefore occurs more often in the first night third. The sleeping people suddenly wake up with loud screams and moaning. From the outside it looks as if they had a bad nightmare and were suffering terribly. In fact, sleepers can't remember anything the next day. It is possible that the sleepers make very powerful stereotypical movements (e.g. stand up and fall back into the pillow with a lot of force). Therefore, it is particularly important to cushion the sleeping environment here. After waking up, the affected people have a hard time orienting themselves. They usually cannot remember any dream images. The next morning there is an amnesia for the nocturnal awakening reaction, so that the effected people hardly have any suffering. The pavor nocturnus is a frightening phenomenon, but it is not actually dangerous. Since it usually occurs in children between the ages of 3 and 7, the suffering is more due to the fears and insecurity of the parents. Therefore, the nocturnal occurrence and especially their harmlessness should be clarified. In most cases, the pavor nocturnus "fades away". Therapy rarely has to be started.

Sleep-related Eating Disorder (7B00.3)

Sleep-related eating disorders are characterized by recurrent episodes of involuntary excessive or dangerous eating or drinking during sleep. Affected people then experience partial or complete amnesia for the nocturnal eating (also with eating attacks) and are unresponsive. Sleep-related eating disorders cause considerable suffering and impairments in family, social, school, work or other important areas of life.

Arousal Disorder in REM Sleep (7B01)

REM Sleep Behavior Disorder (7B01.0)

REM sleep behavior disorder is characterized by repeated episodes of sleep-related complex motor behavior (punching, kicking) with partly very loud vocalizations (screaming, cursing, swearing) during REM sleep. The behavior and speech are usually very aggressive and it can lead to serious injuries to the patient himself or the bed partner. The cause of these episodes is a lack of muscle atony during REM sleep. The next morning, those affected have no memory of the events in the night. The cause of this is a degeneration of specific brain structures. REM sleep behavior disorder is therefore a degenerative brain disease. It has a poor prognosis, as numerous studies show a nearly causal relationship to the development of Parkinson's disease or Lewy body dementia (Galbiati et al. 2019). In addition, studies show that most patients have previously experienced traumatic experiences in their lives (Husain et al. 2001).

REM sleep behavior disorder can only be diagnosed with a detailed medical history and a polysomnography in the sleep laboratory.

Recurrent Isolated Sleep Paralysis (7B01.1)

In recurrent isolated sleep paralysis, the person affected experiences repeated paralysis of the body during falling asleep or waking up. These episodes usually only last a few seconds to a few minutes. Nevertheless, they cause great fear and thus clinically significant suffering. Insomnia can be a consequence. The explanation of this sleep phenomenon already brings a reduction in the suffering pressure to most of those affected.

Nightmares (7B01.2)

Nightmares are dream sequences that are characterized by strong negative emotions such as fear, panic, hatred, anger or shame and embarrassment. They include a very real, pictorial and detailed dream experience with great fear, which usually leads to waking up. As a result, the dreamer may not be able to fall asleep again for a longer period of time or dreams another episode of the nightmare. They occur primarily in REM sleep and last from a few seconds to about 30 min (rarely longer). After waking up, the dreamers can usually quickly orient themselves in time and space.

There is a distinction between idiopathic and post-traumatic nightmares. Idiopathic nightmares have no primary cause. They occur more often in the context of depression or anxiety disorders, but are not caused primarily by them. Typical idiopathic dream themes are persecution, physical or verbal attacks, receiving bad news (illness, separation) or one's own death or the death of a loved one (Schredl 1999).

Post-traumatic nightmares are the result of an actually experienced traumatic situation that has led to the development of post-traumatic stress disorder (PTSD). In these nightmares, the actually experienced traumatic situation is "dreamed" over and over again unchanged and realistically.

To be distinguished from this are anxiety- or otherwise stressful dreams, which are also strongly negative, but do not lead to awakening. After nightmares, the same or similar content is dreamed again. They are experienced as very stressful by those affected and can be accompanied by an increased expectation of anxiety before going to sleep. This can additionally lead to insomnia.

Depending on the frequency and duration, occasional nightmares that occur less than 12 times a year and frequent nightmares (more than 12 times) are distinguished. If nightmares occur repeatedly within a month, this is referred to as acute nightmares.

Nightmares can occur occasionally in healthy people and are not necessarily pathological. Therefore, treatment is only necessary if there is a clear suffering.

Brief Overview of the Diagnosis Criteria of Parasomnias

Sleepwalking (7B00.1)

- Leaving the bed during sleep and walking around usually during the first third of the night
- Empty, blank facial expression, increased reactivity, difficult to wake up
- Amnesia after waking up
- Mostly no impairment immediately after waking up
- No evidence of an underlying mental disorder such as dementia or physical disorder such as epilepsy

Pavor nocturnus (7B00.2)

- Waking up from sleep with a panic cry, severe fear, body movements and vegetative over-excitability
- Duration of episodes: 1–10 min, usually during the first third of the night
- Relative unresponsiveness, at least some minutes of disorientation and persevering movements
- (Partial) amnesia
- No evidence of a physical condition such as a brain tumor or epilepsy

Nightmares (7B01.3)

- Waking up with vivid memories of intense fear dreams, usually with a threat; typically during the second half of sleep
- After waking up, quickly oriented and alert
- Clear distress

▶ If there is distress due to parasomnias, a psychotherapy should be scheduled.

In individual cases, pharmacological treatment can be considered. However, the risks and benefits must be calculated very well, as the use of neuroleptics can cause strong side effects and thus also create even greater distress.

Sleep-wake Disorders, not Otherwise Specified (7B2Z)

Sleep-wake disorders, "not otherwise specified" as well as "other sleep-wake disorders" include all syndromes that are related to insufficient sleep, lack of refreshment and nocturnal sleep phenomena. They include symptoms that are diagnostically noteworthy and important, but do not fit into any of the aforementioned categories or do not meet the diagnostic criteria in full. Sleep disorders that occur in the context of physical diseases (e.g. pain or medication) and substance use are coded here.

In Table 2.4 you will find a clear overview of the sleep disorders and their main symptoms presented in this chapter.

2.3.3   The Diagnostic Process

Screening

In everyday treatment, there is often not much time for long doctor-patient conversations and diagnostic processes. In order to gain an initial overview of whether something is wrong with the patient's sleep, a screening for the corresponding symptoms can be carried out. It is important to note: A screening does not replace a thorough diagnosis. However, it can be helpful in order to rule out or narrow down certain disorders from the outset. In everyday practice, the screening questions shown in Fig. 2.3 have become established. These can be given to the patient as a patient questionnaire FB01: Screening questionnaire for sleep disorders to be filled out and taken home. The evaluation is explained in the overview or in the working material on the worksheet AB 01: Screening evaluation for practitioners. He can then use it to gain an initial indication of which type of sleep

Table 2.4 Summary and overview of the most important diagnostic criteria

Disorder	Leading symptoms	Differential diagnosis
Insomnia	• Difficulty falling asleep • Difficulty staying asleep • Waking up too early • Daytime sleepiness (except for sleep perception disorder)	Sleep apnea syndrome
Hypersomnia	• Excessive daytime sleepiness, possibly sleep attacks • Not explainable by lack of sleep	Seizure disorders, sleep apnea syndrome, depression
Sleep-related breathing disorder	• Snoring with apnea • Excessive daytime sleepiness • Most of the time sufficient sleep duration	Hypersomnia, depression
Circadian sleep-wake disorders	• Individual sleep-wake rhythm not synchronized with day-night change and social rhythm • Can manifest as insomnia and hypersomnia	Insomnia, hypersomnia, affective disorder
Sleep-related movement disorders	• Repetitive, stereotyped, rhythmic movement patterns during sleep	Parasomnias, seizure disorders
Parasomnias	• sleepwalking, nightmares, night movements • sleep drunkenness • partly difficult to awaken	Post-traumatic stress disorder, psychosis, substance-induced
Sleep-wake disorders, not otherwise specified	• catch-all category for clinically significant distress regarding sleep	

Patient questionnaire

Below you will be asked some questions about your sleep. Please answer them in relation to the past four weeks.

1.	Do you need longer to fall asleep in the evening? a.　　　If yes, how long? _______(minutes/hours) b.　　　If yes, how often? _______x (per week)	☐ yes	☐ no
2.	Do you wake up at night? a.　　　If yes, how often? _______x (per night) b.　　　Can you then quickly go back to sleep? 　　　☐ yes　☐ no	☐ yes	☐ no
3.	Do you wake up much earlier in the morning than you would like? a.　　　If so, can you go back to sleep? 　　　☐ yes　☐ no	☐ yes	☐ no
4.	Do you feel like you're not refreshed despite getting enough sleep?	☐ yes	☐ no
5.	Do you snore or have breathing stops at night?	☐ yes	☐ no
6.	Do you tend to sleep during the day and are often up late at night?	☐ yes	☐ no
7.	Do you move around a lot while you sleep?	☐ yes	☐ no
8.	Do you suffer from nightmares or do you sleepwalk?	☐ yes	☐ no
9.	Would you say that you suffer from sleep disorders?	☐ yes	☐ no
10.	Do you feel fresh and rested in the morning?	☐ yes	☐ no
11.	Do you feel tired, unrested or have less energy during the day?	☐ yes	☐ no

Abb. 2.3 Screening questionnaire for sleep disorders

disorder may be present. The corresponding copy templates will be made available to you for download in the working materials.

Overview
To 1., 2. and 3.

- If the patient responds to one or more of these questions with "yes"
- and indicates a frequency of 3 times or more per week

- and has a (re) sleep latency of 30 min or more,

the patient probably suffers from insomnia.
To 4.
If the patient responds to this question with "yes", a possible hypersomnia may be present.
To 5.
If the patient responds to this question with "yes" and question 4 also with yes, a

possible sleep-related breathing disorder may be present.

To 6.

If this question is answered with "yes", a possible circadian sleep-wake disorder may be present.

To 7.

If this question is answered with "yes", a possible sleep-related movement disorder may be present.

To 8.

If this question is answered with "yes", a possible parasomnia may be present.

To 9.

The patient's subjective assessment of sleep also provides information on the possible presence of a sleep disorder.

To 10. and 11.

Daytime sleepiness is usually present with any form of sleep disorder. In addition, it is a non-specific symptom and can have many causes. If this symptom occurs isolated, a thorough comprehensive physical and psychological examination should take place.

Anamnesis

In the anamnesis, the patient's subjective assessment of sleep as well as the onset and course of the medical history are queried. Certainly, data such as a polysomnography or actigraphy can provide more objective sleep data, but they do not give an overview of the patient's suffering. However, this is an essential diagnostic criterion and must therefore be subjectively recorded. If discrepancies arise between the perceived sleep and, for example, the daytime fitness, additional diagnostic procedures may make sense.

As already mentioned, the diagnosis of a sleep disorder is not difficult in itself. However, in order to plan the therapy, the overall symptomatology including all accompanying symptoms and possible comorbidities must be recorded. A thorough anamnesis is therefore important. It should include the following points.

Specific Sleep Anamnesis

- Beginning of the disorder and special life situations, changes, diseases as well as medication at the beginning of the disorder
- Duration and course of the sleep disorder as well as the accompanying symptomatology
- Subjective bedtimes, collection with a sleep diary (see working materials for download)
- Condition and behavior before going to bed, collection with an extended sleep diary (see working materials for download)
- Number and type of nocturnal wakefulness (standardized questionnaires such as PSQI, RIS, sleep diary)
- Mood and performance during the day
- Increased propensity to sleep and fatigue during the day (standardized questionnaire ESS)
- Sleep-wakefulness structuring of the day
- Sleep-promoting and sleep-inhibiting behavior
- Psychophysiological level of arousal, emotional, cognitive and motor tension
- Sleep expectation anxiety, rumination tendency, disturbance perception
- Sleep hygiene conditions
- Parasomnic symptoms (nightmares, night terrors, sleepwalking)
- Sleep in childhood and adolescence

The Q02: Patient Anamnesis Questionnaire shown below can be given to the patient to take home. You will find this questionnaire for use in everyday practice in the working materials for download (Fig. 2.4).

In addition, biographical data are collected in the anamnesis interview, on the way in which the patients have grown up, on their family and school time, etc. It is also asked whether other diseases are present or have been present in the

1. What type of sleep disorder do you have?
☐ Difficulty falling asleep
☐ Trouble sleeping through
☐ Early Wake
☐ Nightmares
☐ Sleepwalking
☐ I sleep relatively well per se, but I am not well-rested.

2. How long have you had sleep disorders?
Since_____________(weeks, months, years)
What was the beginning of your sleep

☐ creeping
☐ suddenly
☐ episodic
☐ other: ____

3. Was there a particular event or stressful/ distressing time when your sleep disorder started?
☐ no, everything was as usual

☐ yes: ____

4. Have your sleep disturbances changed recently, e.g., have they been more severe or milder in their symptomatology?
☐ no, they have remained the same

☐ yes:
☐ episodic fluctuating
☐ they have become worse lately
☐ they have become better lately
☐ other: ____

5. What was the course of your sleep disorder?
Events with dates, age, persons involved, etc. Ask about the course so that you can imagine exactly how the sleep disorder has developed up to the present day.

6. Do you take sleeping pills?
☐ never
☐ occasionally ☐ regularly

　　　　Preparations, dose, duration:____

7. What symptoms do you feel after one or more bad nights?
☐ Exhaustion
☐ Lethargy
☐ Inertia
☐ none of the above
☐ other symptoms: ____

8. Do you have one or more of these problems after bad nights?
☐ Lack of concentration
☐ Memory disorder
☐ worse learning ability
☐ poorer problem solving ability
☐ less creativity than usual
☐ poorer receptivity and/or understanding of facts
☐ easy distractibility
☐ disjointed thoughts
☐ many thoughts that I can hardly grasp
☐ worse orientation than usual
☐ less willpower
☐ Other symptoms:

Abb. 2.4 Q02: Patient Anamnesis Questionnaire

9. Do you increasingly feel any of these moods on days following one or more bad nights?

<table>
<tr><td>□ Depressiveness</td><td>□ Impulsivity</td></tr>
<tr><td>□ Mood swings</td><td>□ I rather withdraw</td></tr>
<tr><td>□ Aggressiveness</td><td>□ Satisfaction</td></tr>
<tr><td>□ Inner restlessness</td><td>□ Serenity</td></tr>
<tr><td>□ Anger or irritability</td><td>□ Balance</td></tr>
<tr><td>□ Fear</td><td>□ I generally feel joy in life.</td></tr>
<tr><td>□ Disgust</td><td>□ I enjoy social contacts</td></tr>
<tr><td>□ Mania or euphoria</td><td>□ other: _______________</td></tr>
<tr><td>□ Panic attacks</td><td></td></tr>
</table>

10. What have you already tried to improve your sleep?

(e.g. relaxation training, therapeutic or medical treatment, herbal preparations, teas, etc.).

____

11. Where exactly is your level of suffering?

(e.g., daytime fatigue, lying awake in bed forever, not being able to perform).

____

Abb. 2.4   (continued)

past and how they were treated or are currently being treated, or whether another family member also has sleep disorders. Subsequently, specific questionnaires can be used to accurately record sleep behavior and sleep quality.

In our sleep health practice, we use the following protocol for the initial anamnesis interview (AB 02: Protocol for the initial interview) for the initial interview, which is also available for download in your working materials (Fig. 2.5).

Questionnaires

In clinical practice, three questionnaires have established themselves to record the severity of symptoms, sleep quality and daytime sleepiness.

The Regensburg Insomnia Scale (RIS)

The Regensburg Insomnia Scale (RIS) captures the manifestations of insomnia and is particularly suitable for measuring therapeutic changes. With only 10 items, it inquires about cognitive and emotional aspects of sleep, such as acoustic hypersensitivity, sleep perception and sleep anxiety of insomnia. Based on the answers of the affected persons, a rapid cross-section of the disease dynamics and its severity can be recorded.

The Pittsburg Sleepquality Inventory (PSQI)

The Pittsburg Sleepquality Inventory (PSQI) gives an overview of the general sleep quality of the person concerned. It contains 19 self-assessment questions which are summarized in 7 components. They can each take a value between 0 and 3 points, which are added to a total value between 0 and 21. The following are queried:

Dr. **Carolin Marx-Dick**

EXPERTIN FÜR
SCHLAFGESUNDHEIT

WS02 - Protocol for the initial interview (with medical history)

Name / ID: Date of birth: Date (today):

Life circumstances (marital status, children, finances, profession...)

Sleep disorders

☐ DFA (difficulty falling asleep)   ☐ STD (sleep though disorder)   ☐ EW (erly awaking)   ☐ Daytime fatigue   since when: __________

Start: ☐ sudden   ☐ episodic   ☐ creeping

Tied to event/stressor? Which one?
____

Other. Sleep phenomena: ☐ Nightmares   ☐ Sheepwalking   ☐ Snoring

                                   ☐ CPAP/ Apnea   ☐ other: ___________

The sleep   to bed: __________   Fall asleep: __________

                     Wake up: _______   Rise: _____

Further information about sleep: (CPAP, snoring)

Day Fitness: ☐ good   ☐ exhausted   ☐ Daytime sleepiness   ☐ neurocogn. deficits

other restrictions: _______________________
Energy level:

Anamnestic history (key data, years, age, events, persons involved, biography, critical life events,..)

Daily routine and structure:
Early / Strat into the day:

Morning:

Noon: (break?)
Afternoon:

Evening:

Fig. 2.5 Protocol for the initial interview with anamnesis

Dr. **Carolin Marx-Dick**

EXPERTIN FÜR
SCHLAFGESUNDHEIT

WS02 - Protocol for the initial interview (with medical history)

Before going to bed:

- -

in bed:

Symptoms (physical and psychological, spontaneously reported)

☐ Tensionl Cramps	☐ Less willpower	☐ Inertia
☐ Nausea/dizziness	☐ Lack of concentration	☐ Lethargy
☐ Hot flash/cold shiver	☐ Jumbled thoughts	☐ Anger / Gereoztheit
☐ Inner restlessness/nervousness	☐ Easy distractibility	☐ Irritable bowel/stomach
☐ Physical exhaustion	☐ Mood swings	☐ Depressiveness
☐ Digestive problems/vomiting		☐ Headache

Medication (preparation, dose, since when, time of taking, prescribed?)

Sleeping pills: ☐ regularly   ☐ occasionally   ☐ never   _______________

other:

Where exactly is the pressure of suffering?

What are the therapy goals?

Suicidality?   ☐ yes   ☐ no   Extraneous danger?   ☐ yes   ☐ no

Notes, Masterpoints:

Fig. 2.5 (continued)

- Sleep quality
- Sleep latency
- Sleep duration
- Sleep efficiency
- Sleep disorders
- Sleep medication consumption
- Daytime sleepiness

The Epworth Sleepiness Scale (ESS)

The Epworth Sleepiness Scale (ESS) captures how likely it is for the person concerned to doze off or fall asleep in different situations, or how tired he or she is in these situations.

Other Diagnostic Measures

Diagnostics in the Sleep Laboratory

In the sleep laboratory, a so-called polysomnography is carried out. Various physiological values are recorded over the entire night using targeted derivation procedures. During the sleep laboratory night, heart activity, respiration, oxygen saturation, muscle movements, snoring and brain activity are observed.

▶ Not all patients with sleep disorders need to go to the sleep laboratory. Patients with insomnia only need a sleep laboratory diagnosis in rare cases.

Patients with nocturnal apnea, daytime sleepiness of unknown cause or nocturnal movement disorders should be examined in the sleep laboratory with a polysomnography.

Many patients are anxious about what to expect in the sleep laboratory. Therefore, it is important to inform them well. The Information sheet 01: "The Diagnostics in the Sleep Laboratory" provides the most important information. It is available for use in your everyday practice in the working materials for download.

Measuring Heart Rate Variability

Heart rate variability (HRV) is a method that was originally developed for the field of biofeedback. It measures physiological processes in the body and makes them visible to doctors,

therapists and patients using complex evaluation software. The derivation of heart rate variability can be carried out in a very simple way, e.g. with a sensor on a chest strap, adhesive electrodes on the chest or electrodes on both wrists. The diagnostic use of HRV allows the detection of a variety of physiological processes in the body. This apparative and non-invasive diagnostic procedure is currently being intensively researched. The measurement of HRV already belongs to the standard diagnostics in stress-related cardiovascular diseases. Since it is a very cost-effective and easy-to-use procedure, it could in future partly replace the elaborate and expensive polysomnographies (PSG) in the sleep laboratory.

Larger studies showed significant agreement between HRV-based analysis and polysomnography data (e.g. Decker 2009) in a variety of sleep-related parameters. Thus, with the HRV examination, the transitions between wakefulness and sleep, i.e. the respective effective sleep times, could be calculated. With the HRV, the onset latency, nocturnal and early morning awakenings can therefore be detected and clearly distinguished from the sleep times. It can therefore be used for the uncomplicated and safe diagnosis of insomnia and especially for paradoxical insomnia. In addition, the proportions of the sleep stages Non-REM and REM sleep could be represented in the same quality as in a PSG.

Due to the differentiated regulation of the autonomic nervous system in deep and REM sleep, solid statements about sleep quality are possible (Penzel et al. 2018). Respiratory-related changes in HRV can be evaluated in such a way that sleep-related respiratory disorders can already be reliably detected using this method. Thus, the measurement of HRV can be used in the diagnosis of the widespread sleep apnoea syndrome.

Heart Rate Variability in the Therapeutic Process

HRV compares changes in heart rate. It captures a variety of parameters. The most important values include adaptability, recovery capacity, activity of the parasympathetic and sympathetic. In addition, the general regeneration capacity can be determined using HRV measurement, that is, how well the body copes with stress and recovery phases or how quickly it changes from load to relaxation. This allows conclusions to be drawn about the quality of sleep. Healthy people can also read the individual parameters of the measurement quite easily to see how fit, stressed or rested they are.

In sleep therapy, patients and therapists encounter these parameters very often, because the cause of most sleep disorders is mental overstimulation and physical underuse. A joint evaluation of sympathetic and parasympathetic activity and general regeneration capacity with the patient can therefore provide important information for the therapeutic process.

However, the heart rate is subject to various influences that can be consciously controlled and changed. In the relaxed state, the heart rate has a great deal of variability, while in stress it remains rigid at a high frequency and is therefore hardly adaptable.

One important influence on the heart rate is the breathing. When inhaling, the filling lung always presses a little on the heart. This makes the pulse briefly faster and the heart rate more even. When exhaling, this pressure decreases, the pulse becomes slower again and the heart rate increases its variability. This simple effect has the impressive name "respiratory sinus arrhythmia". In this way, the HRV rises and falls slightly with each breath.

These fine changes are controlled by the autonomic nervous system and thus have a major impact on the sympathetic (fight or flight mode) and the parasympathetic (relaxation and social engagement). In turn, they control breathing, heart muscle, digestion and distribute stress hormones in the body. This mechanism can be used in reverse to consciously control sympathetic and parasympathetic reactions and thus specifically to the underlying therapy of sleep disorders. The effect of breathing and relaxation exercises, yoga and meditation, conversation and anger topics can be made visible in this way.

Smartwatches, Sleep and Actitrackers

Many patients already own a "smartwatch" or fitness tracker. In addition to displaying various fitness parameters, such as distance covered, number of steps, times of physical rest, etc., many of these "watches" can also make statements about sleep. They have programs that promise to record sleep, and they also give valuable tips for better sleep. The technology used is derived from the measurement of heart rate variability. The pulse can be used to derive a pulse rate variability. This in turn can be used to approximate heart rate variability, and thus an estimate of sleep and wake times as well as REM and non-REM sleep can be made. Another mechanism used is actigraphy. Here, the analysis of the movement patterns of the wearer is used to determine whether the person is awake or asleep.

As with all electronic devices, there are good and less good products. In some studies, the data generated were compared with values from polysomnographies. The deviations were within an acceptable range, so that values from smartwatches can be included in the diagnostic and therapeutic process with the appropriate caution (Penzel et al. 2018).

2.4 Common Comorbidities

Sleep disorders in general and insomnia in particular rarely occur in isolation. In most cases, people with sleep disorders have symptoms that go beyond sleep symptoms. It is estimated that more than 50% of patients with insomnia also have an additional psychiatric or psychological disorder (*Ford and Kamerow* 1989). These mental disorders can be the cause of the development of sleep disorders. At the same time, however, sleep disorders can also be the cause of mental disorders.

2.4.1 Affective Disorders

Affective disorders are characterized by a pathological change in mood, drive and/or emotionality. Disease patterns within this group of disorders include depressive and manic episodes, which vary in their duration, frequency and severity and therefore require different diagnoses and therapies. They can be accompanied by anxiety or psychotic symptoms. The trigger of affective disease phases is often stressful life circumstances. It is also assumed that certain hereditary factors cause an increased predisposition to affective disorders.

Depressions represent a significant risk factor for the development of insomnia, but can also be a symptom of insomnia (*Bhaskar et al.* 2016). Long-term studies show that the risk of developing depression is 5 times higher in people with existing sleep disorders than in the healthy comparison group (*Chang et al.* 1997). More than two thirds of depressive patients have sleep disorders. Persistent sleep disorders also increase suicidality in depressed people. Those affected often have the problem that they cannot come to rest and cannot sleep through the night due to the over-activations (hyperarousal) of stress-promoting physiological mechanisms in the evening. These physiological patterns are also found in patients with chronic insomnia, which can explain the high comorbidity of both disorder patterns.

▶ Patients with bipolar disorder and isolated mania often suffer from circadian sleep-wake disorders. Sleep deprivation and hypersomnia can in turn trigger manic episodes.

2.4.2　Anxiety Disorders

Anxiety disorders are characterized by an unrealistic and excessive feeling of anxiety. Often, those affected avoid the situations, thoughts or objects that trigger anxiety. Since anxiety disorders are characterized by incorrect or exaggerated reactions of the body and the resulting strong over-activation of the autonomic nervous system, those affected often experience very strong physical symptoms, such as palpitations, nausea, dizziness, high blood pressure, etc. The causes of anxiety disorders are multi-factorial and characterized by neurobiological factors (altered brain metabolism), psychological factors (e.g. traumatic childhood memories) and genetic predisposition.

After affective disorders, anxiety disorders have the second highest comorbidity with sleep disorders (Bhaskar et al. 2016). The over-activation of the nervous system characteristic of anxiety disorders has evolutionary origins and provides the physical resources necessary for escape. Against this background, the strong comorbidity of anxiety and sleep disorders can be explained by the fact that our ancestors have learned to defend themselves quickly and effectively against night-time threats or to flee. For these behaviors, a moderate activation of the body was necessary and deep sleep was not possible.

Patients who have suffered from sleep disorders in childhood are more likely to develop anxiety disorders in adulthood. In addition, many people with an anxiety disorder have significant difficulty falling asleep and staying asleep (Saletu-Zyhlarz 2014).

Generalized anxiety disorder often goes hand in hand with insomnia due to the excessive tendency to worry. Worrying cause increased muscle tension (Borkovek et al. 1991). This tension prevents (re-)sleeping.

Nocturnal breathing pauses in the context of a sleep-related breathing disorder can trigger intense anxiety, panic and panic disorder. The gold standard treatment for sleep apnea syndrome is nasal ventilation by continuous positive airway pressure (CPAP). Patients receive a nasal or nasal/mouth mask through which room air is blown into the throat under increased pressure. Wearing the mask and the unusual air supply can lead to suffocation anxiety, air hunger and panic. The practice of mask tolerance with therapeutic support shows good efficacy here.

2.4.3　Stress and Adjustment Disorders

Stress and adjustment disorders are reactions to stressful life events, a prolonged period of severe stress, or a particularly drastic change in familiar living conditions. The symptoms typically show a mixed and changeable picture. Those affected have difficulty relaxing and often suffer from severe feelings of being overwhelmed, pronounced exhaustion, disorientation, and reduced attention and concentration. Since stress and adjustment disorder is characterized by physical overactivity, physical symptoms often occur, such as pain, sweating, or heart palpitations.

▶ Stress and adjustment disorders can be both the cause and the consequence of a sleep disorder. They are one of the most common comorbidities.

Post-traumatic Stress Disorders

Post-traumatic stress disorder (PTSD) arises as a delayed reaction to a subjectively very stressful event (trauma) of different duration, which is perceived by the affected person as exceptionally threatening and of catastrophic proportions. Typically, those affected experience their trauma repeatedly through intrusive memories (flashbacks) and/or nightmares. They describe lasting feelings of apathy, emotional numbness, joylessness, fear and depression. On the physical level, PTSD is characterized by a strong vegetative over-excitability with increased vigilance, which occurs especially in combination with trauma memories.

There is a strong comorbidity with parasomnias, especially nightmares and insomnia.

It is currently assumed that PTSD is the cause of sleep problems, as many sufferers experience a basic physical overactivity with increased vigilance and muscle tone.

2.4.4 Obsessive-compulsive Disorders

Obsessive-compulsive disorders are characterized by obsessive thoughts and/or compulsive behaviors that sufferers experience as very burdensome and uncontrollable. While obsessive thoughts are intrusive and often experienced as repulsive or threatening thoughts, compulsive behaviors are characterized by repetitive behavioral stereotypes. These behaviors are greatly exaggerated (e.g. washing compulsion) and in part have no relation to the original purpose (e.g. pressing light switches in a specific repeating pattern). Usually, sufferers try to suppress their compulsions. However, this increases the subjectively experienced anxiety and tension and reinforces the compulsive behavior.

This comorbidity is also bidirectional: Obsessive-compulsive disorders generate increased muscle tension, which disturbs a restful sleep. Not infrequently, compulsions have to be carried out exactly before going to bed, such as creating order, aligning couch cushions and curtains, etc. However, people with sleep disorders also develop rituals that are supposedly beneficial for sleep, such as excessive movement, meditation, sequences of evening rituals, nutrition, etc. If these are not carried out completely and at the right time, the sleep disorders occur (also in the sense of self-fulfilling prophecy).

2.4.5 Addiction Disorders

Addiction or substance abuse disorders are caused by an extraordinary desire for a particular substance or activity. They can vary greatly: as an addiction to alcohol, drugs or medication. However, there are also non-substance-related addiction disorders such as gambling addiction. Through a misdirection of the reward system in the brain, the addictive substance activates messenger substances that trigger well-being, relaxation or euphoria. These pleasant states create the desire to have more of them. People with a genetic predisposition or specific conditioning, such as model learning in childhood, are particularly vulnerable to addiction.

In substance-related addictions such as alcohol, drug or medication abuse, sufferers experience a strong desire to consume the corresponding substances. In addition, they have great difficulty controlling or stopping the use of the substance despite the harmful consequences.

With long-term use, the body develops tolerance for the relevant substance, so that the effect of the corresponding addictive substance decreases and a higher dose has to be consumed for the desired effect. If the substances can no longer be consumed or the consumption is interrupted, severe physical and mental withdrawal symptoms occur.

In non-substance-related addictions such as gaming, mobile phone use, social media use, gaming, sports, sex or work, a partly enormous body tension arises when those affected cannot live out the addiction. This increased basic tension in turn leads to sleep disorders.

Addictions usually involve a huge amount of time to procure and consume the substances or to carry out the addictive activities. In an intact life with professional and social obligations, time periods must be created for the realization of the addiction. This often comes at the expense of night sleep.

The comorbidity of addictive disorders and sleep disorders is also bidirectional. Addictive disorders can develop as a result of sleep disorders. Studies have shown that a significant proportion of patients with sleep disorders consume cannabis (approx. 10%; Shibley et al. 2008) or alcohol (30–40%; Shibley et al. 2008; Saletu-Zyhlarz 2014) in order to sleep better. Insomnia is thus a significant risk factor for the development of an addictive disorder.

Conversely, an existing addictive disorder can be a significant risk factor for disturbed sleep. Insomnia, for example, often persists even after long-term abstinence from the addictive substance (Crum et al. 2004).

Unfortunately, the use of hypnotics is still often the first treatment approach. Before other measures are taken, the patients receive sleeping pills that are also addictive.

Even supposedly "harmless" over-the-counter drugs or modern non-benzodiazepines develop tolerance after a few weeks and thus worsen the symptoms.

2.4.6 Eating Disorders

Eating disorders are very serious illnesses in which the way of dealing with food and the relationship to one's own body are severely disturbed. Different types of eating disorders are distinguished: anorexia (anorexia), bulimia (bulimia), eating attacks (binge eating disorder) and obesity (obesity).

All forms include behavioral disorders in which regular food intake is severely disturbed. For a long time or in phases, too little or too much is eaten. In addition, a constant mental and emotional engagement with the topic "food" plays a central role. Those affected often have psychosocial problems and a distorted attitude or a disturbed subjective perception of their own body. Eating disorders can lead to severe health impairments in the long term.

The comorbidity with sleep disorders lies in the interfaces to hunger or satiety, the anger about "bad" eating behavior and the psycho-physiological and hormonal dysregulation caused by hunger or vomiting. Hunger awakens the "survival mode" of our body and keeps us "alert". Too large meals have to be digested while awake and thus prevent a restful sleep.

In the "Night Eating Disorder" eating and sleep disorders meet directly. It is characterized by sleep disorders with night eating in the longer wakefulness. This can lead to uncontrollable eating attacks. In part, large meals are taken at night and fasted during the day.

2.4.7 Pain Disorders

Pain and sleep disorders occur very often comorbidly, as the regulation of pain processing and perception has many parallels to sleep. Sleep disorders interfere with pain processing and pain or its treatment interfere with sleep. Many sufferers of pain disorders therefore know this vicious circle.

Many vital functions take place during deep sleep, and unconsciousness is absolutely necessary for this. A person can only be awakened from deep sleep by a pain stimulus or a noise that is louder than 80 decibels (e.g. loud traffic noise or a lawn mower). Consequently, one does not fall asleep with pain, and the processes that should expire cannot take place. Lack of deep sleep leads to a deterioration of all neurocognitive functions, the breakdown of the immune system and stress regulation, and thus also to a lowering of the pain threshold. In turn, this leads to a more sensitive perception of pain, which in turn exacerbates the pain disorder. In addition, the immune system transports inflammatory cells away at night, so that painful inflammation of all kinds can be alleviated and healed.

According to a healthy sleep architecture, a person moves into light sleep or short wakefulness at night. These position changes are very important in order to avoid stiffness or pain the next day due to one-sided positioning and the associated strain on muscles and joints. However, with pain in the musculoskeletal system, this change of position cannot take place smoothly, which in turn leads to further pain. In addition, the pain caused by night-time movement can lead to an increased awakening reaction, resulting in sleep disorders.

Pain medication can also cause sleep disorders. Therefore, it is advisable to look at the patient's medication in detail and, if necessary, develop a sleep-promoting or at least non-sleep-inhibiting medication and administration plan for the patient in consultation with the treating physician. The use of alternative pain therapy should be given more consideration in the event of a comorbid sleep disorder. Measures such as physiotherapy and movement therapy, a balanced diet and stress management also have a positive effect on the switching quality.

2.5 Dealing with People with Sleep Disorders

People with sleep disorders often have an extremely high level of suffering. They often experience the symptoms every night and feel the effects every day. Often, worries about sleep accompany patients throughout the day. In addition, there are catastrophic (mis-)information from the media, which additionally makes people afraid that they will soon get serious physical and mental illnesses in addition to the sleep disorder. It is not uncommon for them to be not taken seriously for their complaints. Sentences like "If you're really tired, you'll sleep" are reported by many patients. These concerns and the resulting suffering should therefore be taken very seriously and picked up by the treating physician. A first sensible reaction in the therapeutic conversation is therefore the validation of the patient's situation and suffering. Being taken seriously already helps many sufferers a little bit.

2.5.1 Difficult Therapy Situations

In the course of a psychotherapeutic treatment, there may always be situations that the patient or even the therapist finds unpleasant and difficult. This is especially true in the field of sleep disorders, because here, as already described, a large theoretical knowledge exists in the majority of patients and the visit to the therapist is often the last resort for the affected persons. In addition, many patients assume a somatic disorder picture.

Unrealistic Goals

Many patients want the "old" sleep back, the one they had before their sleep disorder. They expect to be able to sleep through the night again after therapy, 7–8 h a night, to be well rested and fit the next day. This is a nice idea, but it is often not realistic for most people with the workload they have, and for other reasons. It is important to define realistic goals for treatment together with patients. Often, intermediate goals or individual stages are helpful to primarily solve the most pressing problems and then think about the next steps. The main goal of therapy is to reduce suffering as much as possible. This does not always have to mean symptom-free.

In view of the fact that sleep disorders can occur episodically from time to time, the symptomatology is rather to be recognized as a seismograph for the general mental and physical stress. In therapy, therefore, it is rather a question of triggering a process of salutogenesis from a disease treatment. The goal is to help patients move from a disease management, which many of them practice dysfunctionally for years (e.g. taking hypnotics, excessive sports program/bed rest, social withdrawal, etc.), to a health management. The self-efficacy of the patients is required. Doctors and therapists cannot "make patients healthy" (Fig. 2.6).

The Impatient Patient

The causal, sustainable therapy of sleep disorders is, in contrast to the use of psychopharmaceuticals, rather slow. In individual cases, the first therapeutic success can be achieved after only a few sessions. However, positive changes usually occur gradually, with more and more good nights appearing over the course of the week. It is important to highlight these sometimes very small successes and make them visible again and again. Patients should be made aware of this at the first consultation that their situation will not change in the short term.

Therapists should also pay attention to their patients' use of sleeping pills. It is very tempting for those affected to know that with the taking of a single small tablet, the sleep problem is "solved" for the current night. By means of psychoeducation on psychopharmaceuticals and sleep architecture, they must be made aware of how these drugs actually work. The goal of the treatment should be to sensitize the patients so that they recognize the necessity and also the desired rewarding result of the treatment and

endure it. The treatment goal is always the long-term alleviation of suffering and symptoms. This cannot be achieved by medication.

The Patient Who Knows Everything and has Tried Everything

Since sleep disorders usually have a chronic course and many sufferers have been treated primarily with pharmaceuticals in the past, numerous patients—as already mentioned—are very well informed about the disorder. Although the aim of psychotherapy is also to encourage the patient to self-help, the therapist can only help the patient to sleep better if he or she is actively involved in the therapy or actually implements the proposed changes in everyday life. Patients often report that they have already tried this or that technique unsuccessfully and want to "finally experience something new". Unfortunately, sleep disorders cannot be alleviated in the short term. Usually it takes a lot of patience until the first improvements occur. In contrast to self-help, the patient is continuously motivated in psychotherapy to consistently implement the proposed interventions over a longer period of time. It is important to explain the current and subsequent therapy steps to the patient in a transparent manner so that no false expectations arise. Often, topics that are not directly related to sleep disorders, such as stress management, bullying, conflicts, work or relationship problems, accompany the therapy. The therapy can then move very far away from the actual topic. However, it is necessary to deal with these accompanying symptoms, as it is not possible to sleep well with worries.

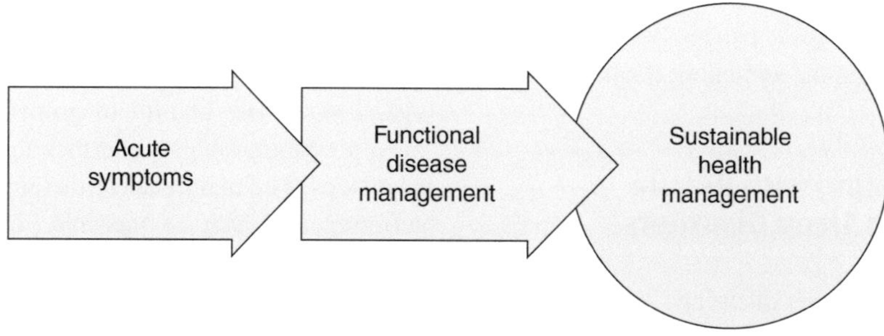

Fig. 2.6 From illness to health

Nevertheless, the red thread must not be lost throughout the therapy and must always be visible to the patient.

The Patient Who Questions the Competence of the Therapist

Since patients often have a wide and deep knowledge of sleep disorders, it can happen that the competence of the therapist is questioned. There are always new remedies and aids for sleep disorders, which are to be sold expensively to customers—well marketed. These include herbal preparations, special pillows or blankets, sleep drinks and much more. As a scientifically working therapist, it is not possible to keep an overview of this variety of offers. Many patients are initially disappointed when the therapist does not know everything the patient reports. Therefore, it should be checked together which remedies and aids are actually useful and which are rather money-cutting. Here the appeal is addressed to the therapist: Be open to new things! A therapist can also learn from his patients.

No Improvement in Well-being

Patients are used to living with their sleep disorder and adjusting their entire day to it. If the sleep disorder now disappears, a important part of life is suddenly missing. Paradoxically, despite the declared need for help, it is very difficult for some sufferers to give up familiar dysfunctional behaviours and ways of thinking, even if they stand in the way of treating the sleep disorder. Therefore, it is important to sensitise the patients again and again for all small therapy successes and to make them aware of them. Dysfunctional behaviour can be replaced by self-caring behaviour to strengthen the patient's well-being.

▶ Many sufferers have a sleep perception disorder (paradoxical insomnia) in addition to the actual insomnia.

This means that patients estimate their sleep much worse than it actually is. With the help of diaries, which are kept regularly throughout the course of therapy, the changes can be documented and thus draw attention to the success of the therapy. The use of apparatus measuring methods of sleep, such as via smartwatches, can support this.

A very frequently observed phenomenon is that despite the enormous pressure of suffering, the patients do not consistently and permanently implement what they have learned. They expect an immediate therapeutic success with the short-term use of the methods and are impatient. It is important for both the patient and the therapist's assessment to give the methods "a chance" and to apply them over the agreed period of time. The techniques used should be modified so that they fit well into the patients' everyday lives and do not overload them. "Mini-interventions" that only take a few minutes can be the ticket here.

It can also happen that a patient expects to be healed by the therapist. He may have no understanding and perhaps no motivation to be active himself. In this case, it must be continuously made clear that psychotherapy does not work like a pill that can be taken and then sleep well and without side effects forever. It is important to strengthen the lack of self-efficacy in these patients. With the first self-controlled successes, this is specifically confirmed.

There are people who find it difficult to open up. In these cases, the therapist should not press, it takes time here. As a rule, those affected open up when they are ready. Until then, the success of the therapy will by no means be diminished, they can still benefit from the therapy continuously, for example by discussing the obvious problems objectively and studying methods.

If undiscovered substance abuse or an addiction disorder is not detected, the therapy elements offered will hardly take effect. If, despite careful control of all accompanying symptoms, no therapeutic success is achieved, this point must be checked again more closely. In general, it is always important to be well informed about drug use and not to lose sight of it during the course of therapy. The feeling of shame due to consumption can only be countered with trust. Therapists are subject to a strict duty of confidentiality, which can be explained to the patient again in such cases. It must be made clear that without absolute openness on this topic, no therapeutic success will be achieved.

Many patients have a supply of sleeping pills at home that can be very dangerous if overdosed or if the wrong combination of preparations is used. In this respect, a conservative attitude is recommended: rather ask once too often than once too little.

Insomnia can be so stressful that patients become suicidal. Therefore, the current suicidality is always to be asked and by no means to be underestimated! If acute suicidality is present, an admission should be made or the emergency doctor should be called.

2.5.2 Common Personality Aspects in People with Sleep Disorders

Certain personality traits favor dysfunctional behavior and thus represent a risk for the development and maintenance of sleep disorders. Each personality trait is basically positive and can be beneficial in special areas. However, they can also disturb a relaxed and restful sleep. In the therapy everyday life some patterns can be observed again and again. Therefore, it can make sense in therapy to recognize these properties and to find ways together with the patient to influence them.

Perfectionism

Perfectionism is a personality trait that many patients with sleep disorders show. In many situations, it seems desirable at first, as it leads to good performance. Perfectionistic people have a high need for control, strive for perfection and register errors very precisely. However, these properties lead to high expectations and demands on oneself. Unfinished tasks attract great attention and anger. This creates a high level of tension during the day that can hardly be reduced at night.

In order to sleep well, the feeling of satisfaction, "to have accomplished something today", is worth its weight in gold. A bad night creates pressure to sleep better the next night. But despite the fatigue, perfectionistic people have the claim to do everything and always show full performance. Many of them find it difficult to switch off their plans, unfinished tasks and worries when falling asleep. Just the observation that they cannot fall asleep can generate anger and frustration and increase inner tension again. Thoughts like "I can't even sleep" are not uncommon. In therapy, it is therefore crucial to question perfectionism, to convey acceptance of mistakes and to create moments without pressure in everyday life as well.

Excessive Need for Harmony

People with a great need for harmony can quickly get into a vicious circle of excessive demands and poor sleep. Unlike people with a tendency to perfectionism, social pressure arises for people seeking harmony. The children have to be picked up from school and driven to sports, the colleague needs another document and the friend needs help moving, and finally the husband is waiting at home for a delicious dinner. Some people find it difficult to refuse others a request, they think that certain things are expected of them. They of course gladly take on all tasks and put their own needs behind. And so their own sleep is also impaired. Many patients report simply not being able to "finish" in the evening. They can only finish their everyday tasks late, which on the one hand causes the point of fatigue to be exceeded or simply too little time to sleep or to previous shutdown. Here too, in therapy, it should be questioned how much one has to give to others and how much one can admit to oneself. Communication training and the invitation of the partner into a therapy session can be very helpful in learning to set boundaries and to question whether certain things are actually expected.

Often sleep disorders occur as a reaction to stress or psychological crises. In this case one speaks of psychoreactive insomnias. In dealing with stress and crises, personal aspects can act protective (resilience) or intensify the stress and support the development of a psychoreactive insomnia.

References

American Academy of Sleep Medicine (2014) International classification of sleep. Disorders Diagnostic and Coding Manual. (ICSD-3)

Bhaskar S, Hemavathy D, Prasad S (2016) Prevalence of chronic insomnia in adult patients and its correlation with medical comorbidities. J Family Med Prim Care 5(4):780–784

Borkovec TD, Shadick RN, Hopkins M (1991) The nature of normal and pathological worry. In: Rapee RM, Barlow DH (Hrsg) Chronic anxiety: generalized anxiety disorder and mixed anxiety-depression. Guilford Press, New York

Chang PP, Ford DE, Mead LA, Cooper-Patrick L, Klag MJ (1997) Insomnia in young men and subsequent depression. The Johns Hopkins Precursors Study. Am J Epidemiol 146:105–114

Crönlein T (2010) Schlafstörungen: ursachen erkennen und behandeln – gesund leben. Compact

Crum RM, Ford DE, Storr CL et al (2004) Association of sleep disturbance with chronicity and remission of alcohol dependence: data from a population-based prospective study. Alcohol Clin Exp Res 28:1533–1540

Decker MJ (2009) Validation of ECG-derived sleep architecture and ventilation in sleep apnea and chrinic fatigue syndrome. Sleep Breath 14(3):233–239

Dilling H, Mombour W (2013) Internationale Klassifikation psychischer Störungen: ICD-10 Kapitel V (F) Klinisch diagnostische Leitlinien. Hans Huber, Bern

Ford DE, Kamerow DB (1989) Epidemiologic study of sleep disturbances and psychiatric disorders. An opportunity for preven4tion? JAMA 262:1479–1484

Galbiati A, Verga L, Giora E, Zucconi M, Ferini-Strambi L (2019) The risk of neurodegeneration in REM sleep behavior disorder: a systematic review and meta-analysis of longitudinal studies. Sleep Med Rev 43:37–46

Grobe TG, Steinmann S, Szecsenyi J (2019) Schriftenreihe zur Gesundheitsanalye. BARMER Bd. 14

Husain AM, Miller PP, Carwile ST (2001) REM sleep behavior disorder: potential relationship to post-traumatic stress disorder. J Clin Neurophysiol 18(2):148–157

Marx-Dick C (2020) The dynamic modell of sleep disorders – a therapy-tool for cognitive behavioral therapy for non-organic sleep disorders. Am J Psychiatry Neurosci 8(1):6–11

Ohayon MM (2011) Epidemiological overview of sleep disorders in the general population. Sleep Med Rev 2:1–9

Penzel T, Glos M, Schöbel C, He Z, Lufka O, Fietze I (2018) Telemedizin und telemetrische Aufzeichnungsmethoden zur Diagnostik in der Schlafmedizin. Somnologie 22:199–208

Riemann D, Baum E, Cohrs S et al (2017) S3-Leitlinie Nicht erholsamer Schlaf/Schlafstörungen. Somnologie 21:2–44

Roth T et al (2007) Insomnia: pathophysiology and implications for treatment. Sleep Med Rev 11:71–79

Saletu-Zyhlarz G (2014) Insomnie und Folgen von Schlafstörungen. psychopraxis neuropraxis 17:12–14

Schlack R, Hapke U, Maske U, Busch MA, Cohrs S (2013) Häufigkeit und Verteilung von Schlafproblemen und Insomnie in der deutschen Erwachsenenbevölkerung. Ergebnisse der Studie zur Gesundheit Erwachsener in Deutschland (DEGS1. Bundesgesundheitsblatt 56:740–748

Schredl M (1999) Die nächtliche Traumwelt: eine Einführung in die psychologische Traumforschung. Kohlhammer, Stuttgart

Shibley HL, Malcolm RJ, Veatch LM (2008) Adolescents with insomnia and substance abuse: consequences and comorbidities. J Psychiatr Pract 14:146–115

Storm A, Marschall J, Hildebrandt S, Sydow H, Nolting HD, Burgart E, Woköck T (2017) Gesundheitsreport 2017. Analyse der Arbeitsunfähigkeitsdaten. Update: Schlafstörungen. Beiträge zur Gesundheitsökonomie und Versorgungsforschung (Band 16). IGES Institut GmbH, Berlin

World Health Organization (WHO) (1946) Verfassung der Weltgesundheitsorganisation. New York

World Health Organization (WHO) (2022) International Classification of Diseases Eleventh Revision (ICD-11). Geneva

Therapy Concept for the Holistic Treatment of Sleep Disorders 3

Contents

3.1	**Background**	68
3.2	**Formal Structure and Framework Conditions of Therapy**	69
3.3	**Development of the Disorder Model**	71
3.4	**Modules of Cognitive Behavioral Therapy**	72
	3.4.1 Module: Psychoeducation	73
	3.4.2 Module: Medications, Alcohol, and Drugs	76
	3.4.3 Module: Bed Rest and Sleep Restriction	79
	3.4.4 Module: Day Structuring	85
	3.4.5 Module: Interpersonal Social Rhythm Therapy	90
	3.4.6 Module: Light as Therapy	92
	3.4.7 Module: Shift Work	94
	3.4.8 Module: Stress Management	98
	3.4.9 Module: Sleep Hygiene	102
	3.4.10 Module: Stimulus Control and Psychohygiene	109
	3.4.11 Module: Cognitive Techniques	113
	3.4.12 Module: Behavior Change	119
	3.4.13 Module: Perfection and Control	121
	3.4.14 Module: Paradoxical Intervention	122
	3.4.15 Module: Sleep Deprivation—Wake Therapy	123
	3.4.16 Module: Relaxation Techniques	125
	3.4.17 Module: Sexuality	130
3.5	**Nightmare Therapy**	131
	3.5.1 Background of Nightmare Therapy	131
	3.5.2 Preparation of the Nightmare Therapy	132
	3.5.3 Module Nightmare Variant 1: Solution of the Dream Conflict in the Waking State	133
	3.5.4 Module Nightmare Variant 2: Nightmare Modification	134
	3.5.5 Module: Dream(-Trauma) Therapy with Eye Movement Integration (EMI)	135
3.6	**Third Wave of Behavior Therapy**	135
	3.6.1 Background	135
	3.6.2 Module: Acceptance-Commitment-Therapy of Insomnia (ACT-I)	137
	3.6.3 Module: Mindfulness	143
	3.6.4 Module: Hypnotherapy	150
3.7	**Mind-Body-Medicine**	156
	3.7.1 Mind-Body Therapy	157
	3.7.2 Modules of Body Psychotherapy	157

	3.7.3	Module: Yoga-Psychotherapy	159
	3.7.4	Module: Meditation	164
	3.7.5	Module: Sleep-Promoting Nutrition	166
	3.7.6	Module: Movement and Sport	172
3.8		**Manual Procedures**	174
	3.8.1	Background	174
	3.8.2	Hydro- and Thermotherapy	174
	3.8.3	Acupuncture	177
	3.8.4	Marmatherapy	177
3.9		**Neurotherapy**	178
	3.9.1	Therapy Module: Eye Movement Integration (EMI)	178
	3.9.2	Module: Polyvagal Therapy	182
3.10		**Pharmacotherapy: Opportunities and Risks**	188
	3.10.1	Benzodiazepines	190
	3.10.2	Barbiturates	191
	3.10.3	"Z-Substances" (Non-Benzodiazepines)	191
	3.10.4	Melatonin	192
	3.10.5	Antihistamines	194
	3.10.6	Antidepressants—Off-Label as Hypnotics	195
	3.10.7	Neuroleptics—Off-Label as Hypnotics	196
	3.10.8	Anxiolytics	196
	3.10.9	Cannabinoids (Tetrahydrocannabinol, THC)	197
	3.10.10	Orexin Receptor Antagonists	199
3.11		**Phytotherapeutics**	200
	3.11.1	European Medicinal Plants	200
	3.11.2	Ayurvedic Medicinal Plants	201
	3.11.3	Herbal Medicines from Traditional Chinese Medicine (TCM)	201
3.12		**Dietary Supplements**	202
	3.12.1	Background	202
	3.12.2	Cannabidiol (CBD)	203
3.13		**Placebo**	205
3.14		**Relapse Prevention and Follow-Up**	206
	3.14.1	Relapse Prevention	206
	3.14.2	Aftercare	206
References			207

▶ This chapter presents the therapy concept for general practitioners, psychiatrists, neurologists and psychotherapists. The multimodal concept offers 30 therapy modules from the field of cognitive behavioral therapy, the third wave of behavioral therapy, the treatment basics of mind-body medicine and neurotherapy. It contains protocols, questionnaires and Information sheets as well as instructions for practical exercises that can be worked out together with the patients or given as homework. Examples of situations with patients are given, which can serve as a template and be individually adapted in the treatment of other patients.

3.1 Background

Cognitive behavioral therapy is the current gold standard for the treatment of psychologically caused sleep disorders. The S-3 guideline for non-refreshing sleep/sleep disorders clearly provides that all non-medicinal procedures should be exhausted first before treatment with hypnotics should be considered. However, everyday treatment looks different: Most of the time, the prescription of hypnotics is the first treatment approach. With this I do not want to make any accusations against my colleagues. The patients come in very stressful situations and have a high level of suffering due to the sleep disorders. A rapid relief of the symptoms is in the mutual interest. However, a drug therapy always only acts on the symptom and never on the cause Therefore, it should only be used temporarily to avoid psychological and physical dependence on hypnotics.

Sleep disorders are often chronic, which means that those affected often suffer for decades. During this time, many sufferers inform themselves in detail about the disorder and, not least thanks to the information available on the Internet, become experts in their own illness. This means that they have already tried a lot and need new ways of dealing with their sleep disorder on the one hand and the motivational support of the therapist on the other hand in order to try out already tried measures again, specifically and in the long term. Unfortunately, the non-medicinal treatment of sleep disorders does not lead to noticeable effects immediately. Sport as a therapeutic agent can take up to 4 months to have a positive effect on sleep.

▶ *It is particularly important that therapists differentiate themselves from pure self-help in their therapy. The theoretical content should be individually tailored to the patient, his everyday life and his value system.*

Even cognitive processes, beliefs, and multiple experienced negative examples manifest the symptomatology and can be very hindering in the therapeutic process. The patients should then be encouraged to find solutions in the Socratic dialogue, which can lead to a sustainable adoption of theoretically justified behaviors and their integration into everyday life. The knowledge that the patients have acquired themselves is thus picked up and, in the best case, the understanding of their situation and likewise their motivation to pursue discussed solutions in the long term is reinforced. In this context, behavioral exercises are given for testing in everyday life and can be discussed in the following session with a view to everyday suitability and the effect of the exercise on the patient's sleep, and if necessary adjusted.

Patients should be encouraged to continue to do things even if they initially fail. A key content of therapy and an important task of the therapist is the ongoing motivation of those affected.

In order to supplement the theoretical knowledge about sleep and sleep disorders, this guide presents many useful therapy components of cognitive behavioral therapy, the "new wave" of behavioral therapy, and for the first time also holistic treatment with approaches from mindbody medicine and their use based on different criteria. Sleep and thus also sleep disorders always affect body and mind. Therefore, targeted and holistic therapeutic measures can and should be taken at all points of human behavior, thinking, feeling and experience, as well as biological, hormonal, physiological and metabolic processes.

The order of the theory moduls and the respective offer for the patient should be handled flexibly, depending on which deficits and needs have been uncovered in the preceding sessions. The repetition of individual aspects is desired and can be considered unproblematic, as repetition creates consolidation of the content and, in particular, people with sleep disorders suffer from memory deficits. It is important that implementation in everyday life and the possible automation of new habits and behaviors takes time. Sleep does not improve abruptly or in the short term, but it often takes several weeks to months until a sustainable improvement is noticeable for the patient.

The procedure according to this therapy concept is exemplarily illustrated by 5 detailed *case studies (7 Appendix)*.

3.2 Formal Structure and Framework Conditions of Therapy

The therapy components presented below are suitable for both individual and group settings and have been tested in inpatient, partial inpatient, and outpatient settings. The theoretical background was conveyed to the patients alternately and repeatedly. Overlaps and repetitions were seen by those affected as helpful. People with sleep disorders often report cognitive deficits and, in particular, memory disorders. The repetitions ensured that the content was understood, retained, and above all applied.

The most important concern of this book is to enable therapists and doctors to awaken in the patients the understanding that only they themselves can be responsible for implementing the therapy elements in everyday life. The actual therapy takes place at home, at work, or in leisure time between sessions. It is important to adapt all exercises so that they can be implemented over a longer period of time for those affected.

It is recommended to have a flipchart with different colored pens ready for a therapy session in order to visually clarify certain topics. Many patients like to take notes during the sessions. It is beneficial if the patient can also take notes. New in this book are worksheets and Information sheets that have been developed in the long-term treatment of people with sleep disorders. They are integrated into the book for viewing and as a copy template. These materials are provided for you to download as a printable version.

The didactic structure underlying this guide is designed to make as many of the offered contents immediately available to the patient as possible. Therefore, the theoretical background should be repeated and interwoven into the corresponding everyday situations whenever it fits the therapy topic. On the one hand, this allows the patient to practice the respective technique and to elaborate his knowledge about the disorder, on the other hand, the techniques become more accessible and applicable. The Socratic dialogue between patients and therapists is the royal road to self-responsible therapy. It should also be used here. If the patients can derive the justification of the individual techniques themselves, this secures the understanding and increases the likelihood that they will be taken into account in everyday life.

A key component of therapy is the feeling of certain elements. Therefore, the patient should not only be told what and how to do it, but it may and should also be tried out actively in the respective therapy sessions in approaches. It has been found to be helpful to provide patients with role-playing, mindfulness, and relaxation exercises to show how different situations feel, what thoughts and signals arise.

The treating physician should not think for the patient. A therapy session does not have to be round—on the contrary: a certain and also tolerable unrest in the patient at the end of the session promotes progress in therapy between meetings. The more content and above all practically the patients work out for themselves in everyday life, the more sustainable the therapy success.

Therapists for sleep disorders should master various exercises, such as progressive muscle relaxation, autogenic training, elements of yoga, meditation, mindfulness or guided imagery. They do not have to be experts in this, but it is helpful to have gathered personal experience and understand the principle of action. Practicing together in the therapy session makes the treatment approach concrete and lowers the threshold to carry out this exercise again at home.

For each patient, a system-immanent and comprehensible language should be chosen. People affected by sleep disorders can be found in all age and educational groups. In everyday practice, various cultural backgrounds and religions can be significant. A good therapist or doctor is able to empathize with his patients. For a sustainable treatment success, it is essential for the treating physician to immerse himself in the patient's system as well as possible and to take into account both his language and his behavior when individually adapting the therapy content. Above all, the use of the appropriate vocabulary (e.g. youth language with adolescents, simple and short sentences with people with lower educational levels, technical terms and foreign words with academics) creates greater trust and understanding of the patient towards his therapist.

The treating physician should create an atmosphere that is pleasant and above all free of fear for the patient. Going to the doctor or psychotherapist is difficult for most people, especially if they have had nothing to do with psychotherapy before. Most affected people only come to therapy when there is really no other way.

Therefore, particular attention should be paid to the initial consultation. Here the patients have to be received and guided. For example, longer rhetorical pauses by the therapist are inappropriate and unnecessarily unsettle the affected person. The patient should be shown a lot of appreciation and should be signaled that he is actively listened to and that a framework is offered in which he can develop trust in the doctor or therapist. It is helpful to address the patient's suspected feelings and then give him time to think and talk. Especially at the beginning of the therapy, relieving conversations should take place in which the patients have the opportunity to present their often very long path of suffering. The treatment experience shows that this only takes a few minutes. This already promotes the inner experience and the dealing with aspects of the disease.

The therapist should pay attention to a good balance between interest, emotional warmth and directness. In addition, value must be placed on a structured approach and a certain order in the "uncontrollable chaos" , which is described by many patients.

The use of metaphors has proven to be favorable. They promote the visualization of problems and allow a likewise pictorial representation of the solution. The therapy of non-organic sleep disorders can be very laborious for those affected and requires a lot of discipline. Therefore, the development of learning-theoretical reinforcement plans is helpful and motivating. The therapist plays the role of a model for openness and friendliness. He should pay attention to clearly naming observed feelings and thoughts.

Resource-oriented work is also of importance. It must be ensured that the resources used are sustainable and stable. In the therapy of sleep disorders, side effects in the form of disputes with the partner can occur (for example, by setting up a separate bedroom for the duration of the therapy). The task of the therapist is to stand by the patient for the processing and handling of these situations. At this point, the distinction becomes clear again, which must be made in order to make it clear to the patient that a holistic therapy is much more than a self-help guide in the style of the many good self-help guides for sleep disorders.

To give clear guidance and plausible change instructions for everyday situations is the task of the therapist. This is also where the essential difference lies to the available online offers and apps, which are mostly well developed in terms of content and didactics. However, nothing can replace personal contact and social reinforcement. Although scientific studies show good effect sizes of virtual treatment options, the compliance up to the first use and the completion of the entire program is rather poor (Lorenz et al. 2019). The therapeutic goal must be transparent throughout and, above all, comprehensible and meaningful for the person concerned.

> *In addition to all these techniques and theories, the therapeutic relationship is particularly important. A psychotherapist can only treat his patients well if there is a sound relationship. He should like his patients and vice versa.*

During a therapy of sleep disorders, very intimate things are discussed. Only if there is a trusting relationship in which one can also laugh and all emotions are allowed, can there be a sustainable therapeutic success.

3.3 Development of the Disorder Model

In order to plan the therapy, it is important to work out together with the patient how his/her individual symptoms came about. Experience has shown that the disorders are often very complex and that the actual disease may have started a long time ago.

In order to analyse the complexity of the patient's symptoms, it would be ideal to use the model of Mind-Body-Sleep-Dynamics© (MBSD) (Sect. 2.1). With the accompanying, very comprehensive Mind-Body-Sleep-Dynamics© questionnaire, the symptoms of the individual dimensions can be recorded and then evaluated together with the patient. With this information, a corresponding therapy plan can then be developed and a prognosis derived. Working with MBSD© requires a lot of knowledge and experience of the different sleep disorders and the dynamics of all the factors involved. A description of the application of MBSD© would go far beyond the scope of this book.

Even without the use of MBSD©, a disorder model can be recorded in a therapeutic conversation. The screening questionnaire (see Figs. 2.5 and 2.6) can help here.

Very good personal experience has been gained with the explanation of a complex clinical picture using the vulnerability-stress model, as shown in Fig. 3.1. It can also be referred to as a biopsychosocial model because it includes all areas in the explanation. Work out the overview together with your patient. The figure shows an example that you can use as a basis for derivation.

Reprinted with permission: Permission is granted to copy, distribute and/or modify this document under the terms of the GNU Free Documentation License, Version 1.2 or any later version published by the Free Software Foundation

3.4   Modules of Cognitive Behavioral Therapy

The therapy components described below have proven to be extremely effective in the holistic and sustainable treatment of sleep disorders. The components are each self-contained and can be used modularly as part of a treatment for sleep disorders. To increase the therapeutic effect, repetition of the application of individual components within therapy is expressly desired.

To facilitate the use of these components, this chapter follows a clear structure: A short

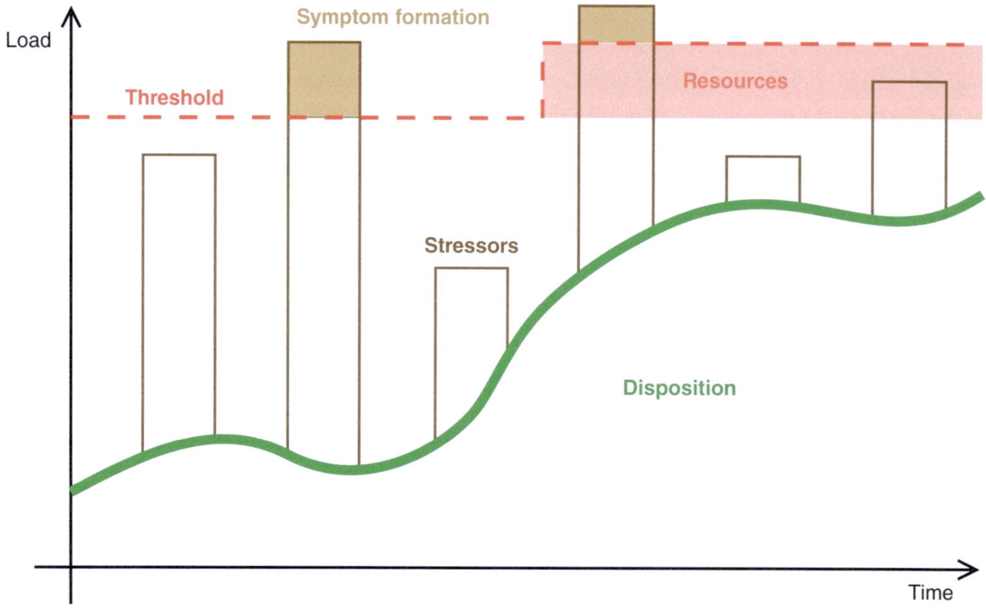

Fig. 3.1 Vulnerability-Stress Model. (© Iroqu)

overview presents the application and indications of the components. This is followed by a detailed description of the professional and theoretical background, and specific instructions are given for the practical procedure and the use of the component within the therapy.

3.4.1 Module: Psychoeducation

Short Overview (Table 3.1)

Background

Psychoeducation is—as with many other disorders—one of the most important therapy components. There are numerous self-help books, websites, online and app-based therapy programs that contain valuable information for a restful sleep. Since many sufferers suffer from sleep disorders for decades, they often have extensive knowledge about sleep disorders. Unfortunately, there are also many myths and false information that can greatly unsettle sufferers and even lead to sleep disorders. In addition, a large part of the theoretical knowledge cannot be applied practically. Often, many different techniques have already been tried, since many of them showed no immediate effect, but were also quickly neglected.

The therapist or attending physician has the task here to provide sufferers with sufficient information about healthy, but also disturbed sleep and to adapt it to the patients and their everyday life, that is, to make it usable. Content can be repeated if necessary (due to possible concentration and reception problems or memory deficits of the affected persons). It is also important to motivate patients to continue to use the methods and techniques discussed in therapy (sleep restriction, nutrition, sport, etc.) even if they do not lead to an immediate success.

If you have read Chaps. 1 and 2 carefully or have specifically searched for information, you know the most important information about healthy and disturbed sleep. The following are the essentials summarized in a nutshell:

Important Facts

Everyone has their own internal clock, their own biorhythm and the optimal bedtime for them. For one it can be at 10 pm, another only goes to bed at midnight. In general, sleep should not be delayed too much and sufficient sleep time should be planned so that there is enough time to experience several sleep cycles and to achieve a recovery effect.

It is important to sleep in the dark because the rhythm-regulating and sleep-inducing melatonin is produced then. If you only sleep when the day has already begun, the production of this hormone is inhibited. This results in a shift of the biorhythm and possibly to a sleep disorder.

What Sleep Disorders are There?

There are over 80 different sleep disorders. Therefore, it is necessary to inform and educate patients about the diagnosis made and also about suspected diagnoses. For those affected, it is always helpful if they realize that they are taken seriously as a person and that their relationship

Table 3.1 Short overview Module: Psychoeducation

Indications	Any form of sleep disorder
Contraindications	Unknown
Effectiveness	Very well documented
Working principle	Enlightening about the structure, function and disorders of sleep facilitates the implementation of a sleep-supporting behavior Dissolving possible dysfunctional cognitions and assumptions about the topic of sleep allow a modification of subjective perception and attitude towards it
Treatment requirements	Knowledge about the topic of sleep and its disorders
Treatment goal	Patient is the expert of his sleep disorder, deep understanding of sleep and its disorders, derivation of realistic treatment goals, relapse prevention

is built on a basis of trust. It is critically important at this point to note that many affected people, especially on the Internet, look for further information that is not always correct. This should be discussed in therapy, false information and expectations should be corrected. Since further research by the patients during therapy cannot be ruled out, they should be encouraged to contact the treating physician with their findings and any questions that arise.

The Dynamics of Sleep Disorders

An individual disturbance model must be developed for each patient. In doing so, a wider circle should be drawn around the actual sleep disorder, as causes often lie in completely different areas of life. Commonly involved factors can be found in the professional or family context, in an exciting phase of life, in living conditions, and in other physical illnesses. Most of the time, there are "good reasons to sleep badly". All aspects of daily life that keep us "awake" in the truest sense of the word can be.

The Mind-Body-Sleep-Dynamics© model (Chap. 2, Sect. 2.1. Mind-Body-Sleep-Dynamics©) was developed as a help in creating such an individual model, with which different levels of experience and behavior can be mapped in a holistic way.

Sleep Phases

Sleep stages and phases are ideally worked out and explained to each individual on a flipchart, as shown in Fig. 3.2. If a complete hypnogram were presented to the patient in a therapy session, such as in Chap. 1 (Fig. 1.2), the complexity of it could easily exceed his or her ability to grasp it. Therefore, while everything important should be mentioned, it should not be gone into too much detail. One way to sketch the sleep architecture can be found under Fig. 3.2 For the patient individually important aspects must be emphasized and explained. This promotes the development of realistic expectations, while at the same time reducing false perceptions of nocturnal sleep. A hypnogram can serve as a orientation in the patient's own sleep cycle.

The nocturnal sleep is divided into different phases by the depth of sleep, which become visible based on brain activity in the EEG. The following describes the sleep phases in the normally typical sequence (see also Sect. 1.1).

Awake State

A relaxed awake state precedes the onset of sleep. The electroencephalogram (EEG) shows upstrokes in the alpha to beta frequency range of 8 to 13 Hz.

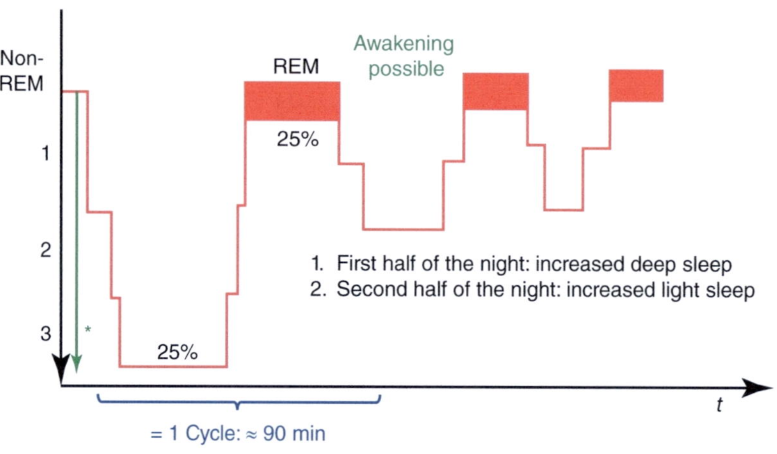

Fig. 3.2 Sketch to explain the sleep architecture during a therapy session (on the whiteboard)

Stage I (NREM 1)

The first and lightest sleep phase arises from a relaxed state of wakefulness. It only lasts a few minutes, sometimes only seconds. It is part of the process of falling asleep and at the same time the first stage of the NREM phase. At this point, those affected still have a relatively open range of perception, which is why it is sometimes not possible to identify this stage as sleep. Thoughts and images of the day then pass before the mental eye and can resemble a state of wakefulness. For those affected by sleep perception disorders, this experience is problematic because they feel they are awake all the time.

Muscle twitching can occur as the muscles relax during light sleep. This sleep phase is often described as feeling like you're falling.

The eyes move slowly and aimlessly (SEM, slow eye movement). The brain waves are predominantly characterized by theta activity with a frequency of 4 to 8 Hz. This sleep mode is the initial or final point of the sleep cycle that occurs several times during the night.

Stage II (NREM 2)

Sleep deepens in this stage. The eyes hardly move at all, the muscles are hardly tense.

The brain wave frequencies increase and, in addition to theta activity, show sleep spindles with a frequency of 8 to 15 Hz.

If dreaming occurs in this phase, it is usually very reality-based. If there are psychological conflicts that cannot be processed during the day, they usually return in this sleep stage. The more serious the conflict, the more often the dream content is repeated as reality. In the worst case, this distraction prevents deeper sleep from being reached. The sleeper cannot switch off, which greatly reduces the recovery value of the night's sleep.

Stage III (NREM)

In this sleep phase, the person reaches the state of deepest sleep. Only now does the physical and mental recovery go into high gear. Deep sleep is especially important for memory formation and regeneration of the immune system.

In the stage also known as the delta phase, the brainwave frequency is only 0 to 4 Hz. The body is in a state of complete relaxation. Breathing and heart rate are very slow and regular. The muscles are slack, and the eye movements are minimal.

Waking up from deep sleep is the hardest, often it takes minutes to get oriented again. If one falls asleep easily again, one may not even remember having been awake.

REM Sleep

During REM sleep, most and the most intense dreams are noticeable, which is why this sleep stage is also called the dream phase. Nevertheless, REM sleep is not as shallow as the measured brainwave curves could suggest. On the contrary, REM sleep is comparable to deep sleep in terms of sleep depth.

Eye movements are particularly pronounced in this phase. Pulse and breathing rate are increased and irregular. In the EEG, alpha and beta waves as well as low-frequency theta waves can be seen. Brainwave activity is higher than in the waking state, the frequency is between 4 and 13 Hz.

The facial expressions of the dreamer change depending on the dream situation he is in. Those who are woken up from REM sleep can remember their dreams particularly well.

On a physiological level, the dream sleep resembles the waking state of the human being. However, the skeletal muscles are usually completely relaxed. The sleeper is in a kind of paralysis. This prevents the movements that are carried out in the dream from actually taking place. The eye movements are an exception, because they are controlled by special nerve fibers.

The first REM phase of a sleep cycle lasts about 10 min, the second is twice as long. Towards morning, the dream phases have lengths of around one hour. Some long sleepers dream uninterruptedly for up to 2 h. With a sleep duration of 7 h, half of the dream phases are in the last two sleep hours. Individual sleep time plays a role.

Homoeostasis

The sleep-wake rhythm in humans is subject to the principle of homeostasis (Sect. 2.2.1). During the day, sleep pressure builds up, at night it is released. In the same way, fatigue increases during the day and decreases at night. A disturbed homeostasis therefore inevitably leads to a disturbed sleep of the patient. The following checklist should provide orientation in this respect.

Checklist for a disturbed homeostasis

- The sleep pressure is not high enough in the evening/at night.
- The patient has not exhausted himself enough during the day.
- The patient has slept during the day (a power nap of no more than 20 min is allowed, as it does not reduce the sleep pressure).
- The patient falls asleep in front of the television in the evening, interrupts the sleep to go to bed, and has already reduced part of the sleep pressure with the short nap.
- The patient has sleep interruptions, that is, one falls asleep and wakes up again (for example, due to noise, light) and then cannot fall asleep again because the sleep pressure has already been reduced to a certain extent.

To adjust or maintain homeostasis in patients, some rules must be followed:

Checklist for setting and maintaining homeostasis

- Regular bedtime and wake-up times
- No naps late in the day, powernaps before 2 pm are allowed
- Active daily life (exercise, errands, cognitive performance, etc.)
- Consideration of age and life situation

Procedure

For a successful therapy, it is important that your patient knows the most important basics of healthy sleep:

- The sleep architecture (for download: Information sheet IS 02: The architecture of healthy sleep)

- The homeostatic process (for download: Information sheet IS 03: The homeostatic process)
- The cortisol and melatonin course of a healthy adult

If you have enough time, it is advantageous to explain the theoretical content in your patient conversations using a flipchart. Alternatively or additionally, you can take the respective Information sheets home.

It is important to adapt the scientific background knowledge to the situation of your patient. Use appropriate and system-immanent language. Use situations for explanation that the patient is familiar with in order to find himself in the theory. Then draw conclusions and parallels together with your patient to the experience of the patient's symptomatology. This can then lead to interventions that he can try out in his everyday life.

▶ *It is important not only to offer the content, but also to make it usable for the patient.*

3.4.2 Module: Medications, Alcohol, and Drugs

Overview (Table 3.2)

Background

The therapy component of drugs, alcohol and drugs is intentionally shown under the first therapy components. As my mentor so aptly put it: "If addiction is in the boat, you can't get ahead in therapy." Therefore, at the beginning of therapy, a possible addiction should be considered and therapeutically planned.

A widely spread problem among sleep-disturbed patients is the use of sleeping pills. Most of these preparations may only be taken regularly over a short period of time, as tolerance can develop and they are addictive. The affected persons then have to take more of the substance to achieve the same effect. Nevertheless, there are always patients who take benzodiazepines,

Table 3.2 Overview Module: Medications, Alcohol, and Drugs

Indications	Sleep disorders, especially in known medication, alcohol, or drug abuse, dissimulation regarding this topic
Contraindications	Not known
Effectiveness	Very well documented, analogous to psychoeducation
Working principle	Information about a topic improves understanding thereof and facilitates a change in behavior
Treatment requirements	Therapist's knowledge of the psychological and physical effects of medications, alcohol and drugs
Treatment goal	De-stigmatization, clarification, increased motivation

sedative antihistamines or the newer non-benzodiazepine hypnotics zaleplon, zopiclone and zolpidem for years. After discontinuation of the medication, the sleep disorder can deteriorate drastically.

Overall, increased alcohol consumption is observed in people with sleep disorders. Alcohol has a sedative effect at first, which makes falling asleep easier. However, alcohol destroys the sleep architecture as a whole, and sleep is not restful. Alcohol can suppress deep sleep because the first half of the night is used for alcohol metabolism. In the second half of the night, (REM) sleep is also disturbed due to withdrawal symptoms. This can lead to arousals and longer periods of wakefulness, nightmares and other psychovegetative symptoms. Do not forget: Alcohol is a poison and makes you physically dependent.

A beer, a heavy red wine, a schnapps or even marijuana can make you very tired and help you fall asleep at first. If these substances are abused permanently and for the purpose of falling asleep, an addiction can develop quickly in addition to the sleep disorder. After discontinuation of these substances, the sleep disorder is often more pronounced than before.

Substances and medications are therefore no solution. They only relieve the symptoms and do not cure the cause. Especially when alcohol or drugs are used as "medications", there is a great risk of addiction. Dysfunctional cognitions and behaviors are then favored: "Without my beer I can't sleep."

Procedure

Substance abuse and addiction are very sensitive topics and are usually not discussed openly. Therefore, it is essential that practitioners have no fear of touching these topics. Patients with addiction are also patients who are responsible for, but not to blame for their illness. It is important to pick up the patients where they are, neither to play down the disease nor to bring it dramatically to the fore. The potential for addiction should be made aware of without leading to catastrophization or feelings of guilt.

It has been found to be advantageous to raise the topic of *use of substances* in the anamnesis conversation together with other possibly delicate topics such as sexuality. If these topics are included in routine diagnostics, therapists often feel more secure. Ultimately, this self-awareness is also felt by the patient.

▶ *If an undiscovered dependency problem exists in the therapy of sleep disorders, the entire therapy can be severely impaired.*

A step-by-step approach has the best chances of success:

Development of Motivation

The first step in the treatment of an addiction is to gain the patient's insight into the disease and to develop the necessary motivation for therapy by means of psychoeducation. Only when the patient himself is convinced that there is a problem does it make sense to initiate a corresponding therapy. The primary goal in the further course of therapy is to achieve (temporary) abstinence. Depending on how severe the addiction is, it can make sense to carry out a stationary detoxification and addiction therapy before continuing outpatient. Abuse of drugs, alcohol and other substances can usually be handled well in an outpatient setting. It is advantageous to inform the patients first of all why self-medication with substances does not improve, but rather deteriorates, sleep disorders. The patient should then credibly agree to try abstinence. If you still have doubts that the patient is insightful, it would be better to wait with the beginning of the corresponding interventions until the patient is motivated to face the abuse or addiction. Starting the abstinence phase too early can lead to it not being maintained. This failure can have a lasting effect on the self-esteem, sleep and overall well-being of the patient.

Possible Physical Detoxification

If there is a dependence on benzodiazepines or a long-term dependence on non-benzodiazepines, a doctor must be consulted for detoxification, especially in older people. Sudden withdrawal can have serious consequences, such as cardiovascular disorders or withdrawal symptoms such as anxiety and panic, sleep disorders, restlessness, tension, severe mood swings, sweating or tremor. This can lead to a relapse of the symptoms that originally led the patients to the medication.

Therefore, a gradual withdrawal according to a fixed plan is necessary. Usually, the dose is slowly reduced until it is completely withdrawn. In case of severe dependencies, it may be necessary to replace the relevant benzodiazepine with another medication with a shorter half-life or better dosing options (e.g. drops) at first. Benzodiazepines are among the substances that are most difficult to withdraw because they can

also cause withdrawal symptoms long after the actual detoxification.

In case of short-term abuse in younger patients without pre-existing conditions, a cold withdrawal, i.e. the immediate withdrawal of the substance, is possible. However, if you have any doubts about this, it is always better to consult a doctor.

Psychological Detoxification

If the patient wants to make a serious attempt at abstinence or has completed the detoxification, you should set a specific period of time during which nothing is consumed. This should not be too long at first, e.g. until the next appointment in one or two weeks, in order to be foreseeable for the patient. One of the slogans of Alcoholics Anonymous is "One day at a time". For people with sleep disorders it should be "One night at a time".

Often it makes sense not to start with the withdrawal of sleep medication at the beginning of therapy. Patients are afraid of losing control over their sleep again and therefore the fear of having to stop taking the sleep medication immediately when they go to the therapist. In practice, it has proved to be advantageous to use a few therapy sessions at first to establish first intervention approaches in everyday life before the sleep medication is "taken away".

It is important to show the patient that they are also able to fall asleep and maintain it without substances.

Aftercare

In order to stay abstinent or to consume alcohol only for enjoyment and sleep medication only as needed, it is important to keep this topic alive in therapy and to sensitize the patient for it. However, a successful end of therapy can also consist in the targeted use of an appropriate medication. Therefore, it should be discussed in therapy when such a moment is and how often, for example, a Z-substance may be taken (maximum 6 times per month).

3.4.3 Module: Bed Rest and Sleep Restriction

Overview (Table 3.3)

Background

The key to a good night's sleep is to live in harmony with your body's natural rhythms and the cycle of day and night. For many people with sleep disorders, this rhythm is disturbed. Therefore, the first step in treating sleep disorders is to find the "right" time to go to bed and get up. These times should be as close as possible to the patient's natural bedtime and wake-up time. To find out in what rhythm the patient is at the beginning of therapy and what times he or she uses for sleeping, the patient must keep a sleep diary for a certain period of time (at least two weeks). In many cases, it becomes clear from these records that the patient's total time in bed, that is, the time the patient spends awake and asleep in bed, is much longer than the patient's actual sleep time. For many reasons, it is important to equalize the total time in bed with the actual sleep time.

Sleep restriction is the right and at the same time one of the most important therapy components at this point. The use of this technique should be considered for every patient from the beginning of therapy. With sleep restriction, regular bedtimes are introduced into the patient's everyday life from the beginning, and these are adapted to the patient's daily rhythm in the course of therapy. Consideration should be given to school and work hours, the care of relatives and pets, and other tasks.

Sleep restriction creates increased sleep pressure during the day by reducing the total time in bed and, to some extent, the sleep time. After a certain period of adaptation, this makes it easier to fall asleep and favors a more compact sleep with higher deep sleep proportions. When this method is used as a single treatment, for example, an average percentage improvement in sleep latency of 59% was observed immediately after the end of the intervention and 42% at 1-year follow-up.

There are "sleep schools" or therapy manuals (Müller and Paterok 2010), which are based solely on this concept. The method was first used by Spielman et al. (1987). Its effect could be replicated in many follow-up studies.

The reason for the high effectiveness of sleep restriction lies in the change of typical behaviors of patients with sleep disorders: The bad sleep at night leads to the fact that the patients try to make up for the perceived sleep deficit and fatigue in some way. Their strategy is usually an extended bedtime, catching up on sleep when tired during the day, and a reduction in

Table 3.3 Overview Module: Bed rest and sleep restriction

Indications	Sleep and/or sleep disorders, early waking, hypersomnia, paradoxical insomnia
Contraindications	Activities with high accident risk during the day, caution with bipolar disorder and hypersomnia
Side effects	Temporarily increased daytime sleepiness, transient mood deterioration, induction of euphoric mood, increased irritability
Effectiveness	Very well documented
Working principle	According to the biorhythm and regular bedtimes are the basis for a refreshing sleep Short-term sleep deprivation leads to faster, continuous and deeper sleep (Borbély et al. 1981) regular, limited sleep times strengthen the homeostatic sleep pressure, daytime sleep or wakefulness in bed are prevented and the depth of sleep is increased
Treatment requirements	Knowledge of sleep protocol analysis, sleep restriction method, good patient motivation
Treatment goal	Find the patient's biorhythm Improved sleep efficiency (quick falling asleep, continuous sleep), increased sleep depth, regular sleep rhythm

daytime activity. However, this behavior often leads to a strong variability of the sleep process due to significantly longer bedtimes, often causing a subjective feeling of loss of control over sleep behavior. It is possible that the patients fall asleep quickly, but it can also happen that they lie awake for hours or wake up again and again and only fall asleep again very late or not at all.

For a large part of the patients it is not understandable at first that it is precisely these behaviors that lead to the development and maintenance of sleep disorders. The reduction of sleep pressure by a longer afternoon nap increases the probability of waking up at night with additional problems falling asleep again. The resulting wakefulness in bed is typically spent with worrying and worrying about sleep or not being able to sleep. There is a physical tension that in turn prevents falling asleep. The patient leaves the bed after a non-refreshing night, feels impaired in his well-being and performance, applies his strategy again and gets caught up in a vicious circle that can lead to a permanent sleep disorder.

Persons with sleep disorders often tend to spend significantly more time in bed than they actually sleep. In addition to the actual insomnia, in the sense of a significantly shortened sleep time, this can lead to a sleep perception disorder, a paradoxical (subjective) insomnia. For example, if a person spends 14 h in bed every day, but sleeps only 7–8 h of these 14 h, the person concerned is awake for 6–7 h in bed. This time can be experienced as very stressful, and despite sufficient sleep time, there is a feeling of suffering. At this point, the person concerned needs to be informed.

The aim of bedtime and sleep restriction is not only to increase the sleep pressure for night sleep. In addition, it has the effect of referring the patient back to his individual biorhythm. Through everyday demands and a torn sleep-wake rhythm, the biorhythm of the affected persons has been disturbed. By keeping a sleep diary as part of the therapy, a first impression can be gained of when the sleep phases usually take place.

There are so-called "owls" and "larks", that is, night owls and early risers. These chronotypes are not solely due to habits and lifestyle. They are based on evolutionary and genetically anchored rhythms of hormone levels and other body functions that should be taken into account when determining bedtime.

Furthermore, it should be noted that the night does not end too early. Especially in Germany, the working day starts very early. If early shifts begin well before dawn, that is, before 6:00 a.m., and patients have to get up as early as 4:30 a.m., these physical and psychological burdens are rather experienced as night shifts.

In addition, it is repeatedly discussed that school starts too early and that children are neither rested nor able to perform. Going to bed earlier would not make any difference here, because the individual's biological rhythm would not make the children fall asleep earlier. Many adolescents have sleep disorders during this phase of life due to their individual, healthy biological rhythm not matching social requirements. There are already some projects in which upper secondary school students are given a flexible time zone within the first lesson. They can decide for themselves whether they would rather sleep a little longer or prefer remedial lessons.

But not only duties, such as shift work, early work and school start times disturb the sleep-wake rhythm. There are people who cannot sleep at night and want to make use of this time. They therefore begin to develop dysfunctional behaviours, such as housework, homework, social networking via the Internet, etc. Once they have become established, such patterns are difficult to break. Especially among adolescents and young adults, such a shift can be found, for example, by playing computer games all night and sleeping during the day in order to be able to continue playing the next night.

The aim of bed and sleep restriction is to make the person concerned automatically associate their bed with sleep. The previously familiar fear of not being able to sleep or lying awake and worrying should be interrupted.

Procedure

In order to capture all the necessary parameters for the introduction of a bed or sleep restriction, it is necessary to carefully analyze the patient's sleep diary. For this purpose, the patient should keep a sleep diary over a period of two weeks, in which the time of going to bed, the time of turning off the light (from here the patient tries to fall asleep), the subjectively estimated time of falling asleep (the patients should not look at the clock here), possibly the times and duration of waking up during the night, the final time of waking up and finally the time of getting up are requested. The recording of the day's activities and energy levels at different times has also proved to be favorable in order to quickly recognize patterns in the patient's experience and behavior. An example of how such a sleep diary can be designed is shown in Fig. 3.3.

These data are then either entered by the patient at home or together during the therapy session in color in the worksheet WS 03: Sleep Diary Diagram (Fig. 3.4) as in the example below. The respective times of going to bed are marked with black, the times of turning off the light (which corresponds to the time from which the patient tries to fall asleep) are marked with blue. Red marks the *felt* time of falling asleep, green the time of waking up and violet the time of getting up. The points are then connected by lines, as shown in the example. In this way, for example, the effective sleep time can be easily distinguished from the bedtime. With the help of the workshee WS 04: Evaluation of the sleep diary diagram you will receive help with the interpretation of the data (Table 3.4).

Based on this data, the effective sleep time can be calculated. Here it should be noted that patients with sleep disorders often underestimate their sleep (Crönlein 2013). However, since psychotherapy is primarily about the subjective well-being of the patient, their subjective statements are sufficient. Technical support, by an Actiwatch, a sleep app, etc., is not necessary. In addition, it is not necessary for patients to constantly look at the clock when keeping a sleep diary. This often disturbs the sleep of those affected. The list of subjectively perceived times is usually sufficient for therapy planning.

After the patient has kept the sleep diary for at least two weeks, the first sleep-restrictive measures can be introduced. Before introducing them, it is important to inform the patient in detail about the sleep restriction and to motivate him. The following points can be mentioned:

- People with sleep disorders need to stick to regular bedtimes; this is a basic component of therapy.
- Despite the limited bedtimes, the patient has enough time to sleep in total. If sleep restriction takes effect, the effective sleep time is even longer than the current sleep duration. The patient should be shown, based on the current effective sleep times, that the discrepancy is not large.
- Motivation: It pays to persevere. The first effects are usually already noticeable after a few nights.

The restricted bedtime should initially be aligned with the actually occurring sleep phases, even if they do not initially fit completely into the patient's social rhythm. In particularly severe cases, a sick note should be considered. Many sufferers are sick leave anyway due to the sleep disorder. If this is not the case, it is advantageous to start the first phase of sleep restriction on a weekend or free day. It is important here to offer enough strategies so that the patient remains awake and active during the day and does not fall back into his usual behavior pattern. A precise planning of the times before the patients go to bed or after they have left the bed very early is very helpful. At this time they are very tired and don't know what to do with themselves. For staying up late, watching TV, handicrafts, puzzles, walks and light tidying up have proven to be very helpful. It is important here that the patients do not fall asleep, but also not to activate themselfs too much. Meditation, relaxation or mindfulness exercises can be

TB01 - My sleep diary

Dr. **Carolin Marx-Dick**
EXPERTIN FÜR SCHLAFGESUNDHEIT

Week from __________ to ______
Name: _____________________

My day	Example	Mon	Tue	Wed	Thu	Fri	Sat	Sun
Morning activities	work							
Afternoon activities	Shopping, pick up kids, yoga							
Mindful moments	Lunch break: mindful eating, way home: walking meditation							
Did you sleep during the day today? When and for how long?	13:30 30 min							
How easy/difficult was it for you to perform (job, household) today? (1: very easy ... 6: very poor); space for notes	2							

This document was created by Dr. Carolin Marx-Dick and is protected by copyright. It may only be used and passed on for non-commercial purposes as accompanying therapy material for the treatment of sleep disorders. Any editing or modification is prohibited. (Version 0/2022) www.drcarolinmarxdick.de

TB01 - My sleep diary

Dr. **Carolin Marx-Dick**
EXPERTIN FÜR SCHLAFGESUNDHEIT

Week from __________ to ______
Name: _____________________

My evening (before the light goes out)	Example	Mon	Tue	Wed	Thu	Fri	Sat	Sun
Aktivitäten in der letzten Stunde vorm Zubettgehen	lesen, Bad nehmen							
Wie frisch/müde fühlen Sie sich jetzt? (1: sehr frisch; 6: sehr müde)	5							
Haben Sie in den letzten vier Stunden Alkohol zu sich genommen? Falls ja, was und wieviel?	1 Glas Wein							
Haben Sie Schlafmedikamente genommen? (Präparat, Dosis & Uhrzeit)	1/2 Stilnox 22:30							
Wann sind Sie zu Bett gegangen?	22:30							

My morning (right after getting up)	Example	Mon	Tue	Wed	Thu	Fri	Sat	Sun
When did you turn off the light yesterday?	23:00							
How long did it take you to fall asleep after the light went out? (Indication in minutes)	40							
Were you awake at night? How often? How long in total? (Indication in minutes)	2 x 30 min							
When did you finally wake up?	6:30							
How long did you sleep in total? (hh:mm)	6:40							
When did you finally get up?	7:00							
How fresh/tired do you feel? (1: very good ...... 6: very bad)	2							

This document was created by Dr. Carolin Marx-Dick and is protected by copyright. It may be used and passed on exclusively within the scope of its purposes for non-commercial use as accompanying therapy material for the treatment of sleep disorders. Any editing or modification is prohibited. (Version 0/2022) www.drcarolinmarxdick.de

Fig. 3.3 My sleep diary

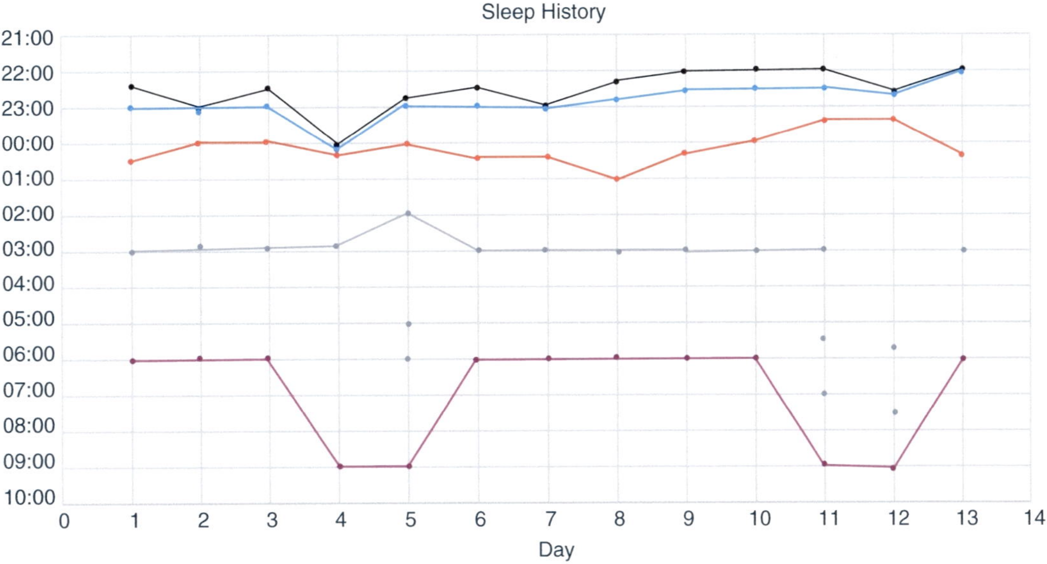

Fig. 3.4 Worksheet WS 03: Sleep chart for sleep diary

Table 3.4 Explanation of results

All lines run relatively straight. This means that there are no large deviations between the individual points of a line (maximum 30 min)	Your patient has a regular day-night rhythm If larger zigzag patterns occur, your patient has a very irregular day-night rhythm. This should be more linear
The blue and red lines run very close to each other (less than 30 min apart daily)	Your patient probably does not have insomnia, even if these lines run in a zigzag pattern If the blue and red lines diverge significantly (more than 30 min) and your patient finds the long awake lying time before sleep very unpleasant, he probably has insomnia If the two widely spaced lines also run in a zigzag pattern, this may be due to the regular day-night rhythm
The red and green lines run parallel to each other (also in zigzag)	Your patient has a relatively constant total sleep time. Unless there are longer periods of wakefulness in between (each more than 15 min), he has a robust night's sleep, especially if zigzag patterns can be seen The total sleep time should show more than 6 h, but preferably 7.5 to 8 h If the red and green lines do not run parallel to each other and have significant fluctuations of more than 30 min, your patient has a very inconstant total sleep time. If in addition there are longer periods of wakefulness in between (each more than 15 min), he also has a very fragmented night's sleep
The green and violet lines run very closely together	Wake-up and get-up times are closely spaced. If your patient has slept long enough that he does not wake up more than 30 min before his desired wake-up time, he does not suffer from early waking. That's very good, because early waking is the hardest to treat! If the green and violet lines are very far apart, significantly more than 30 min, this prolongs the time in bed. If your patient is already awake for a long time and still stays in bed, his body concludes: "Beeing awake in bed is also okay". However, his body should learn: "Bed equals sleep". Even if he regularly wakes up significantly before his actual desired wake-up time, your patient should leave the bed

counterproductive. With positive experiences at the beginning of the day, the overall mood of the day can be lifted and possible stress can be reduced.

It has been shown to be very effective to start with a drastic sleep restriction for the first 2–3 nights (e.g. 4–5 h in bed) in order to build up the greatest possible sleep pressure. The bedtime should be at least 30 min after the average sleep onset. The wake-up time should be at least 30 min before the end of the total effective sleep time (not before the end of the usual wake-up time!).

Even in the drastic nights the bedtime should not be less than 3 h. If the bedtime results in less than 5 h, no more than 2 of these very short nights should follow one another. Subsequently, the bedtime should be extended by 30 to 60 min for the following 5 nights. After one week, the next therapy appointment for debriefing and, if necessary, refinement of the bedtime should take place.

Example Case: Sleep Restriction

Ms. K. reports going to bed every evening between 10:00 p.m. and 11:00 p.m. However, she usually stays awake for another hour and a half to two hours. Then she sleeps for about two hours, wakes up again and lies awake for another hour and a half. This continues until 7:00 a.m. So according to Ms. K.'s subjective feeling, she sleeps a total of about four hours. Since Ms. K. usually doesn't fall asleep before 1:00 a.m., it doesn't make much sense to send her to bed earlier. Therefore, the following bedtime is recommended:

- 1st and 2nd night: Go to bed at 1:00 a.m. (possibly even at 1:30 a.m.) and get up at 5:00 a.m. This corresponds to a bedtime of 4 h, which corresponds to her current effective sleep time.
- From the 3rd night: Go to bed at 1:00 a.m. and get up at 6:00 a.m. This

should be done for 5 nights until the next therapy appointment.

- Ms. K. reports that the first two days were terrible, she felt exhausted during the day, but still held on. From night 3 it actually got better. She even looked forward to going to bed and the moment she could finally go to sleep. She can't sleep through the night yet, but she only needs 30 min to fall asleep.
- Instruction from the 2nd week: Go to bed at 1:00 a.m. and get up at 6:00 a.m. until the sleep disorder has improved.
- At the end of the therapy, Ms. K. has the following bedtimes: Go to bed at midnight and get up at 7:00 a.m. Most of the time the patient is already awake at 6:30 a.m., but she feels rested and recovered.

In addition to sleep restriction, other therapy components were also used. This means that it was not only sleep restriction that led to success. At the end of the therapy, there was still an average of one bad night per week, which Ms. K. could live with.

Crönlein (2013) is rightly warning against prescribing too short bedtimes, because this can significantly reduce motivation and trust in therapy and lead to an early termination. Furthermore, it must be noted that, in particular in the first days of sleep restriction, there is an increased risk of accidents due to pronounced fatigue. This must be discussed in the preparation phase.

In the relevant literature (Müller and Paterok 2010) on the subject of sleep restriction, it is recommended to only then expand bedtimes when no sleep and wakefulness disorders occur anymore. In everyday practice, however, this goal is rarely achievable. Therefore, bedtimes should be adapted to everyday obligations and the social rhythm after a relatively stable phase and, above all, still during therapy. In this way, it is possible to equalize these phases over a longer period of time and thus achieve the best possible result for the patient.

Therapists should feel confident in trying out different configurations with patients and adapting the sleep concept to their needs. However, it must be ensured that bedtimes do not become unnaturally long again.

Procedure for Sleep Restriction at a Glance
Step 1: Recording of the usual

- Time of going to bed (a)
- Time of falling asleep (b)
- Wakefulness during the night (c)
- Time of waking up in the morning (d)
- Time of getting up (e)

Step 2: Calculation of the net sleep time

- Time between b and d minus c

Step 3: Determine the new bedtime

- This should be a total of at least 30 min shorter than the net sleep time
- The bedtime should take place during the night so that there is sufficient sleep time in the dark (even in summer); this causes a better adaptation to the natural circadian rhythm
- If sleep through problems are in the foreground, the corresponding wakefulness should be deducted from the bedtime (a) and this should be moved backwards

It has been found to be favorable to go to bed 30–60 min later than the original **sleep** time (b) in the evening and to wake up 30–60 min earlier than the original **wake up** time in the morning (d). This means a reduction of the net sleep time and should provide a sufficient sleep pressure to stabilize sleep.

The motivation by the therapist or other group members is of great importance in sleep restriction. It is a very strenuous part of the therapy for the patient because he is constantly tired. The patient will have the desire to fall

back into his "old times" or, if necessary, to take a nap. It is important that the patient also endure the sleep restriction for at least 2 weeks without visible success. If, after the first week, with consistent adherence to the restrictive bedtime, no change has occurred, the restriction should be recalculated and possibly further restricted and adjusted on the basis of the sleep diary.

If the desired results such as quick falling asleep and sleeping through show and the patient still complains of daytime sleepiness, the restriction may be loosened. This loosening should be done gradually and very slowly. For example, it is recommended to let the patient sleep 30 min longer in the morning (if the patient wakes up in the morning by an alarm call and not by himself). Such a change should then be observed for at least one week and its effect documented. The sleep restriction is loosened weekly and step by step until the patient feels comfortable with it.

The age of the patient is of great importance in planning the sleeping times. Younger people need more night sleep than older people, whereas there is nothing against a short, but planned morning or midday sleep in the sleep concept and accordingly reducing the night sleep phase in older people. In addition, the basic constitution of a patient should be considered. Less robust or older people may possibly benefit more from a smaller reduction in bed times. In people with (severe) physical illnesses, bipolar or psychotic disorders, only bedtime but no sleep restriction should be carried out.

3.4.4   Module: Day Structuring

Overview (Table 3.5)

Background

▶   A balanced daily rhythm is the key to healthy sleep.

A highly complex hormonal system controls all functions of our body, including the adaptation to the day-night rhythm. There are hormones

Table 3.5 Overview Module: Day structuring

Indications	All types of sleep disorders, but especially in insomnia, hypersomnia and circadian sleep-wake disorders Lack of structuring compulsory and leisure activities, lack of regularity and timing of everyday activities to a sleep rhythm, especially in unemployed and shift work
Contraindications	None known
Side effects	Giving up familiar rituals and everyday routines
Effectiveness	Very well documented
Mode of action	Activities in accordance with the body's natural rhythm are the key to a good night's sleep Structuring the day according to the individual's performance curve and other needs synchronizes the biological rhythms
Treatment requirements	Knowledge of the rhythm-supporting effect of regularity in daily life, methods for learning self-discipline
Treatment goal	Establishing good performance, improved sleep quality Incorporating structuring activities and appointments as well as set periods of time for sleep, meals, etc., independent, disciplined adherence to rules

that activate and wake us up, there are hormones that make us tired and shut down the body, and there are hormones that produce and maintain sleep. Accordingly, this healthy hormone course, it is necessary to plan the daily structure so that we use optimal performance phases to complete important and difficult tasks. In return, the human being needs compensation in the form of positively evaluated leisure activities and periods of rest.

A very complex part of our human "control" is subject to the hormone cortisol. It is commonly referred to as the "stress hormone" and suggests that it is only secreted when we are stressed. But this is far from the case: Cortisol is the hormone that makes us performant in the first place. It has an activating and performance-enhancing effect and thus makes both physical and mental activities possible.

In the morning, if the "cortisol biorhythm" is well synchronized, the highest cortisol secretion can be observed. During the day, the cortisol level then decreases slowly in fluctuations. In Sect. 1.5 the hormones involved in sleep are described in detail.

In addition to the natural course of the circadian rhythm, the cortisol secretion also adapts to the performance demand and to our requirements and wishes. Before an exam or a sporting event, but also while we are doing tasks that require a lot of concentration or effort from us, the cortisol level rises.

So if we want to achieve a lot, more cortisol is also secreted. That is not a problem for our body, because our organism is oriented towards such limited performance and stress moments.

However, if we always want to achieve too much, this is chronic stress, so the performance hormone is constantly pumped into our bloodstream and we have a permanently increased cortisol level, which is also not reduced in the evening. This results in restlessness and sleep disorders.

Therefore, it is essential for a restful sleep and also for our overall health to structure the day according to the natural cortisol course with targeted performance queries.

The secretion of cortisol takes place in a circadian rhythm in healthy people, i.e. a 24-hour rhythm.

A high secretion takes place in the morning and early afternoon. In these periods we are very productive and can work very well mentally and physically.

In contrast, the often very clearly noticeable midday slump. The reason for this is a short-term drop in cortisol levels, which makes us tired and sluggish. In healthy people, the cortisol level drops from around 5 p.m. in the evening and reaches its lowest level in the first half of the night.

The highest cortisol secretion can be observed in the morning, which is referred to as the "cortisol awakening reaction". During the day, the cortisol level then slowly decreases again in fluctuations.

An increased cortisol secretion at night leads to more light sleep, while the deep sleep percentage decreases. Sleep is interrupted more often and causes longer periods of wakefulness and early waking. This makes it less restful.

Procedure

Before beginning this section of therapy, it is important that the patient has been educated about the body's natural rhythms, as well as the natural course of the hormone cortisol and the "sleep hormone" melatonin. The worksheet WS05: Daily Structure and the Information sheet IS04: Hormones that determine sleep (Sect. 3.4.1) can be used to support this. The patient can use this sheet simultaneously for the first sensitization to this topic and on the last page of the sheet, a short screening of a typical day can be carried out by filling out the final table of his daily structure, as shown in … (see Fig. 3.5).

Your current daily structure

To give you a feeling for the many small tasks of the "I just have to ..." variety in your

everyday life, please think through a typical weekday and enter the information

in the table below.

What are your (almost) daily tasks: Work, family, sports, hobbies,

friends, etc.?

What more concrete tasks do you have to deal with (almost) every day: a long commute,

meetings, shopping, etc.?

What still comes up "spontaneously" and thwarts your plans?

How do you feel about it? How much energy do the individual tasks cost you?

What does a typical weekday look like for you?

Your typical weekday Monday -Friday

Time of day	Activities	Mood	Energy consumption
Tomorrow		😃 😐 😟	🔋
Morning		😃 😐 😟	🔋
Noon		😃 😐 😟	🔋
Afternoon		😃 😐 😟	🔋
Evening		😃 😐 😟	🔋
Night		😃 😐 😟	🔋

* on the IS05 information sheet, your patients have more space for their observations.

Fig. 3.5 Your current daily structure

The patient then fills out the diary D 02: My weekdays in preparation for this therapy session by noting his activities for 1–2 weeks.

However, most patients know their daily routines and have all the necessary information in their heads. Now sort with your patient which are actually necessary tasks and how much cognitive or physical effort they require:

> - What daily duties need to be fulfilled (work and errands)?
> - Which meals should be taken and how can they be integrated into the daily routine (break design)?
> - Which social and family duties exist, when and how can they be pursued (children, partner, parents, etc.)?
> - What times are there for self-care (yoga, sports, friends, hobbies, etc.)?
> - What buffer times should be built in?

It makes sense to give the patient the plan worked out in this way in writing to take home with them. Use the worksheet WS 05: My new daily routine for this (Fig. 3.6). This sheet should be placed in a visible place in the patient's everyday life (e.g. on the desk) so that he is reminded again and again how his healthy day should look. The more specific this plan is, especially for the next 3–5 days, the easier it is for the patient to implement it.

In addition, the patient can use the worksheet WS 05: My new daily routine on a daily basis or for particularly challenging days to plan their activities, possibly also enter them retrospectively, and assess their mood and energy level.

It is also very useful to retrospectively record tasks. Often we do things "on the side" that tire us out but do not appear in the list of activities for which we can pat ourselves on the shoulder in the evening. Therefore, activities should also be recorded retrospectively that were carried out without being planned beforehand.

In the following session, which should ideally take place 2–4 weeks later, it is ascertained what the patient was able to implement from the new daily routine and how it went for him. If the patient has coped well, he should be encouraged to continue like this. If there were difficulties in implementation, the therapeutic conversation will work out what the implementation problems were and how the daily routine has to be designed to meet the requirements of a healthy daily routine taking into account all the patient's tasks.

The next step in designing a sleep-promoting daily routine is a rough planning of upcoming tasks and projects. For this purpose, the daily routine worksheet WS 06: My to-do list can be used. Discuss with the patient which larger tasks do not have to be fulfilled daily or have already been done for a long time, such as cleaning windows, sorting out the wardrobe, repainting the bedroom, etc. Plan these larger tasks and projects so that they fit into the patient's life in such a way that it is realistic that they can then be carried out and no longer "haunt" the patient constantly. Unfinished tasks activate our entire nervous system and are therefore very sleep-inhibiting.

Excursus: Designing Breaks

Many people are under the false impression that good performance and extensive breaks do not go together. Quite the opposite is the case: Anyone who wants to show outstanding performance needs good breaks: at the right time, of the appropriate length and with a meaningful break design.

Short breaks improve your work performance.

In the 1980s, an impressive study on breaks during work was published. It was discovered by chance at a large automobile manufacturer that the smokers among the employees worked more effectively: They managed to put together more parts in a shorter time and made fewer mistakes than their non-smoking colleagues. Of course, it was quickly discovered that this positive aspect was not due to nicotine, but to the regular smoking breaks of the employees. From then on, all employees were given regular "smoking breaks". They had to leave their workplace for 5 min every 60 min, preferably with colleagues to get some fresh air. The plan worked, they also worked more effectively. However, there was another very positive aspect to the introduction of short breaks: The number of sick days of the workforce decreased and there was reported to be greater job satisfaction. More breaks create more effective work.

In connection with short moments of reflection and mindfulness, the feeling of stress can already be greatly improved, even if, for example, two tasks are never done

WS05 - My new daily structure

Week from _________ to ______
Name: ____________________

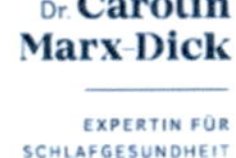

In the diagram below you can see the cortisol, i.e. performance curve, of a healthy person. For optimal performance and restful sleep, it is important to set up your daily routine according to this pattern. In the diagram below , plan all the regular tasks of your daily life for a convenient time when you naturally have enough energy for them.

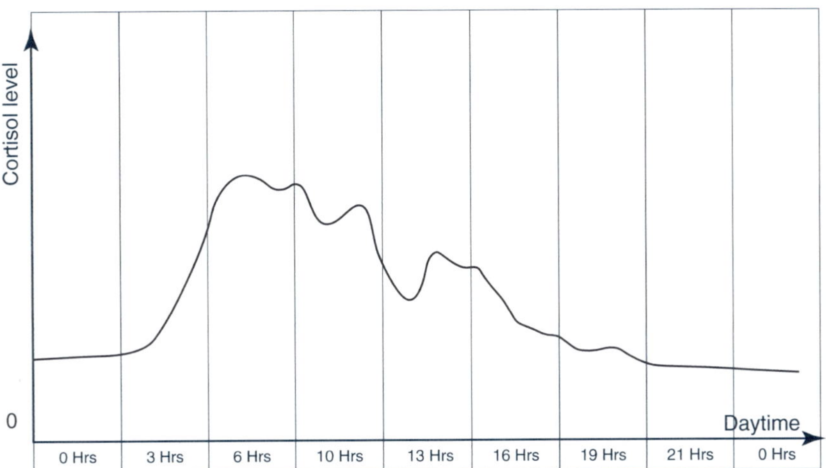

This document was created by Dr. Carolin Marx-Dick and is protected by copyright. It may be used and passed on exclusively within the scope of its purposes for non-commercial use as accompanying therapy material for the treatment of sleep disorders. Any editing or modification is prohibited. (Version 0/2022) www.drcarolinmarxdick.de

Fig. 3.6 My new daily routine

directly one after the other. You don't need minutes of reflection, but (milli-)seconds. For example: You send an email and then take a deep breath. Only then do you look at the next email. The head then has the opportunity to also mentally finish and save the one task as completed and then to approach the next task with more capacity. Taking a moment to focus on the here and now also reduces the feeling of being driven.

What one already perceives as a break, the other still perceives as work. An important finding from work psychology is that a break is everything that is different from work. Most of us are desk workers who don't move enough anyway. You should rather actively shape your breaks, definitely leave your workplace and, for example, take a walk at a fast pace. People who have a physically active job, such as gardeners or scaffolders, should actually put their feet up during their break and regenerate (Table 3.6).

Overtime does not bring any value. Numerous scientific studies have shown that a highly efficient employee, if highly qualified, well-rested and extremely motivated, can perform a maximum of 4 h of full performance per day. In the remaining 4 h, concentration, receptiveness, reaction speed and memory retrieval decline continuously. In a normal 8-hour workday, 50% is therefore "self-administration or tidying up" time, which is very effectively used with less mental and physical effort. Anything that goes beyond an 8-hour workday no longer brings good work quality and therefore no value for itself or the employer. On the contrary: Those who constantly go beyond their limits cannot recover sufficiently in their free time. Burn-out is then a common consequence.

With regular short breaks or longer, active or passive breaks, your patients will maintain work effectiveness over a very long period of time, stay healthy and have much more fun at work.

Table 3.6 Mini interventions in one working day

Good opportunity to	How long does it take?	How often should I do this?
Deep Breathing	Takes 3–10 s	Every 15 min
A moment of mindfulness	Takes 1–3 min	Every 30 min
Short break for tea or coffee, short chat with colleagues etc	Takes 5 min	Every 60–90 min
A real break	At least 30 min	Every 3 h

### 3.4.5	Module: Interpersonal Social Rhythm Therapy

Overview (Table 3.7)

Background

We humans are social beings! The needs for social contact are very different. One needs a lot of time for himself, while the other can not be alone. This treatment of social rhythm therapy was originally developed to support the psychotherapeutic treatment of bipolar disorders. Unfortunately, there is still very little literature available on this topic. Basically, this technique includes an integration of different aspects such as:

Table 3.7 Overview Module: social rhythm therapy

Indications	For all sleep disorders
Contraindications	Not known
Effectiveness	Very well documented
Principle of operation	Humans are a social beings and should maintain regular and balanced social contacts
Treatment requirements	Knowledge of the rhythm- and mood-enhancing effects of social relationships, communication skills
Treatment goal	Building supportive social relationships, balanced integration into everyday life

- Balance of active and passive phases during the day
- Inclusion of social aspects such as family, colleagues and friends

The use of this technique aims to stabilize the entire circadian rhythm—including the biological functions, with the support of the social rhythm. This means: There should be an everyday life introduced with

- regular performance of duties (school, university, work, housework, etc.),
- balanced leisure time (active and less active parts),
- balanced, regular social contacts,
- balanced phases of rest and activity,
- regular meals,
- Observation of the sleep-wake rhythm.

Procedure

First, the patient is asked to keep a diary in which the daily routine, social contacts and the respective mood are queried. Very unstructured, disorganized people find it difficult to keep such a diary. Therefore, only the really important aspects should be collected over a short period of time at first. For this purpose, you can use Diary D 03: Social Rhythm Therapy. Appropriate apps for smartphones and computer programs are already offered as a help.

Based on the diary created, it is analyzed to what extent the currently lived rhythm and the contained social contacts are conducive or rather generate stress, overstrain and negative emotions. Together with the patient, unstable patterns are uncovered and discussed. Subsequently, goals of rhythmization are set and elements, resources and people are sought who can create and support the rhythm. Finally, possible triggers are identified that could take the affected person out of the rhythm.

Then a new daily rhythm is created, whereby the days should be as similar as possible. For example, there should be a small highlight on each day that the patients can look forward to—for example, the favorite series on television with the partner, coffee with a friend, playground with the children, dog walk, etc.

> ▶ *It is important to make sure that the days are not overloaded. The aim of social rhythm therapy is not to plan every second and spend time with other people. Time for oneself is just as important. Boredom may also occur.*

The following aspects must be considered when setting the new day rhythm with regard to social contacts:

- Contacts at school and at work
- Regular meals alone or with others
- Time at home alone or with family
- Designing own rules
- Finding the right balance (How many activity or rest phases does the patient need?)
- Incorporating routines into everyday life (e.g. every Friday I meet …)
- Regular bedtime or wake-up times

It is recommended not to change the entire structure immediately, but to introduce fixed rhythms first, which are expected to have a high acceptance and thus a high probability of success. Based on these successes, further structures can be incorporated into the daily routine. The structure must be adapted to the severity of the rhythm disorder.

A topic that should not be overlooked in this context is *social networking* via virtual platforms. Such communities do not replace real-life contacts. Many people are "addicted" to Facebook, Instagram, Twitter, and the like. They open their accounts every free minute to see what's new. In addition, they communicate with acquaintances via messaging systems such as WhatsApp, Signal, or Telegram. This makes patients virtually accessible for a large number of messages at any time of day or night. All of these messages have an effect on the person and must be processed. On the one hand, this type of communication provides a wealth of information such as "last online", "message read", etc., on the other hand, information that is urgently needed to assess social contacts, such as the voice (volume, melody, speech speed), facial expressions and gestures, remain hidden. People cannot process such stimuli as effectively and quickly via online media as they can with real-life social contacts that have been established for a very long time from an evolutionary perspective. Therefore, this represents a special challenge for perception and stimulus processing. A responsible approach to virtual worlds is very important. This aspect must be discussed individually with each patient and then worked out.

To work on the topic in a concrete way, a specific plan should be developed on how social contacts can be integrated into everyday life in a meaningful way. The worksheet WS07: Planning my social contacts can be used for this purpose. There is the possibility to let the patient work on it alone as homework or to design it together in the therapy session.

3.4.6 Module: Light as Therapy

Overview (Table 3.8)

Background

Light suppresses the production of the hormone melatonin, the hormone that significantly influences the human sleep-wake cycle. Its task is to induce and maintain sleep. During the day, the melatonin concentration is very low due to daylight. A small dose of melatonin taken orally can make a person very tired during the day and even induce sleep. In the evening, the natural melatonin concentration in the body is significantly higher. At night, the melatonin content is highest and, despite decreasing sleep pressure, maintains sleep.

So far, melatonin as a medication for sleep disorders has proven to be of little use, except in the case of jet lag and shift work syndrome. In order to have an effect on sleep induction with melatonin administration, a very high concentration must be supplied, which often causes very unpleasant side effects.

In autumn and winter, the nights become longer and the days shorter. With increasing darkness, melatonin release also increases during the day in the body. This means that you may also feel tired and sluggish during the day. Some mammals go into hibernation or even winter sleep and have adapted well to the changing light conditions in this way. Humans, on the other hand, have to be fully operational even in winter.

The improved use of daylight as well as the use of artificial light can have a very beneficial effect on well-being, whether in summer or winter.

In order to bring the melatonin level into balance in a natural way, the targeted use of light can be used. Mood, fatigue and wakefulness, as well as drive and motivation, can be influenced by certain brightness nuances and light colors. Light can therefore be used very effectively for the treatment of sleep disorders and also affective disorders.

When we sleep is therefore mainly determined by the light. If there were no external cues telling us to sleep, such as light, the human day cycle would be about 25 h long! We would therefore shift our sleeping time one hour backwards every day and "lose" a night's sleep at some point.

Our body is basically well adapted to the natural course of the sun. We see and perceive light through the retina in our eyes. There are 3 types of so-called photoreceptors on our retina that enable us to see: Through the rods we can distinguish between light and dark. The rods are very sensitive, which is why they also register weak light stimuli and thus enable us to see in twilight or at night. However, rods cannot process different colors. This is the task of the so-called cones, more precisely: their three visual pigments for the colors blue, green and red. There is also a third photoreceptor that is sensitive to light and only perceives the brightness of the environment.

Table 3.8 Overview Module: Light as Therapy

Indications	Morning fatigue or lethargy, daytime sleepiness, mood lows, lack of fatigue in the evening
Contraindications	Strong light sensitivity or intolerance
Effectiveness	Very well documented
Working principle	Information about the effects of light on melatonin levels, the body and mood, learning appropriate uses for light
Treatment requirements	Knowledge of the effects of light and their specific use possibilities
Treatment goal	Independent use of natural or artificial light to achieve the desired level of alertness or sleepiness and to influence mood

Procedure

The clarification of the importance of light for the performance during the day and for the control of fatigue in the evening is an important basic element in every therapy of sleep disorders. *The current habits and conditions should be analyzed with the patient in terms of his/her dealing with light. Subsequently, new behaviors in the patient's everyday life are possible.*

First, your patient needs important background information to understand why it is so important to live a life in line with the course of the sun. The information sheet IS06: Light as therapy, which you can give to your patient as a handout, provides essential information about the targeted use of light in therapy.

Our biological day-night rhythm adapts to the course of the sun and therefore lasts as long as the earth needs for a complete rotation around itself.

▶ When the sun is in the sky and illuminates the earth, this means for us that we are awake and activated. When it sets and darkness falls, the hormone release in the human body is switched and a phase of regeneration is possible.

Depending on the position of the sun and the degree of cloudiness, nature provides us with different light spectra. These different wavelengths have different effects on us in terms of wakefulness, fatigue, activity, sluggishness and emotionality.

The different spectra of light are listed below according to their color temperature and their appearance (Table 3.9).

Suggestions for Dealing with Light
- In the evening, dim the light, possibly lighting with candles and lamps with warm light colors
- In the morning, expose yourself to the light consciously, lighting with cold light colors, using bright light

- In phases of fatigue, expose yourself to the light consciously (e.g. in the midday slump), leave the office/workplace as often as possible, even on cloudy days the influence of daylight is sufficient to have an effect
- Also and especially in winter, look at the natural daylight in the sky during the day (even on gray days it suppresses melatonin production sustainably)
- Use daylight lamps
- Pay attention to the color of the light:
  - Warm light
    calming and therefore contributes to relaxation
    can be fatigue-inducing if necessary
    mood-enhancing
  - Cold light
    makes and keeps you awake
    activates and motivates
    but can also cause an irritable mood
- Targeted application of light therapy

  - Take a "light shower" for 30 min every morning in front of a daylight lamp (e.g. during breakfast)
  - Adapt light conditions to the time of day and the intended mood or alertness
  - At night, completely do without light (do not use night lights or turn on the light when going to the toilet)
  - Even a short light exposure can inhibit melatonin production for hours and prevent you from falling asleep again
  - Children should also not use a night light
  - In most cases, there are enough light sources in an apartment for orientation
  - Pay attention to small light sources (LEDs on TV, phone, displays, etc.)

▶ *As with a medication, the patient-individual dose of light should be determined at the corresponding times of the day.*

Table 3.9 The light spectrum and its effect on humans

Light color and brightness in Kelvin	Natural counterpart	Artificial counterpart	Alertness	Inner drive	Emotionality
Red 1000K	Glow		drowsy	barely there	calm, balanced
Bright red 2000K	Candlelight	40 watt bulb	sluggish	slightly present	calm, collected
Orange 3000K	Sunrise	100 watt bulb	rising	slightly activated	relaxed
	Sunset				
Yellow to light yellow 4000 to 5000K	Daylight	Fluorescent tube	very awake	very powerful	balanced
White 6000K	Daylight at the zenith of the sun, moonlight	Daylight lamp with different shades of color	maximum wakefulness	maximum power	balanced to slightly euphoric
Light blue 7000K	Cloudy sky		Very awake	Very powerful	Balanced
Blue 8000 to 9000K	Overcast sky		Awake	Powerful	Balanced
Indigo 10,000K	blue sky		very awake	maximum performance	balanced, slightly euphoric, can be irritable

To implement an individual and time-coordinated lighting plan, there are lamps and light bulbs that can be controlled by an app. Complex smart home systems can reproduce the entire spectrum of daylight and thus ensure optimal use of light. To create an individual lighting plan tailored to your patient's chronotype, commitments and daily structure, you can use the WB 08: My Lighting Plan worksheet.

3.4.7   Module: Shift Work

Overview (Table 3.10)

Background

Human beings are, in contrast to nocturnal animals such as hedgehogs or bats, diurnal. Nocturnal species are equipped with certain features to survive in the dark habitat. Humans do not have such sensory systems and are adapted to being awake and productive during the day and to regenerate and sleep at night. However, many people have to work and be productive at night and sleep during the day to regenerate. For many affected people, this shift in rhythm is not easy, and they develop sleep disorders.

Sleep disorders with such backgrounds have to be dealt with in a special way, since a variety of factors have to be considered. Therefore, it is initially important for those affected to know the physiological effects of the shift in sleep. The most important are:

- No human being is as productive at night as during the day.
- Even if we stay up at night, the circadian rhythm intervenes and deactivates wakefulness cycles and initiates regeneration mechanisms.
- The production of the sleep-inducing and -maintaining hormone melatonin is suppressed in light.
- Therefore, light should be used accordingly in night shifts and very early morning shifts or late night shifts.
- The circadian rhythm synchronizes a variety of physiological control loops that are subject to the sleep-wake rhythm.
- If you keep shifting your circadian rhythm, you will experience feelings of discomfort.
- People who have to work night shifts over a longer period of time have a significantly increased risk of developing a tumor.
- For those affected, so-called forward-rotating systems are favorable, i.e. early shift, then late shift, then night shift and then at least 2 free days. The new cycle begins again with

Table 3.10 Overview Module: Shift work

Indications	Shift work, shift work syndrome, performing private activities during nighttime insomnia
Contraindications	Unknown
Effectiveness	Very well documented
Working principle	Information about the effects of night work on the body and mind, explanation of health-preserving methods
Treatment requirements	Knowledge of methods of behavior modification
Treatment goal	Establish a rhythm adapted to working hours, independent implementation of health-preserving steps

an early shift and so on. Early shifts that start so early that they are actually night shifts for the circadian rhythm are critical. Depending on the type (owl or lark, see above), early rising is associated with a special burden. In general, no more than 3 night shifts should follow one another, as this would put the least strain on the organism. However, this is rarely possible in practice.

Procedure

First, it must be precisely discussed how the current sleep-wake behavior and the shift system (work system) of the patient look. For this purpose, appropriate protocols are helpful to prevent memory distortion. You can use the diary D 04: My shift diary, as shown in Fig. 3.7

Then a pattern in the shift system is to be sought, which is difficult to recognize in some cases because the shift plans are partly created without system. In the more favorable case there are early, late and night shifts or early, middle, late and night shifts, which are each occupied for several days in a row, followed by free days.

Analogous to the *sleep restriction (Sect. 3.3)* as regular sleep times as possible should be introduced. This is best done via a bi- or polyphasic sleep rhythm. This means that there is not only one, but two main sleep phases and possibly 1–2 shorter sleep periods, which are each adapted accordingly. It should be noted that both deep sleep and phases with lighter sleep and REM sleep can take place in the main sleep phases *(information on the sleep cycles, Sect. 1.3)*. The individual sleep times should therefore be oriented towards the healthy sleep architecture and be held in approx. 90-minute stages (e.g. three hours, four and a half hours, etc.). This ensures that despite the fragmentation of sleep all necessary regeneration and construction processes can take place. A check in the sleep laboratory can be helpful.

Contrary to the long-held belief that one cannot "pre-sleep" or "catch up on sleep", it is very advisable for people on shift work to relieve the already existing sleep pressure before the late or night shift by then taking a sleep phase.

The sleep cycles must be set up in such a way that there is still time after each shift to distance oneself from the strain and stress of work before the patient is to sleep.

Case Example: Shift Work
Mr. M. is a 40-year-old nurse practitioner on a 3-shift schedule:

- Early shift: 6:30 a.m. to 3:00 p.m.
- Late shift: 2:30 p.m. to 11:00 p.m.
- Night shift: 10:30 p.m. to 7:00 a.m.

Although the nursing staff tried to schedule five workdays in the same shift and then two days off, this was successful only very rarely, so that the shifts were mixed up and both forward- and

D04 - Diary: My shift diary

Week from ________ to _______

Name: _____________________

Dr. **Carolin Marx-Dick**

EXPERTIN FÜR
SCHLAFGESUNDHEIT

tte note your sleep times and wake cycles in shifts. *Give sleep a school grade (1-6) to assess how restful it was.

Day	Duty/working time	Sleep time	School grade	Mood	Energy level
		B = bedtime; E = slept (approx.); AW = woke up; AS = got up; GSZ = total sleep time.	1-6		
Monday					
Tuesday					
Wednesday					
Thursday					
Friday					
Saturday					
Sunday					

Fig. 3.7 Extract from the diary TB 04: My shift diary

backward-rotating. Mr. M. is more of a lark type, who likes to get up early, and he was allowed to work more often in the early shift. He suffered from sleep through problems and early waking.

If Mr. M. had early duty, he had to get up at 5 a.m. to be on time for work. After the late shift, Mr. M. was at home at 11:15 p.m. and then needed some time to "wind down". He therefore did not go to bed before midnight. On most days, Mr. M. had early and late shifts. As a result, Mr. M. could sleep between 12 a.m. and 5 a.m. on most days.

The following plan with fixed bedtimes was worked out with him:

- Main sleep phase from 0:00 a.m. to 5:00 a.m. on *all* days when it was possible
  - During the early and late shift, on free days, at weekends and on vacation
  - Not earlier to bed on early shifts!
  - Not longer stay in bed on late shifts!
  - Also on weekends and on free days (at least until the sleep disorders had improved)
  - Only exception: night shift

→ Background: This way Mr. M. had the opportunity to develop a fixed biorhythm by the body receiving the clear signal: It is *always* from 0 to 5 a.m. o'clock bedtime.

- The biorhythm can synchronize itself and automate the corresponding hormone cycles
- Second sleep phase
  - For early shift after work between 3:30 p.m. and 5:00 p.m.
  - For late shift before work between 11:00 a.m. and 12:30 a.m.

- For night shifts

  - Before the start of the night shift from about 5:00 p.m. to 8:00 p.m.
  - After work in the morning from about 9:00 a.m. to 1:30 p.m.

This included the rhythmization of sleep as well as a restriction of bed times.

After the sleep disorders had visibly improved, the bed times were again adapted to the needs reported by the patient.

The following bedtimes resulted:

- For early shift: 11:00 p.m. to 5:00 a.m., if necessary, daytime sleep between 3:30 p.m. and 5:00 p.m.
- For late shift: 0:00 to 6:00 a.m., daytime sleep between 11:00 a.m. and 12:30 p.m.
- For night shift: before the start of the night shift from about 5:00 p.m. to 8:00 p.m. and after the end of the shift in the morning from about 9:00 a.m. to 1:30 p.m.

The patient's sleep disorders could not be completely eliminated with this plan, but a rhythm could be identified that the patient feels comfortable with. In addition, other therapy components were used.

The worksheet WB 09: My sleep plan in shift work can be used to jointly develop and integrate the new sleep and wake times. The patient should place the plan worked out in this way in a visible place in his environment in order to be constantly reminded of the sleep plan. Figure 3.8 shows an example of such a sleep plan.

Which service? Duty hours	Main sleep phase from xx to xy Hrs	Sleep phase 2 xx to xy Hrs	Naps and power naps
Early service	00:00 – 05:00	14:00 – 16:00	18:00
Late shift	0:00 – 5:00 Hrs	11:30 – 13:00	-
Night shift	8:00 – 12:30	17:00 – 19:00	At the break: approx. 0 Hrs 15 min

Fig. 3.8 Shift diary

3.4.8 Module: Stress Management

Overview (Table 3.11)

Background

Many patients are thrilled when they are offered stress and time management in therapy. There is great disappointment when it is pointed out that stress and time management does not mean that more tasks are to be done in less time and more effectively. It means setting priorities and crossing certain tasks off the to-do list.

Despite many pending tasks, it is not necessary to be constantly under stress. A sensible approach can help to use the body's natural rhythm and avoid falling into chronic stress, which can actually make you sick.

Cortisol is an important hormone for stress regulation. Like many other processes, secretion is subject to a 24-hour rhythm and is intended to keep people fit and functional. Cortisol has a variety of functions, for example, it increases blood sugar and blood pressure, is involved in immune processes and has an anti-inflammatory effect. Overall, it prepares the body for potential stress situations. It is secreted more during acute stress and thus makes people more responsive. With chronic stress, cortisol is secreted more. If this system is overused, it can lead to fatigue, i.e. physical and mental exhaustion.

In order to counteract this, it is necessary to know the natural cortisol cycle. Cortisol secretion begins very gently in the very early morning hours of the second half of the night. Shortly after waking up, the cortisol concentration is at its highest and is secreted in spurts several times during the morning. In the later course of the day, cortisol secretion decreases. This can be seen, for example, in the midday slump or other small performance slumps, which can be caught by taking a short break or doing another activity. Between approximately 3:00 p.m. and approximately 5:00 p.m., another small cortisol release may occur, which makes the body more efficient again. In the further course of the day, less and less cortisol is provided. In the evening

Table 3.11 Brief overview module: Stress management

Indications	Stress, tension, inner unrest, nervousness, fatigue, listlessness, irritability
Contraindications	Not known
Effectiveness	Very well proven
Working principle	Inform about stress and its physical and psychological effects, identify stressors, inform about methods of decomposition and prevention
Treatment requirements	Knowledge about the topic of stress and coping methods
Treatment goal	Convey a comprehensive understanding of stress, learn methods of coping, integration into everyday life

the cortisol level is vanishingly low, at night it reaches its lowest point.

Many things to do does not necessarily mean to have stress. Only when we perceive the workload as a burden or evaluate it as stress, we feel it in physical and psychological stress reactions. To accommodate all the necessary appointments and tasks in everyday life and stay healthy, it is important to follow the performance curve just described. Individual differences in the cortisol curve depending on the chronotype are possible and should also be considered in therapy. With the diary TB 05: My cortisol curve, the respective cortisol peaks and valleys can be observed and recorded by the patient in his everyday life (Fig. 3.9). A diary allows the observation of one day (so feel free to give your patient several diary sheets so that he can record his cortisol curve on different days of the week; long and short workdays, weekends, holidays, etc.).

The patient should pay attention to when he feels particularly energetic and when he experiences performance losses (cognitive, physical, emotional) and record this in the diaries. It is also possible to determine the cortisol curve by means of saliva analysis. There are various providers who offer test sets for home use. It is important to make sure that at least five samples are taken at different times of the day (buccal mucosa with cotton swab). Only then can a course be recognized. Single measurements do not provide any useful information at this point.

When we are stressed, the body responds with a stress response. This includes a complex hormone release with norepinephrine, possibly adrenaline, dopamine and cortisol. For individual stress moments or situations, our body is made and can cope with them several times a day. However, if we are in constant stress, cortisol is secreted continuously, day and night, and

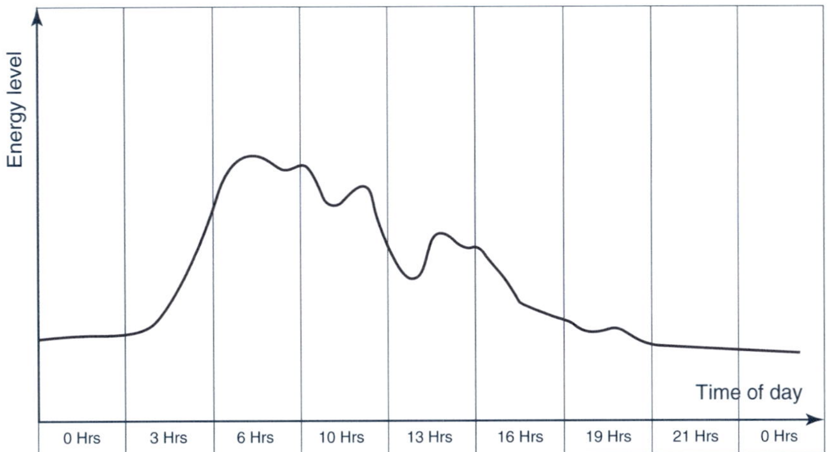

Fig. 3.9 Diary TB 05: My cortisol curve

our natural circadian rhythm is lost. This causes severe sleep disorders and other stress-related diseases. Therefore, it is essential to work out a stress management with the patients, with which the natural course can be restored and maintained.

This means that things that require a lot of mental or physical effort and may be rated as stress should be done at the times of high cortisol in the morning or afternoon. In the later part of the day, the stress level should be kept flatter. Therefore, it is also recommended to confront potentially bad news or social conflicts rather in the morning.

People react very differently to stress. In science, two different types of stress are distinguished:

Stress Type A

A person of stress type A is externally visible that he is under stress. He is under constant tension, is easily irritable, restless, nervous and hectic. He is rather a lone fighter and tries to cope with all tasks alone. Due to the usually permanently elevated cortisol levels, he often suffers from high blood pressure and sleep disorders.

Stress Type B

A person of stress type B rather internalizes stress and anger. He appears to be calm and relaxed from the outside. Often he feels helpless in situations and falls into a trance. Chronic stress leads to an exhaustion of cortisol secretion and can thus cause permanent fatigue and lack of motivation. Therefore, this stress type is at increased risk of depression.

The fewest people can be clearly assigned to one of the two stress types. Depending on the situation, they react differently. It cannot be directly concluded that a person must be under stress just because he has to cope with many tasks.

The feeling of stress is basically subjective. A good daily life and personality structure can be very helpful to stay productive and calm at the same time. Conversely, it is just as wrong to assume that a person who has only a few tasks

to cope with cannot feel this as stress. What is important here is the evaluation of the tasks, the time management, the everyday life and the personality of the person concerned.

Procedure

Identification and Assessment

First, the therapist should make every effort to get a complete picture of the daily demands on the patient. This should be as complete as possible, as small inconspicuous tasks often go unnoticed in the overall balance of the day and are usually not taken into account in the planning of the day's activities. These "small" activities, which are particularly stress-inducing, are often described by patients in their stories with "Then I quickly …

- vacuumed the apartment, tidied up, unloaded the dishwasher, cut fruit, etc.,
- on the way home, did some shopping or other errands,
- called someone in between,
- did two things at the same time (e.g. talked on the phone and drove the car; tidied up and looked after the children),
- generally did everything that should be done quickly or just fit in between."

To record all tasks, appointments and burdens in everyday life, your patient can keep the diary D 06: What I have achieved.

It is particularly important here to recognize dissimulation and to show the patient what they have to do cognitively, emotionally and physically at this point and how high the stress is at this point. So "poke holes" in your patient when you evaluate the diary together. It is particularly helpful for patients if you work with graphics.

Warning Signs

Everyone reacts differently to stress, and just as different can be the early warning signs of chronic over-commitment. Typical signs are:

- Headache, stomach and back pain (especially children tend to stomach pain when the stress level is too high; this is due to the close link between the central and autonomic nervous system)

- Persistent fatigue, which remains after periods of rest
- Loss of appetite and libido
- Drive disorders, joylessness, loss of motivation, loss of sense of meaningfulness
- Sleep disorders

Nowadays it is usually not enough to just keep the balance between work and private life. Many people have leisure stress because they are always reachable or have to attend many appointments outside their working hours. Parents are particularly affected by this. It should be noted at this point that for children it is much more important to have healthy parents than early childhood education at the highest level and to enjoy constant activities.

In leisure time there should actually be free times to be able to react spontaneously or to have buffer times for relief. It is important to know your own limits and to defend them. Patients should be guided to be careful with themselves in contact with other people and—as soon as a bad feeling arises—to find out where it could come from. With the help of social competence training, patients can learn to say no and to protect their boundaries.

► *Perfectionism is bad for the psyche! Man learns from mistakes, so they may happen. It is important for those affected to question their own claim in situations that are perceived as stressful.*

Perfectionism makes you unhappy because it is rarely possible to solve tasks perfectly. In most cases, it is even possible to accept or present an imperfect result. Experience has shown that other people (such as employers or partners) do not have such an immensely high claim as the person concerned. This saves resources and enables a new project. The treating physician and the patient should jointly analyze tasks in which significantly more was done than expected. At the same time, it makes sense to look for projects that have been successful, even though not everything was perfect or one's own claim was not met.

Above all, stress can cause great damage in interpersonal relationships. In order to avoid this, the following strategies can be used:

- Make clear agreements, do not read between the lines,
- Assign or accept responsibilities,
- Work with I-messages in case of dispute (I think …, I feel …, I find …).

Implementation

First, the current stress level in everyday life must be recorded by the patient. This works best with the help of a stress diary, as shown in the diary 07: My stress diary.

This is evaluated in the next therapy session and, above all, attention is paid to unexpected stressors when, for example, a certain activity or a person present (social contact) causes stress in the respective situation. In addition, the energy level should be considered. If unexpectedly much energy is needed here, this should be taken into account in everyday life. After evaluating the stress diary, alternatives are worked out how everyday life can be designed in the future in order to reduce the stress level and still be able to do all the necessary and important tasks.

Generally, a structure of everyday life should be found that is in harmony with the patient's personal biorhythm. Peak performance can only be expected in the respective performance phases, corresponding to the healthy cortisol curve. The other time must be used for regeneration. This does not mean that that necessarily have to be leisure time. It can be used sensibly with physical activities (go to the post office, clean windows, etc.) or mental things (design birthday card, make photo book). A pictorial comparison for this is the management of a field: When monocultures are grown, the soil is exhausted and the yields are lower in the long term. With a sensible change between different cultures, the soil regenerates itself and remains productive for a long time. The same should happen with the "use" of a person. Physical and mental effort should alternate with phases of complete relaxation.

The worksheet WS 05: My new daily routine from *Component 3.4: Daily structuring* can be used to develop the new daily routine. Here you can design a healthy daily routine together with the patient.

Since we humans often hurry through our lives in a more careless way, on "autopilot", we are often not aware of when we actually have stress. When it comes to the subjective assessment of stressors and time pressure, we often overestimate or underestimate the actual amount: Some people always feel stressed. Others do not feel any stress despite a busy schedule. The truth is usually somewhere in between these two extremes. To find out what duties there are in everyday life, how much pressure they create and when the pressure turns into symptom-causing stress, the worksheet WS 10: Stress and Time Management can be used (Fig. 3.10). With this approach, you can work out (early warning) symptoms together with your patient that indicate that the load is too great. Sleep disorders often show very early on that someone is overwhelmed and overloaded.

3.4.9 Module: Sleep Hygiene

Overview (Table 3.12)

Background
In current psychotherapy studies it is becoming increasingly clear that although sleep hygiene is an important basic requirement for healthy sleep, it is usually not sufficient as a sole intervention in pathological sleep disorders. In the long-term practice experience it has become clear that some sleep hygiene rules are even counterproductive, which science has confirmed in recent years. Particular attention should therefore be paid to the following rules:

1. If you are awake in bed for longer than 30 min, you must definitely leave the bed (especially in the case of sleep onset and sleep maintenance disorders).

2. Patients with insomnia are not allowed to have a midday nap.
3. The bed is only for sleeping and for sexuality.

To 1. It should be noted that leaving the bed at night is particularly stressful for those affected. On the one hand, it requires a certain awareness to notice whether 30 min have already passed without dozing off. On the other hand, the patients are lying in bed with a smoldering decision: "Should I get up or not?" Making decisions is a high-performance task for our brain. Depressed people often find it very difficult to make even the smallest decisions. For example, when shopping, they may be completely overwhelmed with the cereal selection. Deciding whether to get out of bed can therefore be extremely stressful, which is known to be associated with a hormonal stress reaction and which can greatly impair sleep. Third, nocturnal awakening can activate the organism and thus create additional wakefulness. Cold exposures, coupled with the unwillingness to get up, can lead to tension instead of relaxation.

Ask the patients how they feel lying awake in bed. If they are relaxed and do not find the situation excessively unpleasant, they can stay in bed. This wakefulness can be used for beneficial mindful moments. To illustrate this, patients can use beliefs such as: "I am lying in my comfortable bed. I have accomplished my day and no one wants anything from me. There is nothing to do. If I fall asleep, it's good, if not, I relax." This cognitive evaluation of the situation as pleasant accompanies the patient into a relaxed state of wakefulness and allows him to fall asleep.

However, if the patients are very restless, tossing and turning from one side to the other, getting stressed, getting angry about the nighttime wakefulness, they should leave the bed and, without turning on the light, gently occupy themselves. A small walk through the apartment, observing the windows of the neighbors, listening to relaxing music or a radio play while drinking a cup of tea can help to calm down and increase the pressure to sleep. If the patients then feel tired again, a new attempt at sleep can be made.

WS10 - Worksheet: Stress and Time Management

Permanent stress can have a negative effect on the development and maintenance of sleep disorders. Establishing good personal time and stress management is therefore a valuable building block n the therapy of sleep disorders.

On the following pages, you are invited to take a close look at your current stress management and improve it if necessary. First of all, try to record as precisely as possible which daily demands in your various areas of life are weighing on you. Try to record even small, inconspicuous tasks, since it is precisely these tasks that are often not taken into account in the daily planning and therefore cause a lot of stress (typical here are things that you do "just quickly", on the way home or on the side).

Job	Family

Social	Budget

1 ______

Free time	______

Fig. 3.10 Worksheet WS 10: Stress and time management

WS10 - Worksheet: Stress and Time Management

Dr. **Carolin**
Marx-Dick

EXPERTIN FÜR
SCHLAFGESUNDHEIT

Now take a moment to consider which of the tasks from exercise 1 you are currently experiencing as particularly stressful. You can then start your personal stress management at these points.

What are your worst stressors? And what makes them particularly stressful (e.g. time pressure, pressure to perform, social expectations, etc.)?

____

Every person reacts differently to stress. That's why it's especially important that you know your own personal early warning symptoms. These alert you when your stress level is permanently too high and prompt you to "take it down a notch".
Typical signs of continuous overload are:

    2 _____

- Headache, abdominal pain, back pain
- Permanent fatigue, which persists even after you have taken a break
- Loss of appetite
- Libido loss
- Difficulty motivating yourself to do something
- No more enjoyment of things that normally give pleasure
- Feelings of futility
- Sleep disorders

Do you know some of these early warning symptoms about yourself? Or can you think of other signs that signal you are overloaded?

____

Fig. 3.10 (continued)

WS10 - Worksheet: Stress and Time Management

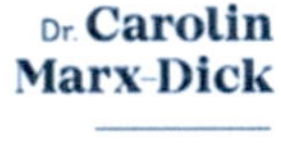

When you're under a lot of stress, it often feels like you have an infinite number of tasks to accomplish, all of which are very important and extremely urgent. This then inevitably leads to a feeling of being overwhelmed.

A first step towards successful time management is therefore to ask yourself which tasks are really urgent and important and which ones can wait or are actually not important at all. It is a good idea to approach this question in a calm moment, since a realistic assessment of the tasks is only possible in a relaxed state.

Try it out! Go through your tasks for the next week in your head (if you keep to-do lists, feel free to use them) and assign the tasks to the areas below. Try to be as realistic as possible and "allow" sick to find tasks unimportant.

Urgent	Important	Unimportant
These tasks do not tolerate any postponement and absolutely must be done next week (e.g. preparing for a professional appointment that is coming up during the week)	These tasks don't necessarily need to be done next week, but are either personally important to you (e.g., getting a birthday gift) or would have dire negative consequences if not done (e.g., filling out a tax return)	These tasks make you feel like you should do them. But if you are completely honest with yourself, it wouldn't be a bad thing if they were just left out (e.g. cleaning out the closet)

3____

With this breakdown, you can now plan which tasks you really need to do next week (namely those from the urgent category). If you notice that you still have some air beyond that, you can sick a few of the important tasks.

Fig. 3.10 (continued)

Table 3.12   Brief overview of module: Sleep hygiene

Indications	To be applied in general, in all sleep disorders, for a healthy lifestyle
Contraindications	Not known
Effectiveness	Often not sufficient as the sole intervention to create restful sleep, but a necessary prerequisite for it
Working principle	In an environment where the patient does not feel comfortable, he cannot relax, certain habits prevent restful sleep
Treatment requirements	Knowledge about sleep hygiene
Treatment goal	Understanding of the mechanisms, motivation for behavior change, possibly moving or rearranging the bedroom

2. It should be noted that a nap (power nap) can help those affected by insomnia to experience the afternoon more relaxed after the midday nap. It is important that this does not last too long (20 to a maximum of 30 min) and is not kept too late (at least 6–7 h before bedtime). This lowers the cortisol level in the afternoon and the patients find it easier to relax in the evening and to fall asleep. The cramp-like staying awake, on the other hand, creates stress, and an increased cortisol release is necessary in the body to get through the afternoon. A power nap of up to 30 min only lowers the pressure to sleep briefly and slightly, so that there is enough fatigue at bedtime to fall asleep. Scientific studies confirm this mechanism (Pace-Schott et al. 2018).

To 3. t It should be noted that reading oneself tired is a much discussed topic in sleep medicine. Basically, nothing should happen in bed except sleeping. The body and psyche should receive a very clear signal through conditioning processes: "In bed we sleep!" However, many people suffering from sleep disorders report that just reading tired in bed leads to shorter sleep latencies and also to shorter wakefulness in sleep disorders. In addition, the patients report that when they are tired on the sofa and go to bed when their eyes are falling, they wake up again during the transition from the sofa to the bed. Arrived in bed, they are awake again and sometimes can not sleep for hours. Of course, the choice of literature plays a role. In this respect, an individual solution should be found for the patient. The tired-reading in bed is very helpful for the restful sleep in many respects:

- It allows patients to notice fatigue so that the time to turn off the light can be found well.
- It binds the thoughts so that stressful brooding loops are interrupted or do not arise at all.
- If patients have to go to bed after reading on the sofa, they will be activated again and finally can not sleep as well.

The background of this rule is the mis-conditioning of many patients that if they stay awake in bed for a long time, the bed is more associated with being awake than with sleeping. However, this conditioning process can be functionally redesigned by the body receiving the signal: "I am in bed and allowed to (read) relax."

Furthermore, in 3. it should be noted that sexuality "may" still take place in bed in terms of sleep hygiene. So it is the exception for the stimulus control in bed. For many people, however, this type of physical proximity is a rather difficult topic. With newly in love, sexuality is often and actively lived. With couples who have been together for a long time and especially in the age group of patients who are particularly often affected by sleep disorders, the topic of sexuality is usually burdened. Different needs of both partners are then, for example, a conflict that is literally taken to bed. The case report of Mrs. and Mr. M.—"Sex ban in bed as an intervention in sleep disorders"—illustrates this dilemma.

▶   *In general, those affected should develop an association that equates the bed with restful sleep. In some cases, it makes sense for all activities other than sleeping (at least for a certain period of time) to take place at another location, especially sexuality.*

In this context, the association bed = sex is not a favorable combination, because sexual activity in the best case stimulates the release of hormones that can lead to strong activation, especially in women. For practice, it should be noted here that the topic of sexuality is often raised as a taboo topic. Sexuality is a sensitive marker for other (psychological) problems. If sex continues to take place in bed, this is again a way to "take problems to bed". Therefore, great sensitivity is required in weighing up to what extent sexual activities (initially) should be banned from the bed. Partners of patients may need to be convinced of this necessity so that no tension is created for the relationship during therapy. Couple conversations create understanding and space for the transformation in everyday life.

Procedure, Rules of Healthy Sleep

To apply the sleep hygiene rules, it is helpful to give the patient the Information sheet IS07: The sleep hygiene rules to take home, accompanied by the homework in everyday life to pay attention to deviations from these rules. The worksheet WS 11: My dealing with the sleep hygiene rules can be used for this. In the follow-up session, it is discussed at which points the patient deviates and how he experiences these deviations. If certain behaviors are rated as critical and sleep-disturbing, these behaviors should be adjusted. However, the general rule is "Never stop a running system" (a belief from information technology), so everything that works can be maintained, as long as it is not harmful, such as substance abuse, etc.

The following are the sleep hygiene rules that I have experienced as helpful in my many years of practice. It is important that these rules are not applied dogmatically and universally. What is poison to one person is medicine to another. When applying the rules, personal needs should always be taken into account.

Circadian Rhythm

1   Try to go to bed at the same time every day and also get up in the morning at the same time. If possible, also on vacation and on weekends.
2   Try to take your meals at the same time during the day. Avoid eating a heavy meal three hours before bedtime.
3   **Siesta!** A power nap is a valuable measure to recharge your battery for the afternoon. If you skip this fatigue, your body has to secrete stress hormones like cortisol throughout the afternoon to stay awake until evening. This can then prevent you from feeling tired and certainly not falling asleep.
    Avoid sleeping late in the afternoon. An exception here is for shift workers. It is good for them to have two longer sleep phases in the 24-hour rhythm.
4   Absolutely avoid dozing off on the couch just before bedtime. Even a relatively short sleep can lead to a significant reduction in the need for sleep and you will not be able to fall asleep for hours.
    Avoid physical exertion 3–4 h before bedtime. The body needs a certain time to calm down afterwards. Before that, light physical activity is best in the fresh air in the evening to be really tired.

In bed

5   Only go to bed when you are really tired.
6   If you cannot fall asleep within 20–30 min of lying down and you are tense, leave your bed again. Only return to your bed when you feel really tired.
    Can you also relax in bed and feel good? Then observe the situation

curiously and feel how nice and comfortable it is to be undisturbed by anyone and just to have nothing else to do but to rest.

7 Avoid looking at the clock at night. The look at the clock often triggers physical reactions such as tension or excitement and robs the last sleep. Until the alarm clock rings, there is nothing to do. Only then is the signal: "Now it starts, the day begins."

8 The bed is only for sleeping! Avoid eating, reading, watching TV or thinking in bed. Only then can a reliable coupling take place: "In bed I am tired and sleep!"

People with sleep disorders should also have no sex in bed. On the one hand, it is not a relaxed topic for some couples, on the other hand it is a very activating activity. There are other nice places for physical love.

The bedroom

9 Electrical devices have no business in the bedroom in principle. In particular, mobile phones and phones emit radiation that can interfere with sleep. For some people, however, falling asleep in front of the TV is a helpful method. This is one of the famous exceptions.

10 Sleep in the dark. Light regulates our wake-sleep rhythm and stimulates hormones that keep the body awake.

11 Supply your bedroom with plenty of fresh air, this promotes the recovery effect of sleep.

12 Sleep in a room that is comfortably temperature, at about 16–20 °C.

13 Noise prevents relaxation and sleep. Therefore, eliminate as many noise sources as possible. Even a very low hum, buzz or tick can steal the last nerve or sleep. Earplugs are very helpful, you get used to it.

14 We spend a third of our day in the bedroom. That's more time than we spend in the living room, kitchen or garden. Your bedroom should be the nicest room in the whole house. Make it so that you like to stay there and you only use it for sleeping.

Interruptions during sleep

15 If you need to go to the toilet at night, keep the light off as much as possible. You will also find your way around in the dark in your own home. If you can't orient yourself in the dark at all, use a very weak night light. A bright light would really wake you up and you would have a hard time falling asleep again.

16 If you are often thirsty at night, put water or unsweetened tea next to your bed. Avoid turning on the light here too. Avoid sugar, green oder black tea and coffee, these stimulate the circulation and make it difficult for you to fall asleep again.

Rituals

17 Come to rest at the end of the day. Avoid doing sports or important things late at night. This keeps the circulation going and you will have a hard time falling asleep.

18 Avoid any excitement in the evening, such as opening important mail, checking emails, arguing, watching very exciting movies or reading exciting books or newspapers.

19 Start dimming the light and the noise level about an hour before bedtime so that your body can adjust to the upcoming night's sleep.

20 A personal good-night ritual of up to 20 min can help you set your internal clock to "sleep".

General

21 Although alcohol makes you tired, it significantly reduces the quality of sleep. Therefore, try to avoid alcohol as much as possible.

22 The same is true for nicotine.

23 Do not drink coffee, black or green tea 4–8 h before bedtime. Try not to drink more than one cup of coffee in the morning and one cup in the afternoon before 3 pm. The stimulating effect of coffee can last for many hours.

Even if many of these rules mean that one or the other favorite habit has to be given up, Patients should in no case live on "economy".

Not only sleep determines the following day, but also vice versa: The day determines the following night. A healthy and pleasant lifestyle that includes activity, work, leisure, nutrition, social contacts and pleasure has a positive effect on sleep and thus on well-being.

3.4.10 Module: Stimulus Control and Psychohygiene

Overview (Table 3.13)

Background

Stimulus control and psych hygiene are important components of maintaining mental and physical health in humans. Depending on the current stress and resilience of the patient, this must be done more or less intensively. The special thing about stimulus control and psych hygiene is: Few people know that there is such a thing, and even fewer know that they can practice it.

Due to the social demands on each individual, we are confronted with tasks and long-term stress that we can sometimes hardly cope with. In today's time, not only emergency doctors have to be available around the clock, but also in the office there can be "emergencies" that could decide the "fate" of the company on Friday afternoon.

However, many people are not only reachable by phone at any time for (bad) news, they also voluntarily confront themselves at any time of day or night via smartphone, tablet, computer or television with new negative headlines, work tasks and feedback as well as personal messages. Due to this constant availability, many of them are put into a permanent tension, as they have to be prepared at any time for new negative headlines, work tasks and feedback as well as personal messages. This behavior can very quickly take on pathological features. In addition to the risks posed by this permanent tension, there is also a high potential for addiction in the use of virtual social networks, news services, computer games and internet shopping portals. In order to stay fit in mind and relaxed, it is necessary to deal very carefully and sensitively with oneself. It is important to notice what this permanent confrontation does to a person.

Paradoxically, a large amount of information on healthy nutrition, sports, health, fitness and related topics is offered via exactly such virtual

Table 3.13 Overview Module: Stimulus Control and Psychohygiene

Indications	Can be used generally, also on healthy people
Contraindications	Not known
Effectiveness	Very high effectiveness
Working principle	Stimulus fasting, conditioning
Treatment requirements	Knowledge of psych hygiene
Treatment goal	Limit psychological stress, break old habits, create calm and relaxation in everyday life

platforms. Psych hygiene, on the other hand, is rarely propagated, although it is just as important for maintaining health. At the beginning of the 2000s, the WHO predicted that by 2020 mental disorders would rank second among health risks, after heart diseases. This development can be seen in Germany. The second most common reason for sick leave is actually mental illness. The most common causes of death are heart disease and strokes (11%), chronic obstructive lung disease (6%), Alzheimer's and other dementias are degenerative or plaques accumulate in/on vital structures, which can lead to death. It seems to be similar in other indsutrialized countries. Stress, overstimulation and overload are almost always the cause (Badura et al. 2020).

Our conscious perception can capture a maximum of 40–50 bits, or about 5 information per second. Our subconscious, on the other hand, can process around 11 million bits of information, or more than a million impressions per second. The ear transmits a million bits, the sense of smell and taste each transmit 100,000 bits (Engelfried and Zahn, 2012). The remaining 9.8 million bits are divided between the sense of sight and body perception. Consequently, we unconsciously perceive almost 1.1 million stimuli per second. Street noise, exhaust fumes, car lights, cell phone ringtones or message tones, coffee smells, electromagnetic radiation, requests from colleagues, and children's screaming are omnipresent for many people. However, our perception system has learned to filter them out. Nevertheless, this information arrives in our brains and has to be processed, even if only to delete the corresponding memory trace.

Overstimulation is the result of such everyday exposure. It leads to physical tension, stress, and all the resulting symptoms, such as burnout, heart attacks, strokes, mental illness, and sleep disorders. Therefore, it is essential for health to be aware of this and to take specific countermeasures. Changes in behavior with regard to media use and everyday life are necessary to cope with this flood of stimuli.

It is also surprising that many people, despite complaints, know what they should change but still cannot manage it. Therefore, self-help, no matter in which area, is often only a beginning. It is necessary to support and motivate patients to take unconventional paths.

Procedure

Most of those affected are not aware that they can be confronted with anything at any time and anywhere. Permanent availability includes work and the tasks and problems waiting there, the entire world political situation, local disasters, and personal news. The constant stream of worrying news has a negative effect on the psyche of the human being.

Therefore, it is first necessary to sensitize the patients to this overstimulation. To assess the current situation of the patient, the following questions can be used:

Leading Questions About the Patient's Current Situation

- What is his home and work environment like? What impressions are there on the respective paths in everyday life (visual stimuli, especially movement, traffic, light, noise, air pollution, etc.)?
- When and how often are virtual platforms or social media used? How does the patient feel about it?
- When is he reachable by phone? How does he feel about it?
- When and how often does he look into his mailbox or open his mail/emails? How does he feel about it?
- When and how often does he look, listen or read the news, follow political discussions, etc.? How does he feel about it?
- When and how often is he personally available for potentially negative news (employer, neighbor, mother-in-law, stock price, etc.)? How does he feel about it?

In order to implement stimulus control and mental hygiene in everyday life, the following strategies can be used from the patient's point of view, which are made available to you as Information Sheet IS08: The Psychohygiene Rules.

Prioritization

"How important is it to me that …?" We cannot cope with all the tasks that are put to us. Therefore, it is necessary to set priorities and first of all to deal with the really important tasks and, if necessary, to cross out tasks that have been on the to-do lists for a long time.

Shut down

Cellphone, computer, telefon, doorbell etc. should be turned off when one does not want to be reachable anymore. Constant ringing and the urge to actively not react to it can greatly increase the level of tension. It is only natural that people affected in these moments think about who the caller might have been and what he might have wanted and whether something bad might have happened. "I should rather …" is the logically following own thought. Already the thought carousel is set in motion and is difficult to stop.

Delete automatic links

Many people have set up shortcuts on their electronic devices that automatically display unread messages from e-mails, open pages from social networks, etc. Social media are designed to keep users constantly online and with notifications to keep the interest alive permanently. Through these mechanisms, it is not possible to decide on their consumption in individual cases, and the person is forced to deal with the notifications and the displayed content.

Make conscious decisions

Affected persons should make conscious decisions about the consumption of news or the availability for other persons.

Limit times/determine times

In therapy, it should be possible to design a time schedule as precisely as possible when and to what extent he deals with things that can be stressful for the psyche. When and how long is the mobile phone used, messages read, online research conducted or communicated via messenger? It is also helpful to decide in therapy when to empty the mailbox at home and when to open and read the letters.

Again, the rule applies: It is not very useful to deliver government mail on Friday afternoon if the next possible clarification appointment is not until Monday morning. It is just as unhelpful to empty the mailbox and then leave the letters unopened. The envelopes and senders can easily give rise to assumptions that set the thought carousel in motion.

It is more favorable, for example, to empty the mailbox every Monday to Friday in the morning. Even important things may "ripen" for 24 (48 on weekends) hours before they are tackled. For example, if people are confronted with potentially bad news in the morning, they have a whole day to clarify. They have time to calm down again by evening to sleep well. These rules initially appear profane. However, such seemingly small things are, according to experience, the biggest sleep robbers.

Say no

Saying no is the most difficult and at the same time most effective way to create free time and relaxation.

Define break times

If possible, set specific and nearly immovable rest periods when your patient will not be available to do certain things if certain emotions have occurred. In these cases, it can be helpful not to answer the phone or open the door "as a matter of principle".

Set rules

In order not to have to decide anew in every situation whether to dedicate oneself to something, such as a call or a message, it is helpful to set very specific rules. It is rather about a moderate handling of

> incoming stimuli in order to avoid overstrain. Of course, those affected must still deal with potentially negative news in their lives. The question is only when and in what dosage.

The assessment of the actual situation can be carried out as homework with the worksheet WS 12: My handling of the psychohygiene rules. Most patients will be sensitized to the problem in this way.

▶ *It must be ensured that after potentially bad news there is enough (day) time to process them or to carry out or plan the execution of resulting tasks. Unfinished tasks are sleep robbers. Individual strategies of psychohygiene have to be developed for each patient. There are exceptions that require immediate action. These should not be suppressed by psychohygienic measures.*

The unconscious overstimulation by the environment (city, office, at home) can be countered by incorporating conscious break periods into everyday life. "Forest bathing" can be just as helpful as finding peace at home with noise-cancelling headphones while taking a soothing bath with your head under water. Here your imagination knows no bounds: Work out possibilities with your patient to escape from everyday life. These measures do not have to be incorporated daily. Once a week would be good to be able to spend 2–3 h in silence.

Excursus: Overstimulation and Hypersensitivity

The people of the western world are exposed to millions of stimuli every day, which they perceive more or less consciously. If we follow a conversation, look at a beautiful picture consciously or enjoy a piece of chocolate, we perceive consciously and thus attentively with all our five senses: seeing, hearing, smelling, tasting and feeling (in the sense of perception). However, we do not consciously perceive most of the information, such as street noise, shadows, smells, tight shoes or just our meals.

The multitude of all these conscious and subconscious impressions constantly stimulate our sense organs and our nervous system. Our head is striving to filter all the information and categorize it as important and unimportant. Unimportant impressions should be forgotten as quickly as possible so as not to burden our nervous system any longer. Important information should finally be stored and easily accessible.

Our body works similarly to a computer in this respect: If many programs are open at the same time, many downloads and inputs are running in parallel, the working memory is full at some point and the processor is overloaded. Then nothing works anymore and the computer crashes. A restart usually helps.

Analogously, it runs in our nervous system: We let several programs run at the same time, e.g. when driving: Most of the time the radio is on, in addition we are talking on the hands-free system and cursing the dense traffic. Driving and obeying traffic rules are added. So an enormous amount of new information is entered into the "computer" (visual sense: red light; auditory sense: "some song" and the voice of your colleague; haptic sense (feeling): tension due to time pressure; olfactory sense: deodorant, car smell and exhaust fumes).

Does that sound like a crazy situation? Yes, this is a crazy state that most of us experience exactly the same or similar every weekday. However, this moment is not experienced consciously, but we suppress a lot of information and simply experience the commute as "stressful". The cortisol level rises and we are in the hamster wheel of our habits that don't let us sleep at the end of the day.

The result is an "overstimulation". For this state there are many synonyms such as "losing nerves", "having no nerves left" or "having the head full". A healthy sleep declutters our head and provides capacity for reception and resistance (resilience) to new stimuli again.

However, people with sleep disorders do not have their heads cleaned up at night. The result is not infrequently a burnout. Every symptom has come to help. The burnout "shouts": This is too much for me, leave me alone! It usually takes months for a person to recover from such an "overload".

In order to protect the psyche from being overwhelmed again, many people develop chronic hypersensitivity, that is, an exaggerated perception of all stimuli.

The overstimulated nervous system of hypersensitive people cannot filter out which incoming information might be relevant. As a result, *all* stimuli are perceived more clearly, in order to then be able to make a conscious decision as to whether this information is useful or not. This leads to overload even faster. Therefore, it is very important for sensitive sleepers to be aware of themselves in their world. This information is available to you in infomrationsheet IS09 Overstimulation & hypersensitivity for output to the patient. To use and integrate these hints, there is the possibility to include the worksheet WS 13: Overstimulation & hypersensitivity together with the patient in the therapeutic process. It can also be given as homework to take home. In Fig. 3.11 you will find an excerpt from the worksheet.

By living a mindful lifestyle, you can prevent everyday overstimulation and overwhelm.

Please reflect on your everyday life and look for situations that are as "crazy" as driving a car.

Situation	Which tasks run in parallel (multitasking)	What senses are engaged
		□ see □ feel □ smell □ taste □ hear

Fig. 3.11 Worksheet WS13

3.4.11 Module: Cognitive Techniques

Overview (Table 3.14)

Background

Many people with sleep disorders complain of increased rumination and constant tension. In many cases, this occurs so intensely that even people who have hardly slept at night are so tense and restless during the day that they cannot fall asleep in the evening despite being very tired.

Our thoughts determine our feelings, and our feelings motivate us to behave accordingly. Above all, the evaluation of certain situations or information often has a negative effect on our mood. This sets in motion a downward spiral that is difficult to control. However, the same dynamics can also be used to improve mood and increase motivation if things are evaluated positively. Therefore, cognitive behavioral therapy starts from a triad between thoughts, feelings and behavior, whereby all factors influence each other (Fig. 3.12).

In principle, it is possible to adapt interventions to change at any of the three vertices. This is most difficult with feelings. Instructing a patient: "Now don't be afraid of going to bed, nothing can happen to you," makes little sense. The patient would certainly like to comply, but how? Thoughts can also be addressed. But here too, the recommendation "Now don't worry too much and just relax" applies that the person affected does not know how to implement this. A higher chance of success can be achieved in the area of behavior. Here, patients can be offered specific behavioral changes and exercises that they can use. The instruction: "If

Table 3.14 Overview Module: cognitive techniques

Indications	Psychophysiological insomnia, increased rumination, catastrophizing, and overly negative perspectives
Contraindications	Not known
Effectiveness	Very well documented
Working principle	Increasing self-awareness and thus the ability to cognitively restructure and change behavior, education improves understanding of mechanisms, finding alternative, flexible evaluations of the situation
Treatment requirements	Knowledge of cognitive therapy, thought and behavior patterns
Treatment goal	Recognizing, classifying and resolving old thought and action structures and consciously replacing them with (more positive, more differentiated) alternatives; training self-analytical/-reflective skills and independent coping with cognitive and emotional crises

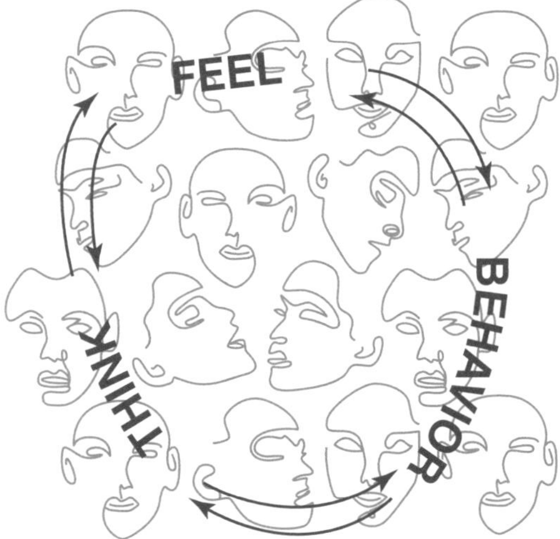

Fig. 3.12 Triad between thoughts, feelings and behavior

difficult. Consciousness slowly switches off, and the person is very receptive to routines like nightly brooding. Therefore, it is important to offer those affected strategies that also work under fatigue and with less effort.

Procedure in General

As with the other therapy components, it is important when using cognitive techniques to discuss in everyday life when and how brooding (thinking/cognition), what the patient is doing at this time (acting/behavior) and how the patient feels (feeling/emotions). Here too, it is recommended that patients keep a diary in everyday life with a focus on capturing their thoughts. Use the diary D 08: My behavior-thought-feeling diary for this. Instruct your patients to note in it daily the situations that seemed difficult, burdensome or stressful to him. At the same time, the diary can be used to record resources by asking your patients to also enter beautiful moments.

Then evaluate the diary with your patient. Lead him through the situations listed therein in the Socratic dialogue, their actions, thoughts and feelings. Many patients can already reflect after filling out the diary which thoughts are hindering and, viewed with a clear mind, make no sense and what makes them feel good and should therefore be done more often. Focus on the feelings of the respective situations. After all, the therapy is aimed at the fact that those affected feel better. In the following, therapy

you can't fall asleep and start worrying, get out of bed and make yourself a herbal tea" can more likely lead to the fact that the person affected drinks tea at night and reports on this procedure and his feelings or the effectiveness of the method.

There are various offers in cognitive behavioral therapy to interrupt brooding loops, such as brooding stop or the brooding chair. These techniques are generally difficult for patients to implement, as they require a lot of discipline and practice. For sleep-disturbed people who want to fall asleep in bed at night instead of brooding, these exercises are much more components are listed for different aspects of dysfunctional thinking.

First, the patient is to be informed about the influence of thinking on mood and behavior. Subsequently, the individual situations of the person concerned are discussed in which he gets into such uncontrollable negative thought loops and phases of brooding, which impair his mood and inhibit positive behavior.

The information from the thought diary can be used, among other things, to develop the structure of the SORKC schema according to Kanfer (Kanfer et al. 2000). It shows the individual components, such as learning processes from possibly dysfunctional behavior and their manifestation in the everyday life of patients. The acronym SORKC stands for:

- **S for Stimulus:** What situation triggers the action chain?
- **O for Organism:** What individual learning historical and biological starting conditions does the patient have?
- **R for Reaction:** which is divided into the 3 basic components of the cognitive triad, namely
  - Cognitions (thoughts): What is the patient thinking in this situation?
  - Emotions (feelings): How does the patient feel in this situation?
  - Behavior: How does the patient behave in this situation?
- **K for Contingency:** How often does the situation presented occur?
- **C for Consequence (engl. Consequence):** What long-term and short-term consequences result from the reactions and behavior in this situation?

This makes it easier for both the patient and the therapist to structure often very complex situations. Table 3.15 shows the example of a patient.

With the help of the worksheet AB 14: Condition Analysis SORKC Scheme, they can work this out individually together with your patient.

▶ *Patients find it very burdensome to be awake. This means: They perceive that they are awake longer than they want to be, and they evaluate this state as negative. This adversely affects their mood and causes a bodily tension which in turn prevents them from falling asleep. A downward spiral is created.*

Cognitive Disputation and De-catastrophizing

The goal of this intervention component is to break the routine of not (re) being able to

Table 3.15 SORKC scheme (case study)

S: Situation	–	Lying awake at night in bed
O: Organismus	–	Increased muscle tone, perfectionism
R: Reaction	Cognition	"Now I can't sleep again, I have to finally fall asleep, hopefully he doesn't come now and want something, I have so much to do tomorrow again"
	Emotion	Powerless, joyless, depressed, overloaded, anxious (fear, the man "might want something")
	Behavior	Pondering, attempt to tire oneself out even more during the day in order to be able to fall asleep at night
	Physiologically	Exhaustion, restlessness, tension
K: Contingency	–	Daily
K: Consequences (Consequence)	–	She remains "the hamster in the wheel", constant tension
	Short-term	Enhancement of the fatigue effect
	Long-term	Constant tension

fall asleep automatically in the evening/night. The first intervention possibility is to prevent the patient from making the often exaggerated negative evaluation of the situation. The evaluation of a situation is an active, although often automated process. First, this automation must be perceived and interrupted in order to subsequently allow functional thoughts to arise.

For example, many people with sleep disorders find it extremely frightening or annoying to be awake in bed. They thus evaluate a rather pleasant situation (lying in a comfortable bed, completely at ease, doing nothing) as excessively negative. It becomes clear that it is not the "being awake in bed" itself that is bad, but rather the evaluation "This is terrible, I won't be able to do anything tomorrow". This emotional evaluation takes place in a thought process and these thoughts in turn lead to feelings like fear and anger. These feelings in turn generate an activating physical reaction, the flight or fight mode. We will certainly not be able to sleep if we are fleeing in fear or fighting in anger. *We think in language!*

Language is a very useful and always available tool. So discuss the specific and literal thoughts that arise with your patient. The personification of the head is helpful in order to build the first distance to the thoughts. For example, ask: "What is your head thinking at that moment?" You don't have to limit yourself to dysfunctional thoughts in the evening or at night in bed, you can also consider general stressful and sleep-inhibiting thoughts during the day.

People with sleep disorders often have irrational beliefs that can be divided into four basic categories according to the pioneer of cognitive behavioral therapy, Albert Ellis:

- Wishes become demands: "I absolutely have to sleep, otherwise …"; "I absolutely have to be fit, otherwise …"
- Global negative evaluations: "I will never sleep well again."; "I will lose my job."
- Catastrophizing: "It's terrible to lie awake at night."

- The belief that negative events cannot be endured: "I will never get through the day."

Often, several dysfunctional thought patterns are pronounced in people with sleep disorders.

The ABC column technique according to Ellis (1979) can be used to break down these thoughts and transform them into a manageable structure. The worksheet WS 15: The ABC Technique can be used for this purpose.

Procedure According to the ABC Column Technique
- Ideas collect—homework evaluate:
- Let the patient describe very concrete and detailed examples of situations. Use the homework D 08: My behavior-thought-feeling diary as homework for your patient in advance of this therapy unit.
- Which situations have arisen? How did that look exactly? Please describe it so that I can see it in my mind's eye. What did you think and feel then? Was that always obvious and easy to tell apart?

Explain the close link between situation and mood, thoughts and feelings, and explore the patient's concrete situations:
Do you always think like this? How do you feel exactly?

- How does this connection of thoughts and feelings come about?
- Why can we change our thoughts and feelings so badly?

Explain the problem using an example (show triangle and close connection):

- Use one of the example situations to explain the respective automation of the feelings and thoughts. Differentiate the thoughts from the feelings exactly. Clearly name the individual feelings and derive the natural impulses for action (e.g. anger makes you ready to fight. When you fight you can't relax.).

- What do you think? What do you feel?

Look for alternative thoughts:

- Together with your patient, look for the simplest explanation for these thoughts and feelings. Check whether they can be used as an alternative.
- De-catastrophize anxiety-related thoughts and discuss alternatives.

Practice and automate:

- Together with your patient, develop exercises for everyday life in which the alternatives can be tried out and practiced.
- Motivate your patient to use these exercises often, adapt the exercises so that they fit well into everyday life and can be automated.

The aim of this therapy module is to have converted the automated evaluations of situations into conscious rational thoughts. The patient should internalize these alternative thoughts (E—effect) to the point where they are quickly and also easily retrievable when tired. Speaking the new thoughts out loud in front of a mirror is a good way to practice.

Dealing with Sleep-Inhibiting Thoughts

There is nothing threatening about lying awake in bed. Those affected know this state very well and also the situation of having to do the pending tasks the next day while being sleep-deprived. Nevertheless, they fall prey to typical cognitive biases that lead to automatically assessing the pending situations as catastrophic, difficult to cope with, and globally negative.

The overview in the table (Table 3.16) gives an insight into nocturnal thoughts and typical cognitive patterns in sleep disorders that can exacerbate the symptoms or actively trigger them again.

Affected individuals should try to accept the situation and evaluate it neutrally or even positively. It is helpful here to work with self-instruction in the form of language: "I am lying here in my comfortable, warm bed. I have everything I need." This means that positive alternatives should be found for the former automatic and catastrophic thoughts, which the affected person learns to think by means of self-instruction (soliloquies). "It's not a big deal to lie awake in bed, this also provides a form of relaxation." With such thoughts, patients are able to relax and eventually fall asleep.

Further information can be found in the sections on mindfulness (Sect. 3.5.3) and paradoxical intervention (Sect. 3.14).

Controlling Rumination

Thinking is, next to sleeping, the main occupation of most people in bed. People affected by sleep disorders are particularly plagued by thoughts and rumination loops. Often, it is not even stressful topics that are spinning in our heads and keeping us awake. Sometimes it's the shopping list that's being mentally completed, or a conversation that still needs to be had, or other small thought loops that fit together and take our attention far away from sleep and to wakefulness. "Unfinished business" are special sleep disturbers, as they require a lot of brain activity and processing capacity. The head wants to make sure that we can finish started or unfinished tasks. He lets them circulate in our brain in endless loops, keeps them active until the time of final completion. Even trivial thoughts and unimportant tasks can lead to physical tension and prevent sleep. Therefore, it is important for (re-) falling asleep to have a "clear" head. With pronounced

Table 3.16 Dealing with sleep-inhibiting thoughts

Cognitive pattern	Description	Example	Alternative thought
All-or-nothing thinking	The situations are only perceived extremely well or badly, instead of interpreting them diversely with "not optimal", "rather pleasant", "endurable" or "not so good"	Because of my *constant sleep deprivation* I don't enjoy life at all anymore	Even though I am sometimes really tired, there are still beautiful moments
One-sided generalization	The attention is limited to single negative occurrences, instead of completely perceiving the situation with positive aspects as well	I haven't slept for weeks	I do sleep badly, but I still get a few hours
Helplessness Attribution	The causes of sleep disorders are seen in factors that cannot be changed	"My sleep disorder is genetically determined."	"Although my mother also suffers from sleep disorders, that does not mean that I have to live with it."
Catastrophize	Negative predictions are made for the future instead of considering other possibilities	"If my sleep disorder does not get better, I will go crazy."	"My body gets the sleep it needs. I hope he gets more in the future."
Overgeneralization	A single situation leads to the conclusion that life in general is being dramatized	"I can't remember anything anymore."	"I'm such a klutz, I left my phone at work."

rumination, the bed is more associated with "Here I am thinking" instead of "Here I am calm and relaxed" through conditioning processes. This conditioning must be interrupted to allow for a restful sleep. However, rumination thoughts can not simply be stopped, which is why known techniques such as the rumination chair (allowing rumination thoughts only on a certain place) or the thought stop (telling his head STOP when rumination thoughts occur) are not sustainably helpful. Both techniques require "wakefulness" in the truest sense of the word and are therefore hardly successful with rumination loops in bed.

Suppressing thoughts requires that they impose themselves even more, that the opposite of the desired effect occurs. Therefore, it is wiser to let the thoughts come and to free them from the rumination loop in the head.

Paper and Pen Method

A proven technique to meet rumination loops is to write these thoughts down. However, this should not only happen in bed, as this would not break the conditioning "In bed I am thinking". Instruct your patients to take a pen and paper earlier in the evening, preferably a diary, and let the thoughts come. If they are then noted, the head receives the signal: "It was written down, so I can now let go of the thought". Of course, there can also be writing utensils next to the bed, which can be used in addition if the thoughts do not stop at night.

Soliloquies

Another very popular method of getting thoughts "out of the head" is to speak them out loud and, if necessary, save them as a voice note on the phone. Speaking the thoughts verbally processes them. Producing language is easy for a non-language-impaired person, but the entire nervous system must perform and synchronize highly complex and fast mechanisms: word finding, semantics, breathing, phonation, etc., with wide parts of the brain being activated. Language production thus supports, for example, the solution of difficult tasks by self-instruction spoken out loud. Also a "self-expression" helps with the emotional processing of experiences.

▶ If these thoughts are then additionally stored in the form of voice messages, the head can finish with the topic, because no memories have to be maintained.

What has been said can simply be heard again the next day. So the head can end the thought loop, so it can come to rest.

You will find more helpful techniques for stopping thoughts in the section "Third Wave of Behavior Therapy" (Sect. 3.6).

3.4.12 Module: Behavior Change

Overview (Table 3.17)

Background

The body gets the sleep it needs, both in terms of duration and quality. If we have physically or mentally exerted ourselves a lot, we need significantly more sleep than if we have spent the day on the couch watching TV. So it is important that we "power down" or get tired. Then the body and mind go into the homeostatic balance of fatigue, that is, sleep. But this is a tightrope walk: If we overdo it and overload ourselves physically and mentally, our body starts a stress reaction that then prevents us from relaxing.

The *sleep hygiene rules (Sect. 3.9)* provide a good basis for identifying dysfunctional behavior and building sleep-promoting behavior. Because even if we are very tired, it can happen that we still do not sleep well.

Typical "behavioral mistakes"
- Irregular wake-up and bedtime
- Irregular meals
- Starting the day in a hurry
- Running through the day like a hamster in a wheel
- No breaks in between
- No mindful moments during the day
- Doing sports too late
- Working too long, including housework
- Late internet research: Even things that are fun can interfere with sleep, such as online shopping
- Late eating, (alcohol) drinking
- Excessive occupation with news, politics and world events
- Rigid adherence to established routines (evening ritual, sport, etc.)
- Basically everything that activates the circulation and thought loops at unfavorable times of the day or excessive/excessive activity

Table 3.17 Overview Module: Behavior Change

Indications	Sleep disorders due to dysfunctional behavior
Contraindications	Not known
Effectiveness	Very well proven
Working principle	By changing habitual behavior, dysfunctional learning mechanisms can be interrupted and replaced by behavior that promotes relaxation
Treatment requirements	Knowledge of techniques for changing behavior and motivation
Treatment goal	Recognize dysfunctional action patterns and consciously replace them with (more positive, more differentiated) alternatives

Procedure

First, dysfunctional behaviors must be identified. For this, the worksheet WS 16: My Behavior—Part 1 can be used both in the therapeutic session and as homework. Then discuss the listed actions. At this point, a psychoeducational therapy unit can take place in which you explain your patient the natural and healthy *cortisol course, as shown in Sect. 1.5.3.* Derive from the cortisol course why corresponding behaviors are unfavorable and then work out alternatives that no longer disturb sleep. In Fig. 3.13 you will find a patient example of these dysfunctional behaviors in everyday life.

Here the creativity of the therapist is required: Everything that interrupts this familiar process is allowed, dysfunctional associations are to be split and new behavior (quick falling asleep) is to be made possible. Examples of such measures are:

During the day:

- Mindful break
- Short relaxation exercises

- Balanced daily routine (especially the start of the day)
- Tasks if necessary postpone or omit
- Avoid compulsive behavior (e.g. evening ritual, sports rituals, etc.)

In bed:

- Lie down the other way around in bed
- Sleep in another room
- Try to fall asleep in a different position (e.g. the stomach sleeper turns onto his back)

Work out these alternative behaviors as concretely as possible and preferably write them down. The worksheet WS 17: My behavior—part 2 can be used as a basis. These action alternatives correspond to implementable behavior and can usually be tried out by the patient in any life situation: *with* sleep disorders, *with* disinterest, *with* anxiety, tired, exhausted, bad-tempered etc. With the diary TB 01: My sleep diary *(bed*

		My "behavioral errors"	How am I doing?
Monday – Friday	morning	I can't get out of bed and press the snooze button quite often	🙂 🙂 😟
	morning	I fall into a hectic pace and work without a break	🙂 😐 ☹
	at noon	I often eat at my workplace	🙂 😐 ☹
	afternoon	I lie on the sofa and watch TV instead of going out and exercising	🙂 😐 ☹
	evening	I fall asleep in front of the TV and then go to bed way too late	🙂 🙂 ☹
Weekend	Saturday	I sleep too long, I move too little	😐 🙂 ☹
	Sunday	See Saturday, I go to bed too late	🙂 🙂 😟

Fig. 3.13 Patient example of the worksheet WS 16: My behavior part 1

and sleep restriction Sect. 3.3) you and your patient can follow the success of these measures and, if necessary, make corrections.

3.4.13 Module: Perfection and Control

Overview (Table 3.18)

Background

Perfectionism is a psychological construct that involves an exaggerated pursuit of perfection that is oriented towards an ideal. From a psychological point of view, perfectionism is not functional and often prevents those affected from actually solving problems. The basic motivation behind this is often the avoidance of a evaluable result. The desire for perfection often has its origin in dysfunctional value systems that are often passed down from generation to generation.

Perfectionism is often found in people with anorexia nervosa, bulimia nervosa or OCD and also in those affected by alcohol abuse, depression and sexual dysfunction.

Many people consider perfection to be desirable. However, the fact is that it is not possible to make everything perfect. By wanting to make everything perfect, there is an over-attention to the task to be done. This already creates tension during the day, which can often not be reduced in the evening and night hours. In addition, there is often the anger about situations or results that are not perfect. Many sufferers of sleep disorders suffer from their perfectionism—at first unconsciously. During therapy, this should be made more conscious and questioned.

The perfectionism of sleep-disordered people includes the precise self-observation with regard to sleep, constant nocturnal checking of the alarm clock, meticulously kept sleep diaries, strict discipline with regard to the consumption of coffee, the admission of certain thoughts or the execution of various activities (sport etc.). This striving for perfection promotes expectations of anxiety and nocturnal frustration.

Personality profile of a perfectionist:

- Increased motivation and strong sense of responsibility
- Fear of failure
- Increased tendency to feel guilty
- Very organized and conscientious
- Highly sensitive to errors
- Very reliable, always available
- Tries to do everything immediately
- Very well informed

The strong desire to control everything plays a big role in the topic of perfectionism. It is necessary to question to what extent control can actually be exercised in each situation. As a passenger in an airplane, you cannot control that it actually does not crash. This is then an unrealistic desire for control. Most of the time, there is only the need to build up a subjective feeling of control. Many affected people are convinced or feel that the perfect execution of behavior and rituals allows them to control the respective situation. At this point, too, there are different dysfunctional patterns of thought that should be questioned.

Table 3.18 Brief overview module: Perfection and Control

Indications	Controlling, obsessive personality structures, perfectionism
Contraindications	Not known
Effectiveness	Increase in self-awareness and thus the possibility of cognitive restructuring and behavioral change
Working principle	Cognitive therapy
Treatment requirements	Knowledge of the techniques of cognitive therapy and behavior analysis
Treatment goal	Encourage the patient to "let go of the reins"

Procedure

The patient's striving for perfection, the tendency to control and the associated dysfunctional behaviors should be discussed with the patient. An analysis of the patient's value system and, associated with it, the patient's reflection on this system, are also important. The therapist should be open to everything and set his own standards back as much as possible. Even if certain aspects are not desirable for him, they could be very valuable for his patient. System immanence is particularly important here.

For example, the ABC schema by Ellis *(Sect. 3.4.11)* can be used for the analysis. For the affected person it is helpful if the different advantages of non-perfect solutions are shown to him, e.g. to come to a result quickly, to invest less effort in a solution, to use less money, time and resources. In this way it can be worked out together where it makes sense to exercise control over the situation and where it is more economical and helpful to trust.

After the cognitive preparation, a restructuring should take place. The patient must feel that no catastrophe occurs if things are not done perfectly and the control over the situation is left to other people. It is favorable to choose everyday tasks for the behavioral exercises for which the affected person usually needs a lot of time and energy. Afterwards it can be worked out together where resources can be saved and how the time gained can be used—ideally for self-caring (euthymic) behavior.

Many patients hand over the control to the therapist at the beginning of the therapy. They take on a very passive role and want to "be healed by the therapist", without being aware that they are themselves actively involved in the success of the therapy. Then it is the task of the therapist to bring the patient out of this passive-waiting position into a willing-to-work phase and thus to activate and subsequently increase his self-efficacy. That is, at the end the patient can control his sleep disorder, and not the sleep disorder controls him. This is particularly effective and plausible when, during therapy, after an initial improvement in symptoms, there is a deterioration in symptoms again and the patient is able to cope with this on his own and using what he has learned so far.

3.4.14 Module: Paradoxical Intervention

Overview (Table 3.19)

Background

In the paradoxical intervention, as the name suggests, the behavioral exercise is in contradiction to the desired therapeutic goal. In the treatment of insomnia, the often-encountered problem is that those affected "try very hard" (to fall asleep again) and spend the entire time they are awake in bed thinking about "finally falling asleep again". This entangles them in dysfunctional patterns of thought, which in turn generate tension and make falling asleep even less likely.

In the context of the paradoxical intervention, patients are supposed to do the exact opposite, namely try not to fall asleep. This usually seems contradictory to most people, but they still go along with it because they cannot fall asleep anyway. At this moment, those affected let go of their "cramp-like" attempts to fall asleep, they surrender to the situation, relax and can fall asleep. This technique is also particularly effective with children, as long as they are able to stay calm in bed.

Even if this intervention does not immediately achieve the desired effect—namely that the patient actually falls asleep—with this exercise everything is turned off that is experienced as sleep-inhibiting: rumination, tension and the fear of not being able to fall asleep. There is a confrontation with the inability to fall asleep and a mindful acceptance of the fact of the inability to fall asleep. Those affected regain control and realize that it is not bad to be awake in bed. What makes it bad are the expectations of having to sleep and the fear of not being able to sleep again.

Table 3.19 Brief overview module: Paradoxical intervention

Indications	Insomnia and sleepwalking, dysfunctional thought patterns: wanting to force oneself to sleep, fear of not being able to sleep
Contraindications	Not known
Effectiveness	Very well proven
Principle of operation	The focus on not falling asleep distracts from the focus on falling asleep, the patient relaxes and falls asleep
Treatment requirements	Knowledge of the paradoxical intervention, existence of a viable therapeutic relationship
Treatment goal	Conscious observation and reflection of the cognitions and behaviors in the sleep and bedtime process, learning the skill to replace them

Procedure

The patient is instructed to lie down ready for bed at the agreed time, turn off the light, close their eyes and *not* fall asleep! The patient should consciously forego familiar rituals such as counting, autogenic training, focusing on breathing, etc. It is important to forego the dysfunctional and also functional habits that have been closely associated with the inability to fall asleep for a long time through "practice". Since the patient is no longer trying to fall asleep, a state of relaxation may occur. The affected person "forgets" that they cannot fall asleep and falls asleep.

▶ *The technique of the paradoxical intervention can be very well combined with a mindfulness exercise.*

3.4.15 Module: Sleep Deprivation— Wake Therapy

Overview (Table 3.20)

Background

Depressions are very often accompanied by sleep disorders. However, the sleep disorder can also be the primary disease and have comorbid depressive symptoms. Both disorders can be treated with sleep deprivation or wake therapy. This type of therapy was introduced in the middle of the twentieth century by the German psychiatrists Schulte and Tölle for depressive disorders (Schulte and Tölle 1971). They showed that in 60–70% of patients, mostly with a typical depression, sleep deprivation had a clearly positive effect.

Even in healthy people, a slight over-excitability and mild euphoria can be observed after a sleepless night. This shows that sleep deprivation can have an effect on a person's drive and mood.

Total sleep deprivation, in which patients are not allowed to sleep at all, is distinguished from partial sleep deprivation, in which patients are woken up after a few hours of sleep and are not allowed to sleep during the second half of the night. There is also selective sleep deprivation, in which certain deep sleep phases are deprived. This is only possible under polysomnographic control in a sleep laboratory.

In the first half of the night, deep sleep takes place mainly with the corresponding recovery and regeneration processes. Sleep in the second half of the night is not as deep anymore, REM sleep occurs more often, and processing and regulatory processes take place more frequently. Depending on the period of deprivation, such processes can be increased or inhibited. It may seem paradoxical that partial sleep deprivation in the second half of the night is often very effective in depressed patients, even though that is when emotional regulatory processes take place. Perhaps in this way, familiar dysfunctional associations are interrupted and a elevated mood follows.

Table 3.20 Brief overview module: sleep deprivation—wake therapy

Indications	Insomnia, subtype sleep perception disorder, (comorbid) depression
Contraindications	Bipolar or psychotic disorders, activities with high accident risk during the day, epilepsy, parasomnias, disturbed breathing due to a sleep disorder, suicidality: extreme caution, with the next sleep the high is abruptly ended (even a short nap can initiate this)
Effectiveness	Very well proven, but only for a maximum of 48 h
Working principle	Shutting down brain activity leads to a decrease in negative, worrying thoughts, balancing of neurotransmitter imbalances in the brain (acetylcholine, serotonin) For patients with sleep perception disorder: confrontation with the feeling after an actually sleepless night
Treatment requirements	Knowledge of therapeutic sleep deprivation
Treatment goal	Improved, brightened mood For patients with sleep perception disorder: better distinction between nights with sleep perception disorder and actual sleep deprivation

The mechanisms of sleep restriction, i.e. an increase in sleep pressure with bedtime restriction, as well as the mechanisms of paradoxical intervention, are effective against sleep disorders. In addition, neurochemical and -physical changes in the cholinergic and serotonergic system produce a mood-lifting effect that lasts up to 48 h. However, there are also reports from patients who experienced a mood-lifting effect for a week. This probably had more moderating causes, e.g. hope for an improvement in depression. After at least 48 h, the patient must sleep again, otherwise other unwanted effects can occur, such as hallucinations, physical discomfort or irritability. To keep the mood-lifting effect going a little longer, it is possible to carry out a sleep phase shift. After at least two good nights, sleep deprivation takes place. On the following day, the patient then sleeps, for example, from 4:00 p.m. to midnight. On the following days, the patient goes to bed one hour later each day until the usual bedtime is reached. This technique falls into the area of partial sleep deprivation. Total sleep deprivation over 36 h with subsequent sleep phase shift for mood stabilization is common. Sleep deprivation can occur 1- to 2- times per week.

Why and how sleep deprivation works is not yet fundamentally clarified. Hegerl and colleagues have examined the mode of action of sleep deprivation more closely, based on the assumption that sleep-disturbed and depressed people suffer from a chronically increased muscle tone, which makes it difficult for them to relax or fall asleep in the first place (Sander et al. 2015). With the sleep deprivation, the sleep pressure is increased so much and the wakefulness in return is so clearly reduced that the patients finally give in to their exhaustion and "have to" stop being depressed. This also promotes sleep quality (Steinberg and Hegerl 2014).

Despite the very good efficacy of the method, it is very controversial because the mood-enhancing effect usually only lasts a few hours. Even a short nap can end the high. Therefore, the main goal of this technique is to show the patient that they are indeed able to feel good and that their body is able to sleep without medication.

People with sleep perception disorder have the feeling of not having slept at all during the whole night. In the sleep stage Non-REM 1 we still have a partial attention, in which we consciously perceive external stimuli, such as noise, light or movement. Thoughts and images of the day flow into the brain processes of light sleep, so that the impression arises that the person is still completely awake. Due to the distorted time perception, the time is perceived as much longer in Non-REM 1. Five minutes can then feel like one to two hours. Deep sleep (Non-REM 3), on the other hand, is extremely shortened. 20 min then appear like a few seconds. This creates the feeling of not having slept at all or not having fallen into deep sleep. Although these people have the feeling of not having slept, they feel fit and productive the next day. As "proof" that they still sleep in most nights, a sleep deprivation can help. After an actually sleepless night, the patients will feel very tired, exhausted and not productive. This difference can help those affected to better understand this special form of sleep disorder.

Procedure

Total sleep deprivation means that the patient does not sleep at all during the night and stays awake until the usual bedtime the following day. This is not easy for the person concerned, which is why sleep deprivation therapies are organized in groups in clinics. During the night, various activities such as games, sports, television and walks are undertaken to suppress boredom and falling asleep.

In partial sleep deprivation, the patients are woken up after a certain period of night sleep. This is difficult in that the affected persons usually wake up and have to stay awake from a deep sleep phase. Overcoming the then experienced sleep pressure is very stressful and requires a lot of discipline. Most patients need support. It is favorable to "get the patients out of bed" with something pleasant, where the imagination knows no limits: A piece of favorite chocolate, a favorite game, a good movie or a night walk under the starry sky etc. are a good reward.

The application of sleep deprivation is also possible on an outpatient basis, that is, at home. However, it is favorable to practice the procedure in the hospital beforehand and make the patient aware of the possible effects. Even with outpatient treatment, the patient should not be alone at night and have support. In order to achieve an effect, it is important that the patient actually stay awake for half or even the whole night.

Again, the more active the patients design the stay awake, the easier it will be for them to actually endure the sleep deprivation.

▶ *It is possible that manic episodes occur as a result of sleep deprivation. Therefore, special caution is advised for patients who are already prone to mood swings. Caution is also advised in the case of latent or acute suicidality.*

The mood may be preceded by an increase in drive, which could lead to suicidal actions. If in doubt, the sleep deprivation treatment should only be carried out under supervision in the clinic.

3.4.16 Module: Relaxation Techniques

Overview (Table 3.21)

Background

A relaxed waking state (alpha activity in the brain) is necessary for a transition from the waking to the sleep state. This is lacking in most insomnia patients. Often these can not relax during the day. The reasons for this are manifold and very individual. In my experience, it is often the case that the patients "run like a hamster in a wheel" through their everyday life, are always available and try to complete all pending tasks as perfectly as possible. In addition, there is the worry of getting everything done on time. Even in leisure time, more and more people are stressed. The leisure time offers and tasks are manifold, and one does not want to miss anything and do everything. Parents are particularly affected, who not only have to think and plan for themselves. Possible buffer times are often used for family duties. But also people in retirement are often "constantly under voltage". Mostly this is a habit transferred from the time of employment. Especially with older, but also with younger patients, the value system plays a

Table 3.21 Brief overview module: relaxation techniques

Indications	Can always be used in combination, tension, chronic increased muscle tone
Contraindications	Any possible physical illnesses, in addition no contraindications known (use less meaningful in insomnia, if already relaxed a lot during the day and pronounced protective behavior exists)
Effectiveness	Very well documented, moderate effect sizes, 30% symptom reduction
Working principle	"Where there is relaxation, there can be no tension" (Jacobson 2002). Relaxation is necessary in order to be able to fall asleep (psychophysiological cycle). Sleep disorders, especially insomnia, are maintained by an increased level of arousal, both on a physical and an emotional and cognitive level (Sanavio 1988)
Treatment requirements	Knowledge of one or more relaxation techniques
Treatment goal	Make the patient as familiar as possible with different relaxation techniques and let him experience the respective effect himself And: Firm adaptation of the exercises into the patient's everyday life

fundamental role. Diligence is a desirable virtue that many want to achieve and maintain. Being lazy, on the other hand, is strongly negative and can only occur in exceptional cases. This attitude can lead to chronic stress, to permanent stress and also to overload.

In order to meet all these aspects, a combination of different therapy components is necessary, such as cognitive therapy, *structuring of the day (Sect. 3.4), mindfulness training (Sect. 1.5.3) and stimulus control & psychohygiene (Sect. 3.10).*

With the introduction and training of relaxation techniques, physical relaxation can be supported and brought about directly in people who are receptive to it. This can be very useful in order to achieve a relaxed waking state before going to bed.

There is a variety of relaxation techniques, which are shown in Table 3.22.

This therapy guide does not go into the individual relaxation techniques in depth, as this would go beyond the scope of the book. Each of these techniques is worth its own book. Particular importance is attached here to the self-experience of the therapists in order to be able to offer individual and problem-oriented techniques to the patients for symptom relief.

Therapists should try out the various techniques themselves with care and experience how individual exercises feel. It is particularly important to give individual indications of how and when patients can use the exercises in everyday life. Undoubtedly, it would be better to practice a technique intensively and have it quickly available, but most of those affected fail to learn a relaxation technique due to the high amount of practice required. In order to achieve a sustainable improvement in symptoms, relaxation exercises must be integrated into everyday life on a regular basis, preferably daily. Through mini-interventions that only take a few minutes and can also be used at the workplace, in public transport, on the playground or even in the car in a traffic jam, the motivation of the patients to use them regularly increases. 3 min of targeted relaxation are better than none at all.

As part of targeted sleep therapy, the aim is not to learn a relaxation technique in a targeted manner, but rather to bring the patient into contact with various techniques. If necessary, one of these techniques can be learned later at another point (e.g. as part of prevention offers from health insurers, in adult education or in a relaxation group). In principle, all relaxation techniques are helpful.

Table 3.22 Relaxation techniques

Name	Working mechanism	Exercise possibilities
Progressive muscle relaxation according to Jacobson (PMR)	By tensing the muscles and then relaxing them, even small changes can be felt	As part of prevention courses offered by health insurance companies, instructions on the Internet or via App
Autogenic training (AT)	The mentally controlled warmth and heaviness feeling leads to relaxation	
Mentally-emotional relaxation techniques		
Fantasy Travel	Relaxation elements (also from other relaxation techniques) are integrated into stories that are experienced in the imagination	Instructions as an audio file on CD, for download, playback on the Internet or via app
Meditation	With the help of guided or free concentration exercises, deep relaxation can be achieved. The goal is to achieve inner mental silence	
Mindfulness	Live consciously in the here and now without judging the situation	
Body-therapeutic relaxation techniques		
Yoga	"Yoga is the stilling or controlling of the modifications or fluctuations of the mind." (Pantanjali; Yoga Sutra). It includes both mental and physical exercises as well as breathing techniques	As part of prevention courses offered by health insurance companies, other course offerings, video files on DVD or on the Internet, instructional videos via app
Qigong	By deliberately using breath, movement and imagination, self-healing powers are activated which can relieve heart, circulatory and nervous diseases	
Tai Chi	"Shadow boxing"; by concentrating on the body and the precise movement, the thoughts are gently brought into the here and now and mental and physical tension is released	

Regardless of which relaxation technique the patient chooses, it must be appealed to the patient's patience: one's own expectations should not be set too high. The awareness should be sharpened that learning a relaxation technique takes time and practice. Even if it has been learned well and used regularly, relaxation techniques are not causal therapies for sleep disorders, as is often propagated.

In addition, the therapist should point out and also pay attention to the fact that relaxation techniques are not only used in the evening to fall asleep, but also to actively and passively structure the day. For example, it can be helpful to do a relaxation exercise during the "Happy Hour", as this will then reduce stress and thus also cortisol production. There are also relaxation techniques and exercises that initially stimulate the circulation, as the blood flow is promoted in the corresponding body parts. Such exercises are not suitable for use in the evening or immediately before falling asleep.

Another important point is the everyday suitability of relaxation exercises: patients with sleep disorders usually have a very busy everyday life.

▶ *When adapting the exercises to everyday life, make sure that using the relaxation exercises does not cause additional stress.*

It should not be expected that the patient will completely learn a relaxation technique. Rather, it is about motivating the participants to use the exercises in small everyday breaks (on the bus, on the way to the daycare center, etc.). It is important to constantly remind the affected people that regular practice is required in order to be able to apply the respective technique in situations where it is needed.

Procedure

The patient should feel and experience the different techniques in small exercises. Various exercises can also be carried out regularly in the sessions so that the patients get an idea of which techniques there are, what possibilities they offer and how individual exercises feel.

The end of a session has proven to be a favorable exercise time: The patients leave the session relaxed (if an effect was felt) and possibly take some of the relaxation with them into everyday life. In addition, this gives each session a structure that is comprehensible for the patients. It is also important here to ask the patients about their individual wishes. This increases the sense of self-efficacy, which is very important for the treatment of sleep disorders. At this point, the patients should be made aware once again that a therapist cannot simply relieve or cure a sleep disorder, but is only in a position to offer the patient the instructions for this.

Relaxation Techniques

- When using relaxation techniques, the time of day should be considered. Some relaxation techniques, especially in the practice phase, stimulate the circulation (e.g. yoga, progressive muscle relaxation [PMR]); for falling asleep at night, autogenic training, imagination techniques and meditation are particularly effective.
- The techniques selected for the patient must be practicable in everyday life. The patient should not feel that it takes too much time to relax; otherwise the techniques will be experienced as too time-consuming and not used.

- Before relaxation techniques can be used to fall asleep, they must be well mastered and experienced by the patient as relaxing and sleep-promoting.
- When learning the individual techniques, the patients do not have to make any extraordinary effort to do everything right. Excessive perfectionism or too high demands on oneself have a negative effect on falling asleep.

▶ *The bed is not for training! Patients should only use the relaxation exercises suitable for falling asleep in bed when they can apply them safely outside the bed.*

Two Short Exercises on Relaxation Techniques

Exercise 1: Quasimodo

This exercise comes from the field of PMR. The muscles in the shoulder and neck area are first tensed strongly, and then the tension is released again. Relaxation should occur. The previous tensioning of the muscles should intensify the perception of relaxation and relaxation itself. It is helpful to breathe deeply to transport more oxygen into the blood and with the blood into the brain. PMR improves the oxygen supply to the brain and has a refreshing effect. In addition, PMR can dissolve all types of tension, cramp, neck and head pain with regular training.

Patient Instructions
- Take a comfortable sitting position, close your eyes.
- We start with the tension phase: The arms are bent and the hands are loose.
- Breathe calmly and deeply.
- Now pull the shoulders up as if the shoulders wanted to touch the ears.
- Push the head back without looking up.
- This creates a cushion in the neck, a small roll of fat. Now concentrate on

this neck roll. Try to squeeze this neck roll together as tightly as possible. Pull the shoulders up tightly and push the head back firmly.

- Breathe deeply and calmly.
- Press the neck roll together very strongly until the head vibrates.
- Now let the shoulders drop slowly and smoothly.
- Slowly let the head hang down until the chin touches the chest.
- Breathe calmly and deeply.
- Keep your chin down, and slowly put your right ear on your right shoulder
- And now your left ear on your left shoulder.
- Do not pull your shoulders back up.
- Enjoy this relaxation phase, enjoy: Where there was tension before, there is now relaxation.

Post-exploration

- Ask the patient how it went.
- Discuss whether the patient was able to let go, turn off and relax.

If this exercise was experienced as pleasant, it can be repeated regularly in everyday life and also in therapy. PMR would then be a good relaxation technique for the patient.

Exercise 2: Let your Head Hang!

This exercise is based on the principles of yoga and can give the patient a first impression of what yoga actually is and how it feels. There are many different types and forms of yoga. In yoga, as it is very widespread in Western culture, three elements are combined in the exercises: on the one hand body exercises (holding and stretching exercises), on the other hand breathing. Deep breathing brings more oxygen into the circulation and moves the body. Stretching exercises are intensified by deep breathing and

the attention is focused on the breath. And the third element of meditation, in which disturbing thoughts come and go, because the attention is always drawn back to the body sensations and the breath.

Instructions for the Patient

- Take a comfortable sitting position, bend the upper body slightly (or more strongly) forward and rest your forearms on your thighs.
- Let your head hang down.
- Try to relax your neck and shoulders completely.
- Let your shoulders hang.
- Breathe deeply in and out. Focus your thoughts on your breathing and feel how the breath comes and goes. If unwanted thoughts come up, gently push them aside and focus your attention back on your breath.

Take your time

- With each exhalation, your head sinks a little lower. It just falls down, only gravity pulls, you are completely relaxed.

Take your time

- Now just focus on your breathing. Let the breath come and go. And let your head hang.

Take your time

- When your head no longer sinks lower and you feel calm and relaxed, enjoy this peace for a few moments.

Take your time

- Now come back slowly, sit up straight, stretch and take a deep breath.

> **Post-exploration**
>
> - Ask the patient how it went.
> - Discuss whether the patient was able to let go, relax and feel comfortable.
> - If this exercise was experienced as pleasant, it can be repeated regularly in everyday life and also in therapy. Yoga would then be a good relaxation technique for the patient.

You will find more relaxation techniques in the sections "Third Wave of Behaviour Therapy" (Sect. 3.6) and "Mind-Body Medicine" (Sect. 3.6).

3.4.17 Module: Sexuality

Overview (Table 3.23)

Background

Sexuality is a very sensitive topic for most people. On the one hand, sexuality is important and does people good, on the other hand it is also extremely susceptible to interference. Therefore, it is always necessary to ask about sexual life and satisfaction in this respect.

Sexuality also plays a big role in the topic of sleep and sleep disorders. In most couples, sex only takes place in bed. Therefore, in addition to the association bed = sleep, the association bed = sex often exists. If the current sexual life is not satisfactory, this problem is automatically "taken to bed". Tension and insomnia can be the result. The case report of the couple M. *(in the service section)* makes this clear.

In addition, sex is a physical activity that gets the circulation going and causes the release of various hormones. This can also have a negative effect on night sleep. Nevertheless, sexual activities can be beneficial to sleep. An orgasm creates relaxation, and to have an orgasm, you have to be relaxed and free in your head. If it is difficult for someone to switch off in the evening and relax, sex (or masturbation) can be helpful.

Procedure

This sensitive topic should be discussed in a system-immanent and safe manner. First information can be collected, for example, using a questionnaire that the patient can fill out at home to approach the topic and also get used to the idea that this area could become the subject of therapy. Take the patient's shame and give him security. Speak openly with the patient about his sexuality in a relaxed atmosphere. Name the things by name or develop an individual language with your patient that both sides feel comfortable with. The more confident the practitioner is with this topic, the more comfortable the patient feels. Sexuality is something completely normal, everyone does it.

If the patient's sexuality is not satisfactory at the moment, sexual contacts should not take place in bed—at least as long as the sleep does not get better. Together with the patient, you can develop ideas and strategies on how he can achieve a fulfilled sexuality outside the bed. Suggestions that the patient can take up are

Table 3.23 Overview Module: Sexuality

Indications	Dissatisfaction with one's own sexuality, tensions in this regard
Contraindications	Not known. Caution with singles: risk of frustration!
Effectiveness	Very high effectiveness
Working principle	Psychoeducation, relief through conversation, classical cognitive behavioral therapy (cognitive restructuring, behavioral exercises)
Treatment requirements	Unbiased handling of the topic of sexuality, tolerance of unusual sexual practices
Treatment goal	Breaking old habits that have a negative effect on relaxation and night's sleep; Use of sexual activity to induce relaxation

just as helpful as discussing possible problems. Couple's therapy can be a great relief and help to talk openly about the topic with the partner.

Often, within a couple, the different demands on the quantity or quality of sex can be a fundamental problem. Sometimes one partner (A) feels significantly less desire than the other, which can lead to enormous tension and conflict in bed. For example, one partner often tries to seduce the other (B) in bed at night. This can cause partner B to go to bed with increased tension because he fears that partner A will reject him and have to endure the resulting disappointment and bad mood. There are many aversive feelings that can even cause or maintain a sleep disorder. So recommend to your patients that they move the sex to another place and also at a different time of day.

▶ *It is important here to promote communication between the two partners. The notification of the respective needs through I-messages is helpful. The patients must be encouraged to talk openly about wishes and concerns. If the sex life is working again, the bed can also be the place of action again.*

The rules of sleep hygiene stipulate that one should only sleep in bed. This should be adapted individually for each patient, as sex can also be helpful for relaxation. Anger is definitely to be avoided in bed, as it causes enormous tension and also prevents people who usually have a good sleep from sleeping.

It is possible to create a relaxed state of wakefulness by means of an orgasm through masturbation. In chronic pain patients, this can even have a positive effect on pain perception, as a large number of hormones are released. For couples with an active and fulfilling sex life, sex can also be a sleep aid until physical exhaustion.

3.5 Nightmare Therapy

The term nightmare (in German Albtraum) comes from Old German and means elf dream. In the Christian church, elves were just as evil as ghosts, demons and the devil. As a "good Christian" one therefore had a natural fear of these figures. Therefore, over time, a nightmare was equated with a nightmare.

3.5.1 Background of Nightmare Therapy

A nightmare is a dream experience that is characterized by strong negative emotions such as fear, anger, sadness, shame, disgust, loss of control, despair, surprise or contempt. It appears to be very real. Often the dreamer cannot distinguish between dream and reality in the dream experience.

Since the transition to the different sleep phases usually results in a total inhibition of skeletal muscle activity, no real movement can take place during sleep. The implementation of the movement representations represented in the cortex is inhibited in the thalamic structures and thus interrupted. Sleepwalking occurs in the transitions between the sleep stages Non-Rem 2 and Non-REM 3. As a rule, it is not a pathological sleep phenomenon.

Dreams and nightmares usually occur during REM sleep and thus usually in the second half of the night and in the morning hours (idiopathic nightmares). If nightmares occur after traumatization, they are called post-traumatic nightmares. In contrast to idiopathic nightmares, they can occur during the entire night, also during non-REM sleep. Another difference is that the dream content in idiopathic nightmares is fictional, whereas the content in post-traumatic nightmares has actually been experienced. The dream then serves the re-experience and the emotion regulation (post-traumatic repetition).

Therefore, dream work can be a very important part of trauma therapy.

Both types of nightmares can lead to a lack of recovery during the night in the same way. The patients may develop a fear of going to bed. This can lead to insomnia because they fear that they will dream badly again. Even if the dreams are not real and quickly forgotten during the day, they can lead to a significant impairment of quality of life and to sequelae and also to chronicity.

Like sleep in general, dreaming also has a variety of functions. Despite centuries of research efforts, we still do not know much about dreaming and base theoretical explanation attempts on hypotheses. Since the actual dream event with its emotions and the pictorial or acoustic experience cannot be transferred to the outside despite modern examination and imaging methods, we are still dependent on the reports of the dreamers. Depending on the personality, dreams can be experienced very vividly, colorful, sensual and eventful. Some people say they never dream. From today's scientific point of view, everyone dreams in REM sleep, even if people do not remember their dreams. However, people who were awakened before REM sleep also reported dreams, so it can be assumed that dreams are possible in every sleep phase. It is certain that semantic memory consolidation and emotion regulation take place in REM sleep and are therefore in close connection with dreaming.

If we sleep and dream well, we wake up refreshed and emotionally balanced the next morning. However, if we experience fearful or stressful dreams, we feel the next morning as if we had actually experienced what we had dreamed.

In the dream, therefore, everything is processed that touches us in any way in everyday life. The subject of disturbing nightmares are therefore things that burden us in everyday life. These burden events can be many years back or highly topical. It is possible that we can hardly

or not establish any connection to the dream content during the day, but mostly there is a link. In the nightmare exposure, a highly individual connection between dream and experienced of the affected person is sought.

Although nightmares can be very burdensome for those affected, they should not be immediately assessed as a pathological disorder. Dreams, as already mentioned, have a variety of functions, so their natural course is also important. So only intervene in the dream action if the affected persons develop a clear suffering pressure.

3.5.2   Preparation of the Nightmare Therapy

There are dreams whose content was so impressive that they are not forgotten. However, most of the time the dream memory fades within a few minutes after waking up. Therefore it is advisable to use a dream diary, which the affected person keeps next to the bed and in which he immediately notes after waking up what his dream was about. Use the diary D 09: My (nightmare) dream diary.

A smartphone can be very helpful at this point, by the nightmares are not written, but spoken in the form of a voice note. Especially after waking up from nightmares, those affected are barely oriented and it can be difficult to reach for a pen and paper. Just saying what was dreamed and saving it on the phone has proven to be very comfortable in practice and provides much more information about the dreams. The resulting dream diary in paper form or as an audio file is then evaluated in the therapy sessions. First, it is important to understand exactly what the patient's nightmares are about, whether there are patterns and repetitions. Analyze the disturbing dreams together with your patients therefore very precisely.

3.5.3 Module Nightmare Variant 1: Solution of the Dream Conflict in the Waking State

Overview (Table 3.24)

Background

One approach to nightmare therapy is to decode the content of the dreams and project the action onto the patient's actual everyday life. Select dream content or a specific dream that is dreamed often or whose elements are repeated in different dreams. The more exemplary the selected dream is, the better other dream content can be generalized by the patient. This could also be dream elements that were relevant in the past some time ago. The head always has "good reasons" to re-activate or not to let go of old events.

Procedure

Ask the patient about the content in such detail that you could write a script about the dreams, then you have captured everything well.

Then look for patterns of behavior and experience, figurative comparisons, feelings, and representatives in people or possibly also (domestic) animals in the patient's everyday experience. Try to abstract the dream content and transfer it to everyday life. Do not rely too much on classic or historical dream interpretation. These are often very far-fetched, may apply to the individual, but are often not specific. Every dream has its individual meaning for the dreamer, which should be found together with the patient.

▶ It is important that it makes sense for the patient. Most patients find it easy to decode the symbolism of the dream with some support.

For example, if your patient dreams again and again of running away from a lion, being very afraid and not moving from the spot while running, it is possible that the occurring lion is the patient's boss, who is actually very nice on the surface, but subconsciously generates pressure. However, it is also possible to want to run away from a task or project (= lion) because one feels that one is not making progress in the project.

The thus uncovered stressors and the emotional experience in everyday life can then be treated in the waking state with the help of all therapeutic methods (depth psychology, cognitive behavioral therapy [also 3rd wave], body therapy, etc.). Dysfunctional thinking and behavior patterns can be restructured and transferred to everyday life. This is usually followed by calmer dreams.

Table 3.24 Overview Module: Nightmare Therapy Variant 1: Solution of the Conflict in the Waking State

Indications	Nightmares
Contraindications	Not known
Effectiveness	Well proven
Working principle	Nightmares are an emotional processing of everyday life. By decoding the dream content, the actual causes can be remedied.
Treatment requirements	Knowledge of nightmare therapy, analytical ability, some imagination
Treatment goal	Recognize stressors in everyday life that lead to nightmares, targeted change of stressors

3.5.4 Module Nightmare Variant 2: Nightmare Modification

Overview (Table 3.25)

Background

This type of nightmare therapy is then suitable for your patient if it is the same dream that recurs with little or no variation. The technique of nightmare modification is also ideally suited for nightmares caused by trauma.

Procedure

A dream diary should also be kept for this technique and the dreams should be analyzed in therapy. With the nightmare modification method, a specific nightmare must be selected for processing and reconstructed in as much detail as possible. If you have selected a specific nightmare, work out the elements that are rated as negative and characteristic as completely as possible. Describe the exact dream experience and make sure that the patient experiences it at night as you describe it. The next step in therapy is to write a dream script. This can be done very well by the patient as homework between sessions. If the patient feels a similar emotional quality when reading or listening to the nightmare script as in the dream, the script is very successful.

In the subsequent conversations, work out alternative content together with your patient for the dream elements experienced so far as negative. These alternatives should be emotionally much less or preferably not at all stressful. They can also be skills and experiences that turn the nightmare into a beautiful dream. There are no limits to the imagination of the patient and therapist here. The patient can be given a magic wand with which he can turn the lion into a mouse in his dream. Another possibility is to give the patient competencies that he can possibly use just as well in everyday life, such as quick-wittedness and cheeky turns of phrase. It is important that the new content fits the patient so that he can identify with it. The alternative action is now integrated into the dream script. The stressful sequences are therefore replaced by the positive developments in the script.

Try out these alternatives afterwards in an imagination if possible. The patient should find and feel his way into his nightmare sequence in his thoughts. Now read the modified nightmare script out loud. The patient should experience how the new action feels. Possible inconsistencies can be identified and adjusted in this way. Modify alternative course of action and elements until they feel consistent for the patient. To deepen the dream experience, a trance can be induced and thus the subconscious made more accessible.

Now comes the practice phase in everyday life. Guide your patient to carry out the procedure independently. Use different media, such as audio recordings, videos, pictures, comics, etc. Dealing with the modified nightmare script should be firmly anchored in everyday life to make it as easy as possible for the patient to practice regularly.

Table 3.25 Brief overview module: Nightmare modification

Indications	A specific nightmare that recurs with little variation
Contraindications	Psychotic experiences of the patient
Effectiveness	Well documented
Mode of action	The distressing dreams are changed so that they are no longer distressing
Treatment requirements	Knowledge of nightmare modification
Treatment goal	Less distressing dreaming, reduction in the number of distressing dreams

In this way, the new dream content is kept present in working memory and can be retrieved more easily during sleep. Patience is also required here. Even if the patients are diligent, it is possible that the first visible results only occur after months. Motivate your patient to stay with it.

Excursus: Lucid Dreaming
The technique of nightmare modification can also be used for lucid dreaming, also known as clear dreaming. When dreaming lucidly, the dreamer is aware that he is currently asleep and his experience is a dream. With this awareness, the dreamer can access conscious memory content from the subconscious and integrate it into the dream. For example, people who dream that they are falling can consciously allow that one can fly in a dream. In this way, the unpleasant feeling of falling is replaced by the pleasant experience of flying.

Many, but not all people can learn to dream lucidly. In the therapeutic context, a central element should be worked out of the dreams, which occurs in many nightmares and never occurs in waking life, or is extremely unlikely, such as running and not getting anywhere, being naked in public, falling, being swept away by a tsunami, etc. The dreamer can recognize these elements as a dream that he can change through his imagination. From a race on the spot, a relaxed break can become, from a nakedness in public, an everyone-is-naked, from the falling a flying, from the tsunami a great surfing wave, etc. Here too, patients and therapists are not limited in their imagination.

The patient should also train this modification as well as possible in everyday life, so that these strategies can be implemented safely in sleep.

Lucid dreaming should not be excessive or for fun. The dream content is important for processing the events of the day, for emotional regulation and memory formation. A permanent artificial influence from outside can disturb these processes and possibly lead to emotional and memory problems.

3.5.5   Module: Dream(-Trauma) Therapy with Eye Movement Integration (EMI)

Since nightmares are experienced as subjectively threatening and burdensome in a pathological sense, almost any therapy can be used that is also helpful in post-traumatic stress disorder (PTSD).

First, a dream diary is used here in spoken or written form. In the subsequent sessions, the dream content is examined for patterns. Unlike the previously mentioned techniques, the found dream experiences, emotions and cognitions are now described with emotionally neutral terms and sentences. If the patient regularly dreams of wanting to run away from a lion and not being able to move, the concrete sentence could be: "I run away and don't get anywhere. The lion is behind me." After 2–3 accurate sentences or word groups have been found in this way, which describe the dream situation well and trigger discomfort or fear in the patient despite their neutral formulation, the EMI exposure session follows.

You will find a detailed description of how sleep disorders can be treated with Eye Movement Integration (EMI) in *Sect. 3.9.1*.

▶   *The instructions for carrying out EMI described here are not sufficient to treat patients with this neurotherapeutic technique. A more intensive, multiday training is absolutely necessary for this.*

3.6   Third Wave of Behavior Therapy

3.6.1   Background

Psychotherapeutic techniques are constantly being further developed in order to do justice to the many different disorders, new trends, world views and social changes. Cognitive behavioral therapy in its current form has emerged in 3 essential stages. In doing so, on parallel branches, many specific and above all practice-oriented techniques were researched and developed to support the respective basic elements.

The Behavioral Phase
The basic assumption of the first stage of cognitive behavioral therapy, which took place in the 1940s to the end of the 1960s, is based on the mechanisms of learning theories. It was

assumed that human (problem) behavior was learned and manifested in habits and could eventually lead to mental disorders. By changing these dysfunctional behaviors, the symptoms of mental illness can be alleviated and even cured. Thus, psychology and psychotherapy clearly took the position of being a natural science, thus giving the starting signal for systematic research. Human behavior is replicable and therefore predictable with certain probabilities. Behavioral therapy developed parallel to psychoanalysis, which follows more of a philosophical principle. There were always controversies between the two streams.

The strength of pure behavioral therapy is that it can also motivate severely ill patients to simple behavior. For example, a severely depressed patient exacerbates his symptoms by not leaving the house and withdrawing socially. It is much easier to then guide the patient to meet with a dear friend outside of his own four walls than to work out cognitively why he feels so bad. Behavior can be "simply" executed. The task of the therapist is to offer appropriate behavior and encourage the patient to just try it out. Often there is (a small) mood improvement and the patient has taken a step forward in his recovery. The weakness of pure behavioral therapy is that the patients are not guided to reflect on why, for example, they withdrew and became depressed. Furthermore, to work purely behaviorally would be like a trial/error learning. That is why it was necessary to include phase two. The so-called cognitive turn came about.

The Cognitive Turn

At the beginning of the 1970s, it became increasingly clear that it was precisely the cognitive processes behind the dysfunctional behavior that had a strong influence on the development and maintenance of mental disorders. In the following 20–30 years, cognitive-behavioral treatment approaches were developed that did justice to this. There was no departure from behavioral approaches. Cognitive therapy elements were added for the purpose of cognitive restructuring. For the first time, the individual disorders were considered in detail and specifically. Targeted cognitive-psychotherapeutic treatment manuals were developed that aimed to guide patients in the reflection of their individual situation and to derive functional behaviors from this. Biopsychosocial models of development for the individual disorders could be derived. This should enable a "change of mind" and a new evaluation of the situation. However, one also came to the limits of cognitive therapy with the cognitive component of psychotherapy. A weakness of the purely cognitive therapy is that symptoms, situations and disorders are "thought through" to a certain extent, which is why it can be difficult for patients to take action. After all, it has to be "right" to act, which can hinder those affected by mental disorders from making progress. Above all, it takes a lot of strength, willpower and not least hope that things will actually improve with the new ways of thinking and behaving to give up established habits. A disadvantageous principle was also that only the current problems are considered and addressed directly in therapy for an effective therapy. The causes of the symptomatology were only included in the therapy for a few disorders, such as adjustment and stress disorders.

Third Wave of Cognitive Behavioral Therapy

In the 1990s, contextual aspects of the respective symptomatology were emphasized more strongly. Instead of wanting to "therapize" the disorder directly, patients should first of all accept it. Especially with cognitive observation and thinking, patients quickly get into their negative "autopilot". They live in their thoughts and, in addition to the few bad aspects of their lives, no longer recognize the many positive moments. Elements of mindfulness have become an important part of modern psychotherapy. Traditional and even spiritual therapy elements are increasingly used. Thoughts and feelings are stripped off, the here and now is important. The therapist and the patient come from the "problem-solving mode" into an exploratory, curious observation mode, according to the principle: "You have to have and get to know a problem before you can solve it." This way of looking can be very relieving, as it allows patients to arrive in therapy first. Empathy and validation facilitate the therapeutic work, as neither disputes nor discussions are necessary, as can happen in cognitive therapy with the well-known "yes—but". The clear strength of mindfulness-based psychotherapy lies in acting from the acceptance of the situation. This made it possible to have a completely new view of mental illness, as each symptom has a function. If you know this function, you will recognize the logic of the symptomatology and can also treat non-changeable facts, the dealing with financial problems, physical illnesses, childlessness etc. psychotherapeutically.

3.6.2 Module: Acceptance-Commitment-Therapy of Insomnia (ACT-I)

Overview (Table 3.26)

Background

The cognitive-behavioral approach (CBT) considers dysfunctional thoughts and behaviors and meets them with methods such as bed and sleep restriction, stimulus control and the rules of sleep hygiene. In addition, patients are instructed to regularly use relaxation techniques to reduce physical restlessness and tension.

From our daily treatment practice, we know that those affected are often people who have a full and thus stressful day-to-day life. It often seems difficult to incorporate additional tasks in the form of regular training of various relaxation and mindfulness techniques as well as physical activities into everyday life.

Even the conscious intervention in dysfunctional thoughts is strenuous and can be poorly automated. It is often not possible to completely and sustainably free the patients from their symptomatology with CBT. Since sleep disorders are often a seismograph for stressful events and difficult life phases, the symptomatology will reappear immediately as soon as there are stresses in everyday life. Therefore, it is more sustainable to work with patients to develop a new perspective from which new, committed options for action arise.

In Acceptance-Commitment Therapy (ACT), the focus is not on achieving a specific goal, but on exploring a possible path to a meaningful life. The focus is away from the disorder-specific symptomatology and towards a life as meaningful as possible. The patient is thus enabled to react flexibly instead of freezing in his symptomatology. The development of these skills makes it possible to act self-competently in other problematic situations and in the event of a relapse.

ACT is characterized by a mindful approach to oneself and one's symptomatology in the here and now. It is about exploring the entire situation, the illness, the symptoms, all the conditions (work, family, finances, housing, etc.) in their entirety at first. This results in committed action to deal with the situation instead of wanting to eliminate it with the pressure of a CBT. This

Table 3.26 Overview Module: Acceptance-Commitment-Therapy

Indications	Insomnia and sleep disorders, especially sleep perception disorders
Contraindications	Psychotic symptoms, suicidality
Effectiveness	From practical experience: very good
Working principle	Sleep disorder and overall symptomatology initially assume, rather than "treat away" them, committed action with the symptoms
Treatment requirements	Solid knowledge of ACT, techniques of mindfulness, self-experience desirable, corresponding conviction and value system of the therapist
Treatment goal	Mental flexibility, solution-oriented, get into action, welcome side effects are quality of life and satisfaction

mechanism is particularly important for people with sleep disorders, as pressure always creates tension and no one can sleep (well) under tension.

▶ With the help of Acceptance-Commitment Therapy, it is possible to build a mindful life environment together with the patient and thus also to let sleep happen as a natural cycle.

Basic Assumptions of ACT

ACT assumes in the sense of acceptance that not all suffering can be avoided in life and that psychological and psychosomatic symptoms occur to signal dysfunction, e.g. overload or misapplication. Sleep disorders often occur as a result of dysfunctional behavior and expectations.

In commitment, the engaged action for change, the patient's insight is reflected that he can improve his symptomatology responsibly. The core of the therapy of sleep disorders, especially insomnia, is the abandonment of the desperate effort to have to sleep.

The primary goal is—in contrast to CBT—not the direct influence on sleep quality, but the acceptance of the sleep disorder as a symptom of a problem complex. The patients are led with the ACT from fixed thinking and behavioral patterns to psychological flexibility. It is not a question of judging and behaving better about the situation, but of looking at things differently and behaving differently, whether profitable or not. This results in a variety of treatment options, which in turn can make use of the techniques of CBT and mind-body medicine etc..

Why is ACT so Helpful?

ACT is not a symptom treatment, but accompanies the patient to a meaningful life. Therefore, the treatment goals of ACT differ from those of CBT, which primarily aim at a reduction or elimination of symptoms.

- ACT facilitates making decisions in the therapeutic process and later in the everyday lives of patients. Making difficult decisions has already led to many sleepless nights.
- The ACT approach provides distance from symptomatology, which is very helpful in sleep disorders. The more thoughts patients make about their sleep, the worse it gets. However, through the "detour" into a meaningful and mindful life, patients still come to much better sleep.
- Patients are motivated by ACT to self-efficacy and thus change mechanisms and willingness to change are activated.
- The use of ACT leads to a better therapeutic relationship. Through accepting the situation, therapists and patients find a consensus from which therapeutic work is done. There are no cognitive disputes and verbal discussions in the sense of "yes—but". The social support of the therapist is used in particular.

ACT comprises six core processes that are recorded, structured and, if necessary, changed with the patients. For this content-related work, therapists may and should draw on their entire therapeutic repertoire, here creativity is required. For the treatment of sleep disorders, all therapy components mentioned earlier in cognitive behavioral therapy are helpful and can be perfectly integrated into an acceptance-commitment therapy. The therapy component mindfulness, which is introduced after this chapter, is essential.

The six core processes can be represented in a hexaflex model: each process is connected to every other and embedded in the patient's overall system. The goal of ACT is to create psychological flexibility and thus enable a healthy and restful sleep (Fig. 3.14).

1) Being aware in everyday life and seeing oneself in one's illness, with symptoms, problems and pain, is a necessary core process of modern psychotherapy. However, mindfulness does not only consider negative aspects of life, but rather discovers resources such as social support,

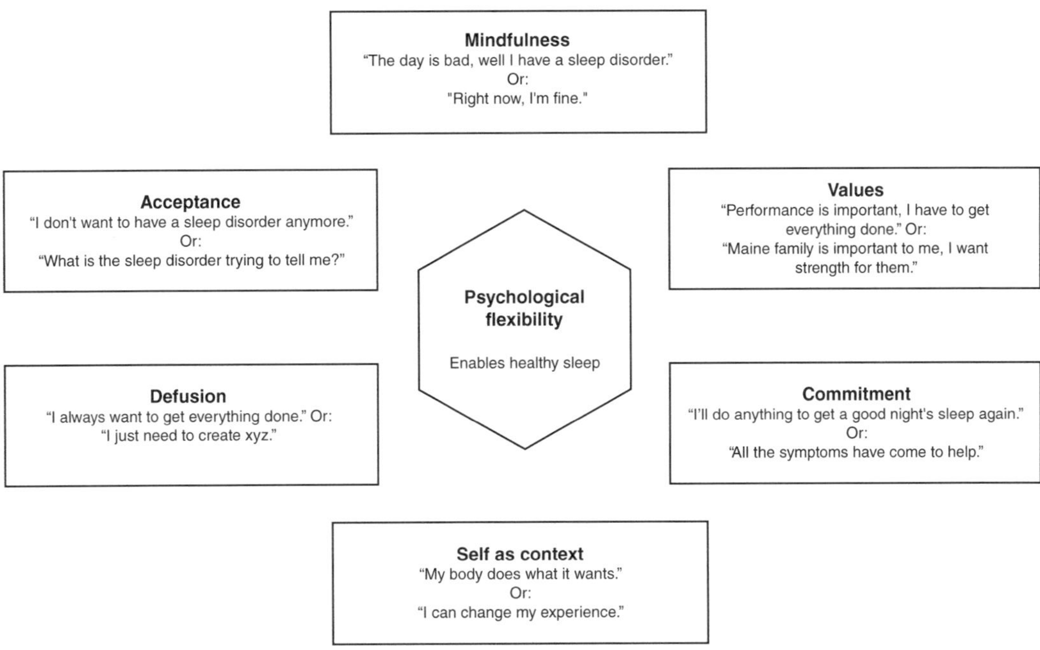

Fig. 3.14 The hexaflex model of non-organic sleep disorders

skills, experiences, resilience, etc., and makes them usable.

2) The acceptance of the sleep disorder and the overall symptomatology allows patients to let go and stop fighting. All previously used techniques, exercises and everyday rules may now be omitted: they have obviously not led to a better sleep.

3) The exploration and disclosure of the patient's fundamental value system allows him to look from the illness to a meaningful everyday life. It is important to remain realistic: we will not be able to be happy and painless all the time. However, it becomes clear that even with one or two bad nights, one can have a beautiful life.

4) Through defusion, the patient's field of view is opened up to something else and new. At first it is not about making things "better", but rather about doing them differently. For example, in the evening not to do autogenic training, then to take a relaxation bath and under no circumstances to watch television. It is about letting go and allowing the patient to fall asleep naturally by doing everything "wrong" in a paradoxical way. They may come to the thought: "Without my autogenic training I can't sleep anyway …". Without this pressure of expectation, relaxation can occur and the patient may fall asleep more easily.

5) It is very important for therapy to bring the patient's self-image closer as a context. Our self-image has been shaped throughout our lives by numbers, such as age, height, weight, etc., and "facts", such as our strengths and weaknesses, personality traits, skills and abilities, etc. With a inflexible and problem-oriented self-image, often dysfunctional emotional and cognitive patterns arise, which become fixed convictions: "I will never sleep well again. Without refreshing sleep I can not live a beautiful life." However, we are not our thoughts or our feelings. Emotions and cognition are rather a part of us. Therefore, one goal of ACT is to enable a flexible self-view and to be able to discover new perspectives again and again.

6) Commitment means "committed action". The task of the therapist is to guide the patient to committed action. The patients can "just do" things without thinking about how good and meaningful they are beforehand. Doctors and therapists can "heal" patients in the rarest of cases. They almost always rely on patient cooperation. From being treated, it becomes an action (Dobos and Paul 2019). Patients become their own doctors, gain self-efficacy and thus self-confidence and self-worth. For therapy this means giving the patient achievable homework and thus showing that he can do a lot without always having a doctor or therapist by his side.

Procedure—The ACT-Matrix

An important therapeutic tool for working out the psychodynamics is the ACT matrix. It is a diagram which captures in the horizontal, to what extent a patient "moves towards his values" (to the right) or "moves away from his values" (to the left). In the vertical, mindfulness is depicted, with which a patient goes through his life. If he lives without mindfulness in the "auto-pilot", this is shown in the downward arrow; if the patient takes his life mindfully with his five senses, this is shown upwards on the vertical axis. These dimensions are shown in Fig. 3.15. Fields 1 to 4 are worked out and filled in during the therapeutic conversation. This can be done in one session or accompanying the therapy process.

First, the sleep disorder, possibly also the overall symptomatology or another selected problem area is systematically analyzed and recorded on this matrix. Figures 3.16, 3.17, 3.18 and 3.19 show examples for this.

First, the current state is recorded, which usually provides information about the current perception of the problem area and possible, mostly dysfunctional coping attempts. Figure 3.16 shows a patient example for this.

In the following therapy process, realistic and above all very concrete solution paths are sought to find a value-oriented everyday life. An example of this is shown in Fig. 3.17.

Many patients with sleep disorders are so limited in their perception and thinking that they see nothing but their sleep disorder and the daytime symptoms associated with it. Therefore,

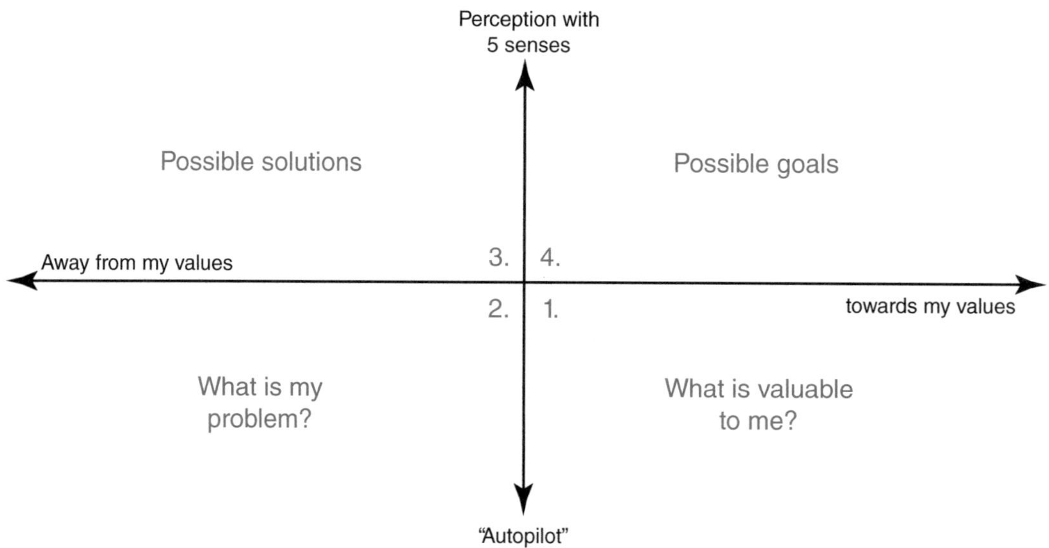

Fig. 3.15 The ACT matrix

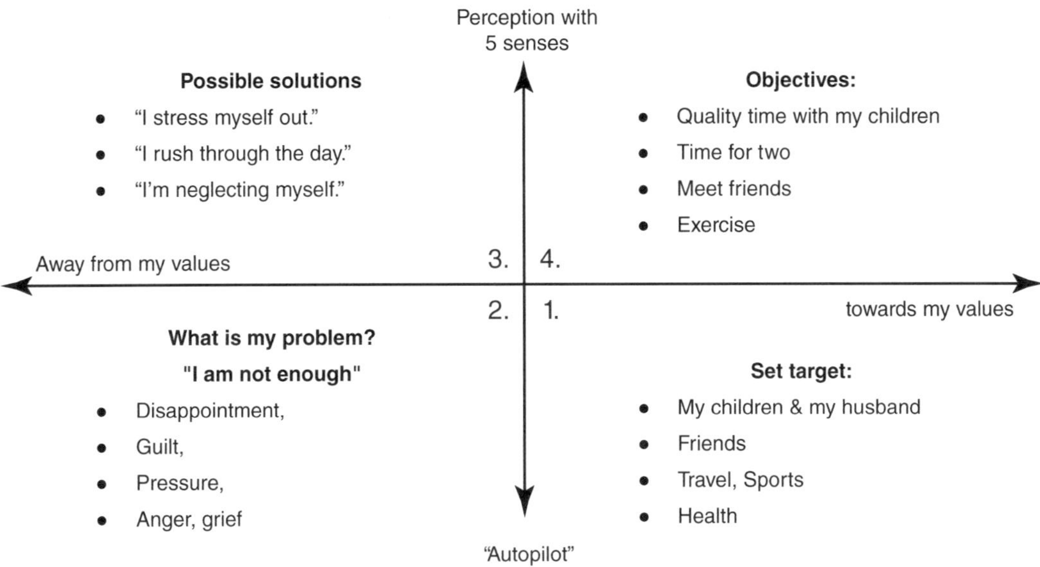

Fig. 3.16 General problem discussion of a patient with sleep disorders

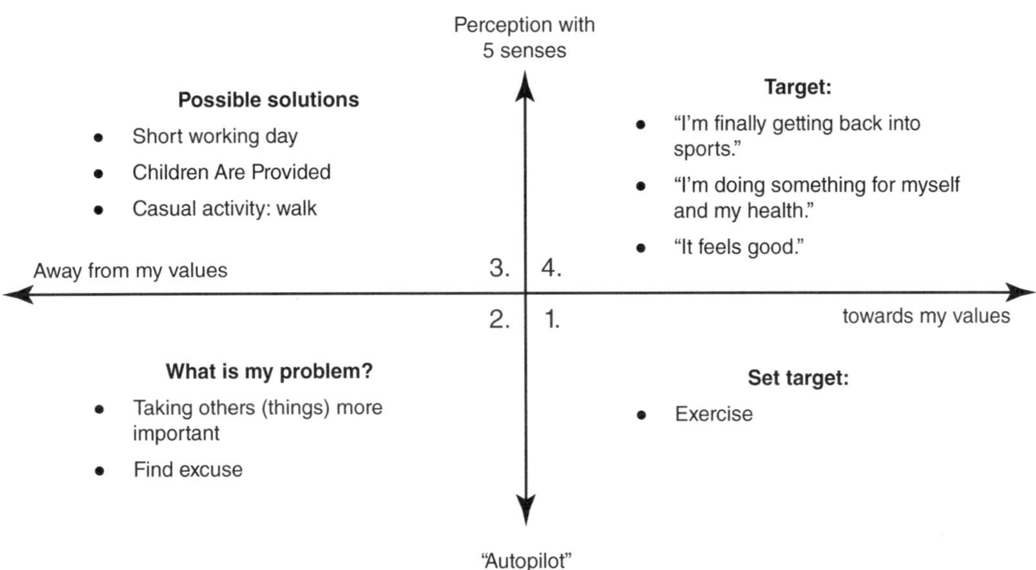

Fig. 3.17 Concrete solution plan of a meaningful action (exercise) of a patient with sleep disorder

they no longer make an effort to engage in meaningful activities and focus exclusively on their illness and what does not work, as shown in Fig. 3.18.

Even if the goal is to alleviate the sleep disorder and the associated daytime symptoms, the first step is to ask the question: "What would you do if you did not have a sleep disorder and

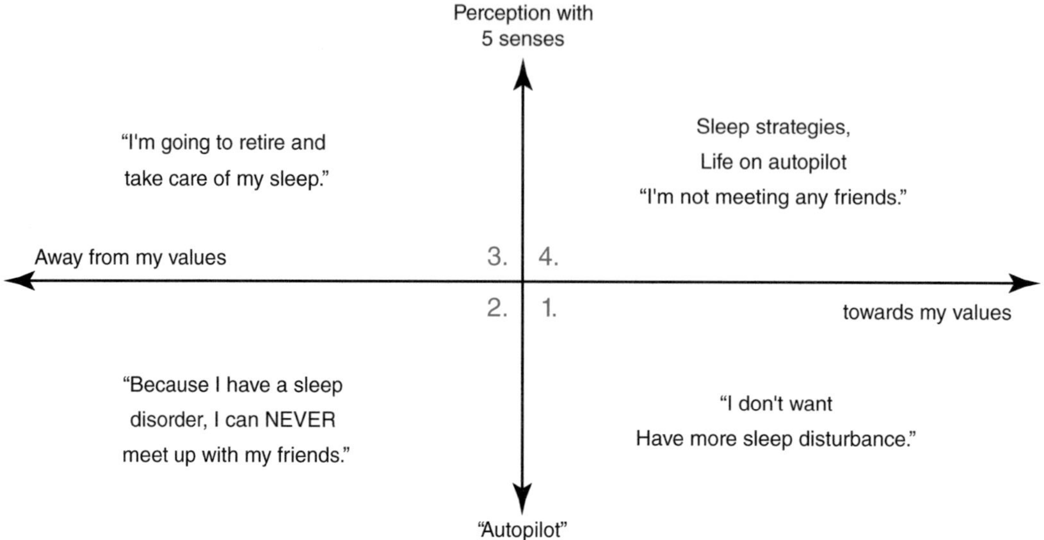

Fig. 3.18 Discussion of a patient's sleep disorder

were well rested?" Figure 3.19 shows the analysis of this question with the ACT matrix and shows how patients with sleep disorders can have fulfilling experiences.

It is important and necessary to work out a concrete starting point from the overall dynamics of the sleep disorder and the associated deficits. From the statement "Because I have a sleep disorder, I can *never* meet friends," it becomes "Even if I have a sleep disorder, I meet a friend today." The patients experience beautiful moments *with* their sleep disorder.

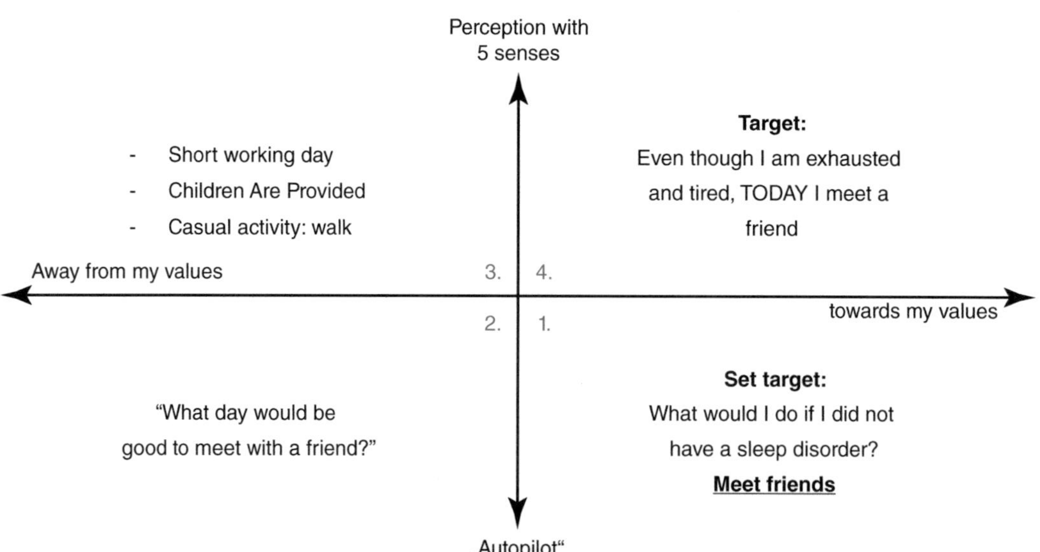

Fig. 3.19 Concrete solution plan of a meaningful action (meeting a friend) with a sleep disorder

Table 3.27 Overview Module: Mindfulness

Indications	Insomnia and sleep disorders, dysfunctional behavioral patterns, rumination in bed and general rumination tendency, stress-related overload, constant circling of thoughts, burden of many unfinished tasks
Contraindications	Psychotic symptoms
Effectiveness	Very well proven
Working principle	Binding the thoughts to the here and now slows down life, promotes the ability to enjoy and distracts from the brooding thoughts
Treatment requirements	Self-experience and theoretical knowledge of the therapist
Treatment goal	Interruption of dysfunctional schemata (thoughts, feelings and behavior), stress reduction, coming to rest, welcome side effects are relaxation and satisfaction

3.6.3 Module: Mindfulness

Overview (Table 3.27)

Note: This module was deliberately written in the first person plural. Doctors and therapists should also practice better self-care. You can also use mindfulness exercises for yourself to, for example, find yourself again at the end of an intense therapy session!

Background

Mindful moments are those in which we consciously direct our attention to the here and now without judging the thoughts, feelings, and situation. We thus come into contact with the living presence of the here and now without fleeing into the past (bitterness) or future (to-do lists).

It is astonishing how little we live consciously in everyday life and how quickly our thoughts jump. These facts apply to everyone equally. Therefore, it is important that therapists who want to use this technique first deal with it in self-experience.

The origins of mindfulness are in Buddhist meditation, the positive effects of which are now well researched. In the third (or new) wave of cognitive behavior therapy (CBT), mindfulness plays a fundamental role. On this basis, numerous new psychotherapy approaches have arisen, which have become and have also been further developed as part of cognitive behavioral therapy. Segal, Williams and Teasdale as well as Kabat-Zinn were the first to take steps in this direction, using mindfulness exercises to prevent relapse in depression and reduce stress (Segal et al. 2002; Kabat-Zinn et al. 1992; Meibert et al. 2006). Mindfulness-based therapy was also taken up in dialectical behavioral therapy according to Linehan and, as already described, in acceptance-commitment therapy according to Hayes (Linehan 1987; Hayes et al. 1999).

Mindfulness must be practiced well at first. Only then it brings inner peace and concentration on the only true moment, namely the here and now. Everything is deliberately considered without judging it. The process is observed of how thoughts, feelings and sensations arise and pass from moment to moment. This gives us a deeper understanding of the reaction to stress and problems and clarity about how and why certain processes take place. Mindfulness training is very successful in combating rumination and rumination loops. Those affected do not have to learn to control their rumination thoughts, which would give them even more attention, but they are allowed to let their thoughts flow, "only" have to learn not to judge them, but to accept them and also to let them go again.

Mindfulness can be Understood as:
- Spiritual principle
- Life principle
- Stress management
- Prevention, aftercare

- Natural scientific element in psychotherapy

Essential elements are:

- Breath
- Body sensations
- Thoughts
- Feelings
- Sounds, visual and tactile stimuli, smell and taste

▶ In summary, mindfulness means:

- Everything we perceive with our senses and cognitively
- Everything is considered intentionally without judging it
- Mindful moments are individual, present-oriented, non-judgmental, exploratory, and also liberating

What is to be Learned?
Concentration

The ability to focus attention on a specific object and maintain it. People with sleep disorders often complain of reduced concentration span. Mindfulness exercises can train concentration.

Mindfulness of thoughts, feelings, bodily sensations

In the treatment of sleep disorders, dysfunctional patterns of behavior and thoughts are to be systematically identified and changed. The mindfulness training should not automatically lead to old, non-functional reaction patterns. The body sends signals, these signals are to convey needs. Due to the high level of stress in everyday life, we often overlook these signals and only act when it is too late, e.g. when a sleep disorder, depression or somatic illness has already manifested. Those affected often report that when they have some free time, they often don't know what to do with it. Therefore, mindfulness exercises should also stimulate the creative thought process for dealing with the perceived situations.

Being present

Being in the here and now! People with sleep disorders often have their heads full of internal to-do lists, worry loops, and fears. The mindfulness exercises are intended to lead those affected away from these automatic thoughts and evaluations and towards a conscious here-and-now experience. Problems can only be solved when they occur! Nevertheless, many people in Western societies tend to make countless thoughts about the different possible solutions beforehand. In these considerations, often factors that influence the situations from the outside (other opinions, help or a change of the overall setting) are not considered. If problems are actually "ripe", their solution is often quite simple. Unfortunately, we all too easily get caught up in "could have, would have, should have" and try to find solutions even though the problem does not need to be or cannot be solved yet. For example, when we travel, we make countless thoughts beforehand about what we will need, whether we will forget something important, find our way around and understand the foreign language. In the stressful situation itself, we are then equipped with a hormone-related "primal over-attention" that lets us master everything we need (e.g. at the airport) without having to think much. Afterwards we are usually very exhausted because body and mind had to perform at peak levels, but in the situation we were fully present and nothing distracted us.

With regard to sleep disorders, the wakefulness in bed that is experienced as stressful can be used actively as a mindfulness exercise. Patients can make use of this time by mindfully perceiving this situation: "I am lying in bed. I feel the mattress under me. I feel the blanket on me. I see outlines of the window. I smell the detergent with which my bed linen was washed. I hear cars driving passing by on the street." The association "awake in bed = stressful and unpleasant" is dissolved and space is created for neutral or even positive associations that are built up as part of the therapy.

Acceptance/Non-Aversion

Many people tend to ponder whether situations and events are good or bad. We often fail to realize that we cannot change the existence of the situation because it is outside our area of influence. It is then advantageous to accept the situation instead of rejecting it. This is usually the case when patients "desperately" try and make a great effort to fall asleep, but they cannot. At this moment, they completely lose control of their sleep behavior. To regain this, it is possible to approach oneself and the situation mindfully and to perceive everything without judging it. In some cases, this is enough to achieve the relaxed state of wakefulness necessary for falling asleep. During the day, situations in which we cannot change anything anyway can be used for mindfulness training, such as when we are stuck in traffic, waiting in line at the supermarket, making coffee, etc.

Letting go

Mindful experience should lead out of the usual dysfunctional spiral of sensations, evaluations and actions. Breathing out is letting go in a natural way. Even negative aspects of our lives serve a purpose. So sleep disorders can be understood as a symptom that something is wrong. Then the cause of the sleep disorder is far outside of sleep itself. If we recognize and also accept this cause/function, we can better detach ourselves from the associated negative feelings and satisfy the need expressed by this function in a functional

way. For this, it is necessary to grasp the entire dynamics of the patient's sleep disorder and his life, to let go of the sleep disorder itself and to look for a solution in a completely different place. An example of this is the effectiveness of the *paradoxical intervention (Sect. 3.4.14)*: If the patient lets go of the desire to fall asleep, he falls asleep paradoxically.

Being instead of doing. There is no goal orientation, no state to be achieved. Therefore, mindful moments can be used well in bed, in the moment of wanting to fall asleep. One *is* simply and has nothing to do anyway.

Procedure

For training at home, the patient should first look for a quiet place where he is undisturbed. The fewer distracting stimuli there are in the room where the practice is taking place, the better it is for mindfulness.

▶ *It is important to note that the upstream mindfulness training should not take place in bed. The bed is for sleeping and not for training. Only when the patient has felt outside how mindfulness feels and he can control it, this technique may be practiced in bed.*

In addition, the bed should not be chosen for mindfulness training, as it is often difficult for those affected to distance themselves from the usual performance thinking ("I have to succeed!"). Later, mindful moments are in principle possible everywhere. The goal of mindfulness training is to create mindful moments not only in the evening in bed, but also during the day to integrate into everyday life in order to build up a balanced rhythm. Mindfulness is also an attitude towards life that—depending on the intensity lived—has an influence on the experience and feeling of the patients, not only on their sleep.

A comfortable sitting position should be taken, preferably without leaning back. At the beginning, the attention should be directed to the breath, the heartbeat, an object or a body part (e.g. foot). If it wanders off, it should be gently redirected. The bodyscan, in which various areas of the body are "touched", is a very popular mindfulness exercise, but already requires a lot of endurance. People with sleep disorders are often very restless and performance-oriented. At the beginning, it can seem endless to be mindful for one or a few minutes. Many patients feel initially overwhelmed because the thoughts just do not stay where they should: with the breath, with the heartbeat or with the foot. That's not bad at all, quite the contrary: it is part of the process of becoming more mindful. If the patient notices that his thoughts have wandered off, that is exactly a mindful moment. Mindfulness training can seem very tedious and difficult: Motivate your patient to stay with it! Healthy sleep is hardly possible in our overstimulated world without targeted mindfulness.

The practitioner should, with reference to the breath, let all thoughts come and go again. All thoughts are welcome, even desired. If we become aware at some point that we are writing the shopping list in our heads, then going through the supermarket shelves in our minds and finally checking our account balance in our minds in case of credit card payment, then we are exactly in this moment mindful!

For example, if we focus all our attention on a foot, feel the sock that envelops the foot, feel the shoe that lies on the foot in some places and perhaps also presses, then we are aware of the pressure in a mindful way, but do not rate the pressure of the shoe on the foot as bad. Pain can also be perceived mindfully without being evaluated.

Since a psychological symptomatology is usually not so "loud" at the beginning, we have to learn to listen to a "whisper". The self-reinforcing cognitive programs (rumination, negative thoughts, dysfunctional attribution schemata) should first be considered mindfully—that is, consciously—and then left again.

You can also be very mindful of yourself and your surroundings when jogging or cycling. Mindfulness does not only mean meditation, but being in the here and now in every situation. There are wonderful and beneficial situations every day that we no longer perceive from "operational blindness". Children are much more mindful than adults, they have an eye for details and discover exciting new things every day. Adults should relearn this with mindfulness exercises.

In order to use mindfulness for upcoming mood swings, stress reduction or even falling asleep, it must be well trained. The goal is, whenever a negative thought or a negative feeling arises, to simply let it remain in the sense of "acceptance", to observe it mindfully and to react to it wisely through "commitment".

In the context of sleep therapy, the aim is not to carry out a basic mindfulness training with the participants, but to introduce them to the topic of mindfulness and make them familiar with it. Show how mindfulness can be learned using short practical exercises and adapt small exercises individually to the problems and everyday life of the patients. The feedback of the participants is the most important teaching medium for the therapist: the patients are the experts! For the instructions, you should formulate open questions that encourage participants to express suggestions, doubts, difficulties and concerns openly. Try to animate the participants to explore their own experiences with interest and curiosity.

- Mindfulness should be practiced regularly
- The exercises should be designed so that they can be easily applied in everyday life
- It is better to practice for three minutes regularly than not to practice at all

- Do not overload your patients by expecting them to concentrate for hours every day; this is not feasible for most of them and is just another stress factor

The core principle behind mindfulness exercises:

- The body sends us signals
- These signals are supposed to convey needs to us
- The perception of these needs has been lost in the stressful everyday life

To introduce the topic, you should collect ideas and find out to what extent there are any previous experiences:

- Do you know mindfulness training? Do you have any experience with meditation?
- What is mindfulness training? What do you imagine it to be?
- Why might it be important for you?

In order to assess how mindful your patient may already be in their everyday life, you can have them fill out the questionnaire FB 03: Self-test: How mindful am I? (Fig. 3.20). It contains certain questions.

It is important to explain in detail what mindfulness training is and how it can be used effectively against sleep disorders. For this purpose, feel free to use nNformation Sheet IS10: Mindfulness.

Sheet 11: Mindfulness Exercises can be given as homework. It offers your patients small exercises for everyday life. Here you will find four short exercises that can be applied directly in the therapy session. This gives your patient a first impression of how mindful moments can feel.

Four Short Mindfulness Exercises

These exercises are very well suited to illustrate to the patient what is meant by mindfulness training. Read the sentences slowly and with a evenly soft emphasis. Leave pauses between the sentences so that the participants have enough time to "feel into" them. The instruction will be particularly good if you repeat the content in your own words.

Exercise 1: The Feet

- Have you thought about your feet today? We trample around on our feet all day and need them for every step, but we hardly pay any attention to them. That's about to change:
- How do your feet feel today?
- How are your feet positioned right now? Are they standing up straight or lying on their side?
- Are your feet bearing your weight right now or are they just lightly touching the ground?
- How do your shoes feel around your feet? Are they loose or tight?
- Are they pressing or are they comfortable?
- Do you have a pebble in your shoe or a wrinkle in your socks?
- Are your feet warm or cold?
- How big do your feet feel?
- How heavy do your feet feel?
- Can you feel your toenails? How do they feel?

Post-exploration:

- How dwas it for you?
- What were you thinking about?
- What did you feel?

I often do several things at the same time.

(1) (2) (3) (4) (5) (6)

Much of what I think and do happens automatically.

(1) (2) (3) (4) (5) (6)

I often have difficulty concentrating.

(1) (2) (3) (4) (5) (6)

I often don't notice the small happiness in everyday life.

(1) (2) (3) (4) (5) (6)

I often don't feel tension until it manifests itself as physical pain.

(1) (2) (3) (4) (5) (6)

Sometimes I'm so lost in thought that I don't even know how I got from point A to point B.

(1) (2) (3) (4) (5) (6)

I often interrupt my conversation partners.

(1) (2) (3) (4) (5) (6)

I often eat so fast that I don't really taste what I'm eating.

(1) (2) (3) (4) (5) (6)

My score: ______

8 to 16 points: You are already very mindful in everyday life, keep it up!

17 to 32 points: You are often not in the here and now. Find mindful moments and experience more quality of life.

33 to 48 points: You run through your life on "autopilot" most of the time. More mindfulness will help you feel better and also sleep better.

Fig. 3.20 Questionnaire FB 03: How mindful am I?

Exercise 2: The Taste Experience
- The patient receives a candy/a piece of chocolate.
- Please take a close look at your sweet:
- What shape does it have?
- What color does it have?
- How is the light reflected or absorbed?
- How does this candy feel in your hands?
- Is it soft or hard?
- Is it rough or smooth?
- How heavy is it?
- Now unwrap your candy and pay close attention to how that feels.
- Is the paper easy to remove?
- Does the paper rustle or is it completely smooth?
- How does your candy look now? What shape does it have, what color does it have?
- Now take your candy in your mouth and taste and feel!
- How does your candy taste, how does it feel?
- Does the candy taste different today than usual?

Post-exploration—please report:

- How was it for you?
- What was different than usual?

Exercise 3: The Simple is Extraordinary—Drinking a Glass of Water

The patient is given a glass of water.

- Please take a close look at your water glass:
- What shape does it have?
- What color does it have?
- How does light reflect in glass and water?
- What do you see through the glass and water?

- What colors do you see?
- How does the glass feel in your hands?
- Is it soft or hard?
- Is it rough or smooth?
- Is it cold or warm?
- How heavy is it?
- Now take your water glass to your mouth and pay close attention to how it feels.
- How does the glass feel on your lips?
- Now take a small sip and taste and feel!
- Take another sip and let it flow slowly and broadly over your tongue.
- How does the water taste?
- Salty, sweet, bitter, sharp, mild, neutral?
- Let water flow between your teeth.
- Now take a big sip and feel it running down your throat.
- Where is the water right now?
- Do you feel it in your stomach?
- Does the water taste different today than usual?

After-exploration—please report:

- How was it for you?
- How did the water taste?

Exercise 4: Sensory Walk (Adapted from Kabat-Zinn et al. 1992)

This exercise can be done very well outdoors. In addition to mindfulness training, it can also be used as a eutony therapy (pleasure therapy) at the same time by enjoying a small piece of nature (if available in the vicinity of your practice) and fresh air. Make sure the patient has enough space in all directions and can not seriously hurt or injure anywhere.

- Now just start walking in the direction you want to go, at the pace you want to go.
- Walk and shake off all the annoying thoughts of everyday life.

- Now focus only on what you see.
- All other stimuli are turned off.

Let the patient walk for a short time.

- Now close your eyes and focus on all the sounds. Listen!
- Let the patient walk for a short time.

Keep your eyes closed and focus on everything you can feel.

- On your feet: are you wearing anything or does anyone touch you?
- How does that feel?
- Let the patient walk around for a short while.
- Keep your eyes closed and focus on everything you can smell.
- Do you smell the furniture/grass/plants/ … ?

Let the patient walk around for a short while.

- Now open your eyes and focus on what you see again.
- What do you see now?
- Do you see things differently than at the beginning of the exercise?

Let the patient walk around for a short while.

Post-exploration—please report:

- How was it for you?
- Could you get into it?
- Please estimate how much time has passed during this exercise.

(Time is often overestimated, which illustrates the deceleration through mindfulness.)

Since many of our patients are used to "running on autopilot" through everyday life, many are not aware that they automatically assess numerous situations as stress-inducing. With a mindful attitude towards these situations, it is even possible to neutralize or even positively evaluate unpleasant moments. Mindfulness exercises in these moments can even serve to relax.

In Worksheet WS 19: Mindfulness instead of stress, it is explained in detail how your patients can find moments of mindfulness and relaxation in everyday life between all the unconscious and stress-inducing situations (Fig. 3.21).

3.6.4   Module: Hypnotherapy

Overview (see Table 3.28)

Background

The term hypnosis derives from the ancient Greek and is derived from *hypnos* (sleep). Therefore, it is hardly surprising that hypnosis can be very effective as a therapeutic agent in sleep disorders. In 1795, hypnotherapy was mentioned for the first time in Scotland by James Braid with a focus on clinical aspects. At that time it was called "concentration of attention and increase of imagination" (Braid 1844–1845). This work was taken up by Milton H. Erickson (1901–1970) and established hypnotherapy in the treatment of mental disorders (Erickson 1954). Erickson is still referred to as the "father" of modern hypnotherapy. He also used these techniques for himself, because he suffered from chronic pain since his illness with polio, and thus improved his symptomatology.

Hypnotherapy is a method with many different applications. For example, it influences pain perception and mood. In addition, coping strategies can be trained and mentally challenging situations can be prepared using suggestion in a safe and relaxed environment. For the therapy of sleep disorders, the achievement of deep relaxation is of great importance.

The clinical effect of hypnosis is based on trance induction and imagination. The patients are put into a deep relaxation, which is often not achievable with full consciousness. Despite the trance, the patients are awake and responsive.

WS19 - Worksheet: Mindfulness instead of stress

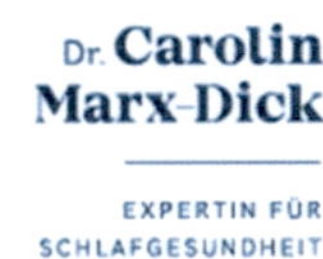

We are used to evaluate everything we perceive automatically and immediately.
Depending on the basic mood, we then evaluate positively or negatively.

For example, if we are cheerful and calm, it is no problem at all if the bus leaves right in front
of us. In UrLaub, if the next bus comes only 2 hours later, we could still eat an ice cream in
peace, for example. However, when we are stressed and in a bad mood, we evaluate the
same situation with a more favorable outlook very negatively, e.g. when the bus drives away
from under our noses in everyday life (even if the next one would already be there in 10
minutes).

In a mindful moment, you are NOT evaluating what you see, hear, smell, taste or feel. You
merely take note of it.

The evaluation is what stresses us the most in everyday life:

Fact	Rating
It's traffic jam.	I hate traffic jams. I want it to go away.
It is raining.	I hate when it rains. I want it to stop.
My best friend has a new boyfriend.	I think he's terrible. I want her to realize that.

1

**To perceive the facts mindfully is to take in a piece of information.
POINT.**

When we add an evaluation, we automatically have to deal with an (unpleasant) feeling.

Next week you can learn how to turn stressful moments into mindful moments by not
evaluating them. In most situations we can't change anything anyway, so no action or
negative evaluation is necessary.

Examples of situations in which you steer through your life in autopilot could be: you have
just run out of coffee and have to prepare new coffee, your computer has crashed and you
have to restart it, your child does not come down from the climbing frame although it is very
late, you have to go to the toilet again, there is a long queue in the supermarket etc.

Fig. 3.21 Worksheet WS 19: Mindfulness instead of stress

WS19 - Worksheet: Mindfulness instead of stress

Please think through your daily life and write your stress triggers in the table

Stress triggers	How do I experience this situation?	What is the actual situation (without my evaluation)?	So I am mindful in this moment.
Car ride to work	*Traffic jam, it's loud, everyone is honking, I'm pressed for time, I'd like to push the cars aside, I feel bad.*	*I am sitting alone in my car.*	*I feel my po on the seat, my hands on the steering wheel, I see the traffic and wait until I can step on the gas pedal again. [or] I accept the situation (since I can't change it anyway).*

2

Fig. 3.21   (continued)

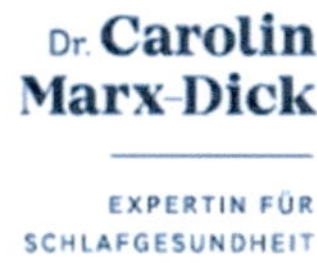

WS19 - Worksheet: Mindfulness instead of stress

Mindfulness and cortisol

A balanced daily routine is important for healthy and restful sleep. Our everyday life is largely determined by the hormone cortisol. It is our performance hormone and enables us to cope with everyday life. Cortisol is often referred to in the vernacular as "stress hormone." The course of cortisol fundamentally follows a natural rhythm. In people with sleep disorders, this rhythm is often disturbed.

Therefore, a day should be designed so that the cortisol level is in a healthy balance. An important information is: negative emotions mean stress. Permanent stress causes disturbed sleep. Therefore it is important to avoid unnecessary evaluations. Because with an (automatic) evaluation you do not change the situation, but only your feeling of the situation. An increased cortisol release starts a stress reaction in your body, which has no benefit, but rather endangers your health and your sheep.

Est is traffic jam! The car is stopped, you can not drive! You could honk, bite the steering wheel, push, swear, yell at people, find out why there is traffic jam, etc.. But you could also turn on some nice music, call your parents, or just indulge your thoughts. There will be traffic jam until it is over.

Design your time mindfully and it will be more enjoyable than being on autopilot.

You will surely ask yourself NOW 😊 how this is supposed to work: only perceiving and not to evaluate. At the beginning it is not so easy either. However, with a little practice you will3 succeed.

Now choose one or more situations that you would like to consciously **perceive** differently in the coming week. Maybe set up reminders to actually remember to be mindful (e.g. cell phone timer, etc.).

Situation: without my evaluation?	So I am mindful in this moment.

Fig. 3.21 (continued)

Table 3.28 Overview Module: Hypnotherapy

Indications	Insomnia, nightmares, pavor nocturnus
Contraindications	Psychotic experiences of the patient or acute mania
Effectiveness	Well documented, depending on the patient's suggestibility
Working principle	The target is the subconscious; thus, unnoticed tensions can be picked up, and relaxation can be helped
Treatment requirements	Knowledge of hypnotherapy
Treatment goal	Solving of subconscious tension, correction of subconscious dysfunctions

Peaceful images are created in the mind's eye, in which the patient should let go of all thoughts, feelings and thus any tension as much as possible. If the trance induction is successful, the patient is relaxed. This state promotes the willingness of a person to change. That is why hypnotherapy is used very broadly to support fundamental changes in life, e.g. in smoking cessation, in addiction or in personality disorders. Increasingly, elements of hypnotherapy are also used supportively in general psychotherapy of affective and anxiety disorders, in psychosomatic complaints and pain, in eating disorders, in obsessive-compulsive disorders, in stress disorders and, of course, in sleep disorders. Hypnotherapy promotes creativity and provides access to new solutions.

With the transition into the trance, consciousness is reset and patients give up a large part of the control. Therefore, hypnotherapy is particularly suitable if there are no intervention options on the surface. Many sufferers find it difficult to give up or change long-established habits. Often they think that this is not possible. With the help of hypnotherapy, patients can learn to feel that there are possibilities. Therefore, this method is also suitable for very compulsive patients who strive for perfection.

The idea of a movement in a trance state can activate corresponding muscle groups and, for example, raise an arm with pure "imagination". But also more complex actions can be "practiced" mentally (Krakow and Zadra 2006). We direct our actions through our thoughts. With the help of hypnosis, we can also cause physical changes or change long-automated patterns of behavior by means of these thoughts. However, the patients are not manipulated, but only functions and mechanisms that are already contained are activated or blocked.

The suggestibility of the patient and a trusting relationship between the patient and the therapist are the most important requirements for the underlying trance induction. However, hypnotherapy should not be used isolated as a therapy equivalent, but should be embedded in a comprehensive therapy.

For patients with sleep disorders, self-hypnosis can be an important tool in everyday life. Often, the lack of relaxation, worries and fears are the reason for the maintenance of sleep problems. With the help of self-hypnosis, patients can apply deep relaxation in everyday life and promote behavioral changes with positive thoughts and key words. However, self-relaxation techniques must be learned and trained before they can be used effectively. Self-hypnosis is not a quick fix. Many patients initially experience failures and bring bad experiences into therapy.

During the trance, changes and expansions take place in subconscious structures. That is, the patient will only notice that something feels different and he may not be able to exactly name what has happened and what has changed. A debriefing of the trance is important. However, it is not necessary and rather disadvantageous to analyze the events during the trance in detail. Release your patient from the session in a "tidy" state as a matter of principle, but also allow for a longer after-effect of the exercise. This can only happen if there are still open internal processes that can continue. In the next session, everything that has happened can be discussed in detail and integrated into everyday life.

Procedure

Since you have already got to know your patient well at this point in time, you should and can design the trance very individually. Try not to read from a script. This introduction to a state of relaxation is the starting point for deepening relaxation instructions and the use of the trance.

Under the use of suggestion, the patient is system-immanent to deep relaxation. This is done by means of communication between patient and therapist. The therapist helps the patient through verbal support to enter a trance state. Often, only a few hypnotherapy sessions are sufficient to achieve an effect. It should be done slowly and gradually. "Practice" first with your patient to enter the trance state, and give him the opportunity to build trust in this technique.

The following phases are necessary for the preparation of the actual hypnotherapy:

Rapport

The rapport serves to build a trusting relationship between patient and therapist. Since hypnotherapy is only embedded as a possible component in the therapy of sleep disorders, the relationship should already be established before the use of hypnotherapeutic techniques.

Focusing

At this point, the patient's attention should be bound in order to gradually turn it away from everyday life and towards internal events. A good preparation for this process are mindfulness exercises.

Trance Induction and Deepening

The attention is turned away from the external to the internal perception. This internalization should be maintained for a certain period of time to stabilize it. This means that the patient should not be torn out of this concentrated exercise at every little distraction (e.g. noise from a passing car). This can be done by continuing the mindfulness inward or quite classically by imaginations on uninteresting ideas (e.g. numbers). Use pictures and metaphors that are tailored to the patient and with which he can identify.

The therapist conveys to the patient his changed consciousness. Here, for example, the therapist can suggest that the patient is completely relaxed, that the eyes can no longer be opened or that no pain is felt anymore etc. The patient should breathe calmly and evenly, feel the relaxation and maintain it.

Trance Induction

Instruct your patient as follows:

- Take a comfortable body position, lean back and allow your eyes to close. Maybe that's right now, maybe later.
- Feel your breath as you inhale and exhale.
- Feel how the chair/sofa supports you, feel the touch with the chair/sofa, the floor, your clothing and your shoes (can be taken off).
- Listen to the silence. What can you still hear?
- Smell in the room. What do you smell?
- Taste the taste on your tongue. What does it taste like?
- Feel into your body, feel the even breathing and the relaxation. Feel how heavy the chair supports you.
- All thoughts are allowed. They are allowed to come and go.
- Feel the relaxation, feel how …

Pacing

The therapist draws on personal resources and individual features of the patient that enable him to anticipate the change. Pacing takes place repeatedly in the hypnotherapeutic process. The patient is accompanied in accepting the desired new and trusting it.

Suggest the Following to Your Patient
- Your bed is a place of rest and relaxation, and you will fall into the same deep relaxation this evening in bed.
- Even if there are still tasks to be done (tidying up, writing e-mails, etc.), you can relax. Offer your patient an authentic fantasy journey into his own home, in which he is relaxed and there may be mountains of laundry or dishes and he is still relaxed.
- You can also be relaxed and fall asleep after an argument.
- You are safe and secure.

Leading

The patient is "led" by the therapist in the desired direction. The therapist intervenes in the behavior to be changed, the thoughts or emotions and suggests a change in previously discussed behavior, thoughts or feelings. In this phase, the actual hypnotherapy begins. It is important to know the exact dynamics or cause of the sleep disorder. Now you can encourage your patients to release the blocks that are not accessible in the clear state of consciousness. This can be the achievement and maintenance of deep relaxation in general ("Look how relaxed you are"), or dysfunctional habits and ways of thinking can be worked on.

Leading and pacing alternate.

Suggest the Following to Your Patient
- It's not bad to lie awake in bed.
- He is also allowed to be awake and relaxed in bed and enjoy the situation.
- Even if the patient feels that he has not slept a wink all night, the body gets the sleep it needs.
- He can endure the tension that arises when he does not complete a task perfectly today.
- Further individual suggestions should be worked out in advance.

The offered fantasy journeys are to be worked out in detail in advance and checked for consistency in the conscious state. In trance, these journeys can penetrate deeply into the subconscious and have a lasting effect.

Reframing

The symptoms and experience are "re-framed". During this treatment phase, a partly very surprising change of perspective of the situation, evaluation or view takes place.

Reorientation

After using the trance, it must be withdrawn step by step. The patient should arrive back in the here and now and orient himself spatially and temporally. Plan enough time for this phase.

Use your own words as much as possible for the instruction of the individual steps. Speak quietly and evenly in your dialect, with your voice melody and your volume. Since your patient knows you, he would be irritated if you suddenly spoke completely differently.

▶ The module hypnosis presented here is not a basic instruction for the performance of hypnotherapy. In order to carry it out in a good quality and safety for the patient, intensive further education offers should be used.

3.7   Mind-Body-Medicine

Mind-Body-Medicine (MBM) is a new and at the same time old holistic view of the human being in his everyday life. It takes into account

- all somatic processes in the body from the perspective of homeostasis,
- all psychological and spiritual processes with a special focus on mindfulness,
- the embedding of the human being in his social everyday life, the corresponding life phase and everyday tasks.

The MBM uses very diverse therapeutic tools that pursue three principles:

- Prevention: The best protection against disease is the preservation of health.
- Salutogenesis: The best way to stay healthy is a balanced lifestyle, including restful sleep.
- This includes a healthy diet and health-promoting behavior, such as sufficient exercise and avoidance of chronic stress.

Conventional medicine has achieved great things in the last century. In particular, emergency medicine, and in diseases that until recently would have been fatal, diagnostic procedures (including early detection), medications and treatment techniques have been developed that can cure, halt or delay the progression of disease and greatly improve the quality of life of those affected. So it was necessary to establish many individual areas in order to be able to do justice to the flood of necessary knowledge and skills.

With the progress of science, the individual disciplines also differentiated within themselves. At the beginning of the twentieth century, the specifications were so complex that the holistic medical consideration of the human being was cut between body and psyche. It experienced a great turning point at this time. With increasing trend, body and "head" diseases were considered separately from each other and hardly any psychosomatic connections were taken into account. Now, at the beginning of the twenty-first century, the reintegration of psyche and body begins with the help of mind-body medicine.

3.7.1 Mind-Body Therapy

Mind-body therapy approaches (mind-body interventions; MBI) are therapeutic interventions that aim at the interaction of brain, soul, body and behavior and the goal of using the mind or the mind in such a way that various interventions have a positive effect on the whole person and lead to an improvement in health. The "National Center for Complementary and Alternative Medicine" (https://www.nccih.nih.gov/) has set itself the task of systematically investigating this approach and developing practice-oriented, multi-professional treatment models. MBI have been increasingly in the focus of scientific interest in recent years in the field of sleep disorders. There is a range of scientific evidence that suggests that mind-body interventions can have a positive effect on sleep quality. In the course of the scientific consideration, above all, interventions such as body psychotherapy, yoga and meditation, movement and nutrition were focused on (Neuendorf et al. 2015b).

Mind-body therapy has a great challenge to meet compared to traditional treatment approaches: The active participation of patients is indispensable, so they must be well motivated and encouraged to "stay with it". Patients are thus quasi their own therapists. They learn the tools for this in the corresponding interventions. However, this also has an enormous advantage: The patients are accompanied from a disease management to a health management. This protects, among other things, preventively against recurrent courses, as is typical for many mental disorders and also sleep disorders.

3.7.2 Modules of Body Psychotherapy

Overview (Table 3.29)

Body psychotherapy is a variety of therapeutic methods that treat mental and physical dimensions of human experience equally. The underlying fact is that the body and the psyche are an inseparable unit. Most body-oriented psychotherapeutic methods use the perception of one's own body as a way of gaining access to subconscious processes. Body psychotherapy works experience-oriented and uses humanistic and depth psychological methods (Young 2006; Geuter 2006).

In therapeutic interest, body sensations and certain body processes that occur automatically and are therefore not consciously perceived are particularly important in body psychotherapy treatment. It is assumed that these experiences

Table 3.29 Brief overview of Modules: Body Psychotherapy

Indications	For all somatic and mental illnesses, for the prevention of diseases
Contraindications	Possible restrictions in the use of individual techniques for specific symptoms; e.g. certain yoga exercises cannot be performed for certain orthopedic diseases
Effectiveness	Very well proven
Mode of action	A holistic adaptation of lifestyle can lead to symptom relief and self-efficacy maintenance of health
Treatment requirements	Knowledge of mind-body medicine
Treatment goal	Holistic health, self-responsible action

often already exist since childhood and shape the physical organization into adulthood. So if, for example, a core conviction such as "I am not enough" arose in childhood, according to the assumptions of body psychotherapy, this will also be expressed many years later and independently of what is actually "achieved" through subconscious body processes and sensations. In performance situations, there may automatically be a physical tension, accompanied by negative emotionality and also the thought of possibly not being enough, although there is no evidence for this. The body psychotherapy approach focuses on changing these internalized assumptions by evoking alternative sensations on the conscious physical level (Geuter 2006; Geuter 2009).

There are a variety of body psychotherapy techniques that can be summarized in three categories:

- therapy through physical touch
- therapy through physical exercise
- therapy with body awareness

The use of specific techniques depends on the respective needs of the patients and must be clarified together in close consultation between therapist and patient (Geuter 2019). It is especially important for psychotherapists to know that patients may indeed be touched in order to allow them to feel, or to guide various body psychotherapy exercises.

Examples of Body-Psychotherapeutic Techniques Recognized by the European Association for Bodypsychotherapy (EABP)

- Hakomi—Experiential body therapy based on mindfulness (Ron Kurtz)
- Integrative body psychotherapy—Integration of body and psyche (IBP, Jack Lee Rosenberg)
- Client-centered talk and body psychotherapy—Integration of talk psychotherapy (GFK, Carl Rogers), focusing (Eugene Gendlin) and body psychotherapy (Wilhelm Reich) and other body-oriented methods
- Body-centered psychotherapy IKP by Yvonne Maurer
- Yoga-Psychotherapy

There are large research gaps in the effectiveness of body psychotherapy for sleep disorders. Some studies have shown positive effects of a body-psychotherapeutic treatment for depression and generalized anxiety disorder (Röhricht et al. 2013; Maurer-Groeli et al. 2005). It could be shown that patients with comorbid sleep disorders can also benefit from a body-psychotherapeutic treatment of the underlying primary disease in terms of sleep quality and sleep latency. There are no overviews of the effectiveness of body psychotherapy for sleep disorders

(Geuter 2019). Therefore, more research is needed.

In order to be able to apply body-therapeutic approaches, it is important to have a deep training in the respective technique. There are various offers for this.

In this book I would like to give you a short introduction to Yoga-Psychotherapy for Insomnia (YPT-I), as I have developed it in my practice for my patients.

3.7.3 Module: Yoga-Psychotherapy

Overview (Table 3.30)

Background

Yoga is a philosophical Indian doctrine that is thousands of years old. It includes a series of different exercises, body positions (asanas), meditation (dhyana) and systematic breathing exercises (pranayamas), which aim to integrate body, mind and soul. Yoga is based on a "body-mind" that performs all functions and processes in a flowing manner. Yoga is therefore the best mind-body medicine.

> **Hatha Yoga, a Classical yoga Stream, is Based on Five Pillars**
> - Asana (body position and movement)
> - Pranayama (breathing exercises and life energy)
> - Relaxation (and sleep)
> - Nutrition
> - Meditation (positive thinking)

These five pillars can be integrated into each other in the sense of mind-body medicine and should be included in therapy as holistically as possible. It is very important not to overburden the patient and to offer the individual elements in small steps, initially with very concrete exercises and instructions in mini-interventions.

Movement and breath are taken up with the basics of yoga. Yoga includes movement, that is, holding and stretching exercises in the asanas as well as dynamic movement sequences in the vinyasas. The strengthening of life energy (prana) takes place through targeted pranayama, that is, breathing exercises. Nutrition is given a separate chapter in this book, which has a huge impact on patho- and salutogenesis. Meditation is intended to lead to positive thinking. The basic function is to accept things, let thoughts flow without evaluation and thus find more serenity.

> ▶ Yoga is not a sleep program that patients go through and then sleep better.

Yoga should be an everyday companion that offers a suitable yoga exercise or sequence as well as a breathing technique for every day and life situation.

Since a sleep disorder affects body and mind and only a union and synchronization can result in a healthy sleep, the described properties of yoga have increasingly come into focus in recent years. In this context, yoga is not only understood as therapy, but also serves to a large extent for diagnosis.

Table 3.30 Overview Module: Yoga-Psychotherapy

Indications	Mainly unrest states, pain, tension and too little mindfulness
Contraindications	Possible restrictions in the execution of certain yoga exercises (e.g. in orthopedic diseases)
Effectiveness	Very well proven
Mode of action	By matching breathing, body exercises and mindfulness, mental and physical rhythms come back to each other
Treatment requirements	Knowledge of yoga therapy (a yoga teacher training is not necessarily required)
Treatment goal	Relaxation, deceleration, enjoyment

There are a number of studies that have examined the influence of yoga therapy on sleep. Especially in patients with depression or remitted cancer, a positive effect of yoga on sleep has been shown (Mustian et al. 2013; Wang et al. 2014). Various clinical studies have also shown positive effects of a yoga practice in patients with insomnia. Accordingly, a regular performance of a standardized yoga routine had a positive effect on the total sleep time, the sleep efficiency, the latency to sleep, the wakefulness after falling asleep and the sleep quality (Khalsa 2004; Hariprasad et al. 2013; Bankar et al. 2013).

The positive effect is mainly due to the reduction of physiological and cognitive arousal, which is increased in patients with insomnia. In addition, the various yoga exercises increase the strength of the respiratory muscles, which results in a higher oxygen saturation and tissue permeability. Since known sleep disorders, such as sleep apnea, are associated with a lower oxygen saturation, yoga exercises can lead to an increased oxygen saturation in combination with improved sleep.

Diagnosis with Yoga

The execution of the asanas (body positions), vinyasas (dynamic exercises), pranayama (breathing) and meditation (attention and cognition) can provide clues to the current symptomatology of the patient. Here, the yoga therapists are dependent on the help of the patients, because they have to feel and name in mindful self-reflection what is happening to them at the moment, both on a physical and on a psychological level. Occurring body symptoms can also be very informative for the diagnosis of mental disorders.

When Performing the Asanas and Vinyasas:
- Tensions with or without pain
- chronically increased muscle tone
- This can be explored in more detail in the therapeutic conversation and additionally treated with cognitive-behavioral techniques.

During the movement sequences:

- Avoiding the exercises or only partially performing, strongly slowed down or accelerated exercise sequence, blockade when continuing etc.
- Blockades in dealing with feelings
- Feeling rushed or extreme (depressive) slowing down
- Through "postures" in somato-psychological expression: body posture of a depressive, anxious, angry, defensive

During the breathing techniques (pranayama):

- Breathing can be used to determine whether natural breathing is allowed and the diaphragm is used or whether breathing is forced through the breathing muscles. This gives an indication of a possible chronic activation of the sympathetic nervous system, i.e. the fight-or-flight mode.

Meditation:

- The meditative part can be used to observe whether and how the patient perceives the moment, or whether cognitive overload and strong tension states occur and "switching off" is only difficult for the patient.

Psychological symptoms:

- Strong feelings and emotional reactions such as anger, despair, fear, disgust, overwhelm, hopelessness, etc. can be shown.
- Expression of this in behavior: Aborting the exercise, remaining or freezing in a position, having to expend great effort to maintain and carry out etc.

- Cognitions: Beliefs (also from childhood development), verbal injuries, but also praise

Physical symptoms/behavior

- Sudden emotional reactions: Crying, screaming, scolding, moaning, whimpering, but also kicking, hitting etc.
- Physical stress reaction
- These physical symptoms and behavioral reactions should be picked up and explored in more detail in the therapeutic conversation. Here, cognitive-behavioral techniques can be very helpful.

Pleasure, joy and relaxation:

- The body is able to relax and perform the movements smoothly and without pain.
- Breathing can flow freely, in relaxation the diaphragmatic breathing and in tension the intercostal breathing is used.
- Meditation: The patient is able to perceive and enjoy the moment in the here and now.

Therapy with Yoga

Yoga for a healthy sleep does not mean doing yoga in bed or in the bedroom. Rather, it is important to take up the various situations and scenarios that the affected persons encounter in everyday life and to offer yoga (-therapy) sequences in order to catch the overall symptomatology of patients with sleep disorders and their comorbidities. Various aspects must be considered here:

People with Sleep Disorders are Often Very Performance-Oriented.
- They have a very full day and have little time to practice.
- They often do things in a perfectionist and under a certain performance

pressure. This can also be seen in yoga and is dysfunctional here.
- In yoga courses it is possible that patients compare themselves with other participants and thus become more firmly anchored in their dysfunctional patterns of thought than released from them.
- They are often not used to doing things for themselves, so they would rather do yoga for "others", possibly also as a favor for you as a doctor or therapist.
- They can hardly feel themselves and their body, do not know their own needs and ignore body sensations. This can lead to injuries.

It is Important to Perform the Right Exercises at the Right Time.

In order to create favorable starting conditions for a good night's sleep, it is not enough to "shut down" in the evening. You should live according to the natural hormonal sequences throughout the day:

- Revive energy and physiology in the morning
- Balance stress and demands during the day
- Regulate energy level, excitement and tension in the evening
- The hormonal cycles described earlier in the book should be taken into account

Requirements for the Yoga Sequences
- The different forms of sleep disorders should be addressed. Each sleep disorder has its own symptoms and thus also different requirements.
- The duration of the sequences should be individually adapted to the patients' everyday life: from 3 to 90 min.

- The effort should also be individually chosen by the patients depending on the form of the day, time and still pending tasks: from very gentle to actually tiring in the evening and shortly before going to bed.
- It is important to pay attention to the respective exercise level of the patients. Many people believe that you have to be or become very mobile for yoga. This is a misconception: No matter how flexible or strong the body is, in yoga it is about the individual perception, which can also happen in very small position changes. At the beginning of yoga therapy, the demand should be very low at first. If the bar is set too high, many patients will have difficulty practicing regularly in everyday life. The power comes with the practice, the mobility is actually genetically anchored.
- The patients should and can learn with the appropriate exercises to feel their body and fatigue in the evening.
- People with sleep disorders, especially insomnia, have a chronically elevated cortisol level, so the yoga sequences should be adapted to the healthy day.
- Yoga should never take place in bed and preferably not in the bedroom. The bed is for sleeping (and tired reading). No training sessions should take place in the bedroom due to conditioning processes. Yoga can stimulate the physiology so that the patients start to sweat.

Good places for yoga exercises can be in the living room and office, preferably on the balcony or terrace. Yoga sequences in nature are very beneficial.

You don't need a yoga mat for all exercises. Many asanas are done standing and some also sitting. Even an office chair can be used as a seat for yoga.

Adaptation to the Different Requirements of the Time of Day
- **Morning Yoga:**
  - In general, one could say that one should practice yoga in the morning as much as possible. Morning yoga will support the awakening and, if a good sequence is put together, allow for a stress-free start to the day. Therefore, the exercises should be adapted to the respective starting situation.
  - On a morning after a bad night, people with sleep disorders need a gentle start to the day. It is then important to arrive relaxed on the mat, but without the risk of falling asleep again. Therefore, meditation should be omitted and rather pranayama, that is, invigorating breathing exercises, should be used to wake up the energy. People with comorbid depression can suffer from a morning low. Here then there is a special requirement: The overcoming to start the exercises must not be too great and sequences should be offered which increase the drive and the mood. A gentle energization with an increase in energy level during yoga practice is favorable.
  - On a morning after a good night, the sequence can be more powerful and prepare for an active day. Here the "sun salutation" known to many is always a good option.
- **Yoga during the day:**
  - In order to enable patients to get started with yoga therapy, it is important to first demonstrate the effectiveness and feasibility in full-time work and family life with mini-interventions. A key component of these short practices is to also encourage

patients to be mindful of stress so that they have the opportunity to feel the difference between the sensations "with mini-intervention" and those "without mini-intervention". Only then does the willingness to incorporate these exercises consistently and intuitively increase: "Now I could do exercise XY, it would do me good." There should therefore be short sequences that awaken and refresh.

- 3- to 5-minute instructions for concentration lapses, neck tension, leaden fatigue, which may possibly be carried out "unobserved" before important meetings, are favorable.
- Relaxation and stretching exercises as preparation for a power nap, which can be very well designed with Yoga Nidra.
- Sequences for an active lunch break should allow you to eat before or after the practice at noon.
- In order to overcome the "mid-day slump" and to activate in the last minutes before the end of the working day and the subsequent leisure time, sequences should also be offered.
- Longer yoga sequences (always taking into account the cortisol level):
  In the time between 5 and 8 p.m. our cortisol level should be adequate and not elevated. These hours are, as already described in the 1st part of this book, our "happy hours". For this period it makes sense to develop yoga sequences that positively influence our emotions. Laughter yoga is very suitable at this point.
- The yoga class in the late afternoon/early evening at home or in the course can be designed with different intentions:
  - Relaxing after work and calming the nervous system

- catching and calming restlessness states after overstimulation and multitasking
- getting energy for the rest of the day
- physical training with muscle building, which may also be sweaty.
- If you are very closely involved with (small) children, you can also do yoga together with the children or as a family.
- **Yoga in the evening:**
  - In the early evening, many sufferers of sleep disorders have to fight enormous fatigue attacks and the associated short nodding off. This causes enormous stress and an increase in stress hormones. Therefore, it makes sense to offer refreshing and relaxing mini-interventions of 3 to 15 min in length to patients for these situations. These can still be integrated into everyday life without completely falling out of family life.
  - After a day's work, many people are plagued by negative emotions such as anger or dissatisfaction. Patients with comorbid depression sometimes experience depressive episodes in the evening. A common phenomenon is then also a diffuse ascending anxiety, for example about the coming night, failure or existential fears. In short: man becomes thinner-skinned and needs yoga sequences that lovingly catch these emotions in self-care.
  - This yoga practice can be accompanied by directed mindfulness exercises and meditations. To be able to end the day satisfied, thoughts of gratitude and the formulation of wishes are of great use. They create distance from the stressful everyday life and guide the thoughts towards a fulfilling life, as described in more detail in Acceptance-Commitment-Therapy (ACT).

It is important to generate positive thoughts about the coming night at this time. Many people with sleep disorders are afraid of the nights. As self-fulfilling prophecies, these fears can actually cause bad nights.

To fall asleep, we need a relaxed state of wakefulness and fatigue. Therefore, in the late evening, yoga sequences are in demand that actually generate fatigue or make it feel with mindful self-holding. In addition, targeted asanas for relaxation, which are mainly contained in Yin Yoga.

Directly before going to bed, there should only be sequences of up to 5 min to leave the day behind and shake it off.

This is where you can specifically loosen tense muscle groups again, such as the shoulder-neck or jaw area. Mentally, satisfaction should then be focused. Here, mantras can be helpful, which can be thought or spoken:

> **Examples**
> - "There is nothing left to do."
> - "Nobody wants anything from me."
> - "I enjoy the peace."
> - "If I fall asleep, it's good, if not, it's also good."

Individual asanas can also be helpful at night to fall asleep again. It is important here to only take a certain relaxing position, to apply a calming breathing technique and above all to turn off the light.

As yoga therapy, specific asanas can also be used to address body symptoms.

The most common causes and symptoms of non-organic sleep disorders include chronic shoulder-neck tension, -cramps, -blockages and -pain. Most people are also professionally bound to sedentary activities, so they often have pain or weak muscles in the back, stomach and hips. With targeted exercises for stretching and strengthening, these problems can contribute to the relief of symptoms. Yoga therapy can also be very successful in jaw tension and teeth grinding.

3.7.4 Module: Meditation

Overview (Table 3.31)

Background

Meditation is a form of mindfulness that is about improving concentration by consciously focusing on perception. Practitioners should be aware of the present moment without making a judgment. The ultimate goal is a sustainable positive change in thinking, feeling and experience.

▶ Mindfulness promotes self-awareness. For example, early warning signs of the body or needs can be better recognized, and action can be taken in the prodromal phase, that is, before manifesting symptoms of illness.

In addition, mindfulness promotes creativity. Through "mindful boredom", people can perceive new impulses for enjoyable action that have a positive effect on satisfaction and, as a result, sleep quality. Through the presence in

Table 3.31 Brief overview module: Meditation

Indications	Restlessness, rumination, neurocognitive deficits, especially in concentration and memory problems
Contraindications	Psychotic experiences
Effectiveness	Very well proven
Working principle	By focusing on the here and now, thoughts and brooding loops are interrupted and inner unrest is alleviated
Treatment requirements	Knowledge of meditation
Treatment goal	Deceleration, improvement of neurocognitive deficits

mindful moments, sleep-depriving loops and recurring thoughts can be interrupted and an over-stimulation of the nervous system can be prevented. In addition, mindfulness teaches to accept the fact that one is not sleeping and not to demonize it. This leads to a reduction in stress, a lower cortisol release and thus promotes sleep.

There is a lot of scientific evidence for the positive effect of meditation on sleep (Nagendra et al. 2012; Black et al. 2015; Neuendorf et al. 2015a). Researchers assume that mindful meditation changes various cognitive and emotional processes that are related to sleep quality. For example, it could be shown that meditation reduces emotional reactivity and rumination while simultaneously promoting the processing of current experiences. This results in better sleep quality and a reduction in sleep disorders and their symptoms (Rusch et al. 2019).

This is based on the influence of mindful meditation on various brain and body functions. Meditation, for example, leads to a regulation of automated excitability, to dysfunctional thoughts and to chronic stress. Physiological measures such as blood pressure, pulse, heart rate and gastrointestinal processes are flexible for the respective requirements. This is accompanied by changes in specific brain regions associated with body perception.

In addition to the generally sleep-promoting effects, recent studies have shown, among other things, the positive effect of meditation programs in the treatment of chronic insomnia. There are also indications that meditation helps people with chronic insomnia to reduce the use of sedative or hypnotic medications, such as benzodiazepines or non-benzodiazepines (Thimmapuram et al. 2020). In addition, many people who meditate regularly report feeling fresher and more awake during the day.

The motivation of the patient is an important factor. There are still many skeptics regarding the effectiveness of meditation. Many people are still of the opinion that this is rather a purely spiritual practice and should not be used as an intervention in the treatment of a disease. There is solid evidence for the effectiveness of Mindfulness-Based Stress Reduction (MBSR), which was developed in the late 1970s by molecular biologist Jon Kabat-Zinn in the USA. Numerous studies confirm positive effects on various somatic and mental illnesses (Dobos and Paul 2019). Sleep was often rated as improved as a side effect. Thus, there were indications that increased practice is associated with improved sleep, reduced sleep disorders and more flexible cognitive processes.

▶ *In yoga and meditation, it is not about believing something, but about experiencing something.*

Another important finding is that with a deep meditation practice, delta waves can be generated in the brain wave pattern. Delta waves only show people in deep sleep (exceptions are brain diseases). This shows that through meditation a deep relaxation can be found which can favor sleep and partly even replace it.

In the classical text of yoga sutra it says that 30 min of yoga nidra can replace a two-hour sleep. Nidra means sleep. This does not mean that yoga nidra should precede sleep, but rather it is a "substitute for sleep" that can be used very well as a power nap during the lunch break. The statement in the Yoga Sutra finds scientific support: If delta activity can be caused in the brain by the deep meditation of yoga nidra, this is equivalent to the deep sleep phase of a sleep cycle, which can last between 80 and 110 min in adults.

Procedure

There are now numerous sound and video instructions on the portals of the health insurance companies, relevant websites (e.g. Youtube) or apps for meditation practice. With the innovation in the statutory health system, so-called digital health applications can now be prescribed and reimbursed by health insurance companies by doctors and therapists. The market is developing at a rapid pace. Due to the usefulness of mindfulness and meditation in everyday life, new products are constantly being developed here.

If you want to lead your patients during a session, it is important to set a goal for the meditation. Rest images, nature, security, etc. are favorable.

An advantage of an individual meditation instruction is that you can pick up your patients where they are: in their very personal dynamics and problems, with their very personal needs and issues. Leading a meditation is not witchcraft. Rather, it is an imagination that aims to capture his senses and focus on a topic. You should speak with a calm voice and slowly. With increasing experience, you are certainly able to offer "spontaneous" instructions during a session. At the beginning you can read the meditations and practice.

Excursus: Working with Mantras
Background:

Influencing thoughts directly is difficult, but not impossible. With the help of "mantras", a helpful thought can be implied directly. In-depth analyses, disputes and discussions are not necessary here. A mantra is something that is repeated: a pictorial pattern, a melody or a sentence, almost like a record with a skip. In psychotherapy, mantras can be used in many places. The meditative painting of mantras or the design of patterns with stones, shells or other materials is relaxation and training of mindfulness in one step. Singing the same syllables or sums of melodies over and over again calms the nervous system. And the "talk" of belief statements transforms words into thoughts. By constantly repeating the words and sentences, they become anchored in memory and can be quickly activated in difficult situations, either purely mental or also as spoken words.

If dysfunctional rumination thoughts are replaced by well-practiced and authentic mantras, the body's activity is slowed down and the sleep process is favored.

Procedure:

It is important that the patients believe the statements of the mantras. So they have to be authentic. It is not about lying to oneself, but about finding helpful thoughts that facilitate the dealing with difficult or stressful situations as well as relaxing or falling asleep.

The catastrophic and stress-inducing thought "If I don't fall asleep right away, I'll stay awake all night" can be replaced with the use of mantras by another, also correct thought: "Even if I don't sleep, I recover." Or: "If I fall asleep, it's good, if not, it's also good."

Mantras should be worked out in the therapeutic conversation. It is important to use the patient's words and to add as little as possible from the outside. Afterwards the mantras have to be internalized, for example with self-talk or even better through meditation with the mantra.

3.7.5 Module: Sleep-Promoting Nutrition

Overview (Table 3.32)

Background

Nutrition is an important factor for our health and thus also for our sleep. Already Hippocrates (around 370 to 460 BC) knew about the need for a balanced diet. He developed lifestyle plans for his patients that included a balanced diet and exercise. There are many different types of nutrition that are said to promote sleep. It is important to understand that not one specific type of nutrition generally has the best effect on sleep, but that nutrition should be individually tailored to the needs of those affected in order to have a sleep-promoting effect. Basically, it can also be said that it is not necessarily about nutrition, but rather about the digestion of nutrients for a restful sleep.

The Microbiome—The Gut Flora

The research of the microbiome, that is our gut flora, is currently in the focus of many research projects. Recently it has been found that gut bacteria have a significant impact on sleep.

Due to intensive research on the gut-brain axis, it could be shown that our microbiome has an influence on the central, peripheral and

Table 3.32 Brief overview module: Sleep-Promoting Nutrition

Indications	Severe exhaustion, feeling of being run down, unbalanced diet, overweight or underweight
Contraindications	None, but beware of certain food allergies or intolerances
Effectiveness	Very well proven
Working principle	By a balanced diet the microbiome (gut flora) is built up and balanced, possible nutrient deficiency is eliminated
Treatment requirements	Knowledge of a balanced diet
Treatment goal	More energy and drive, holistic health, self-responsible action

gut-nerve system via interactions with the immune system, the neuroendocrine system and the vagus nerve (Man et al. 2020). So the microbial metabolism is involved in the production of a large number of important neurotransmitters, cytokines and intermediates such as serotonin, GABA, dopamine, etc. (Li et al. 2018; Yano et al. 2015). These neurotransmitters and hormones regulate the sleep-wake rhythm, vigilance, relaxation, and sleep initiation and maintenance (Farré et al. 2018).

For example, an association could be shown between the composition of the gut microbiota and the duration of sleep (Holingue et al. 2020). The greater the diversity of bacterial strains in the gut, the greater the total sleep time and sleep efficiency. In contrast, with less diverse gut flora, nighttime wakefulness increased (Smith et al. 2019). When comparing the microbiota of healthy subjects and those with insomnia, significant differences were revealed in terms of structure, composition, diversity and functionality (Liu et al. 2019). It is assumed that there are bidirectional connections here, that is, the diversity has an effect on sleep and sleep affects the composition of the microbiome. These interactions also explain why a good night's sleep maintains health, but at the same time can cause sleep disorders and many somatic and mental illnesses (St-Onge and Zuraikat 2019).

On the one hand, insomnia seems to lead to functional and structural changes in the microbiome as well as to disturbed intestinal bacteria interaction. Also, a disturbance of the circadian internal clock can cause an imbalance of the intestinal flora ("dysbiosis") and changes or even the abolition of normal structural and functional fluctuations in the intestine. On the other hand, changes in the microbiome affect sleep. For example, the experimental administration of pre- or probiotics can change the intestinal flora in such a way that it has a positive effect on the natural course of sleep architecture (Liu et al. 2019). Against this background, it is hardly surprising that Farré et al. (2018) conclude that future treatment approaches to insomnia should also focus on positively influencing the microbiome and restoring the relative abundance of

individual bacterial strains to balance. Here, numerous targeted studies are necessary. So far, it has not been specifically examined to what extent the microbiome changes with a cognitive behavioral therapy (CBT). Another key question is whether a targeted sleep-focused dietary change or the systematic use of phytopharmacology can provide added value over existing treatment options in the S-3 guideline "Healthy Sleep and Sleep Disorders". However, practice experience shows clear positive effects of a targeted diet on reduced sleep latency and increased sleep quality as well as less daytime sleepiness.

Already the change of diet causes changes in the lifestyle of the patients. The organization of the procurement of food, the preparation of food and the mindful eating, the structuring of the day through cooking and meals bring deceleration and mindfulness into everyday life, as illustrated in the *case report by Mr. J. in the service section*.

Excursus: Digestion During Sleep

Orexin, a hormone, establishes a fundamental connection between food intake or digestion and sleep. The term "orexin" comes from the Greek language and means "desire" or "appetite." Orexin disturbs sleep by stabilizing the waking state by increasing body temperature, vigilance, and attention. In addition, orexin stimulates the feeling of hunger and thus has an appetizing effect, regardless of whether hunger is present or not. For many people with sleep disorders, a vicious circle arises from a lack of knowledge of these basic biophysical principles: after a late, carbohydrate-rich meal, the orexin level increases and promotes wakefulness. In addition, the appetite is increased. If the appetite is followed, more orexin is released and the cycle begins again. Since carbohydrates greatly promote orexin release, but proteins do not. So it is recommended to restrict carbohydrate intake in the evening and instead rely on foods with higher protein content (Binks et al. 2020).

In general, it can be said that sleep accelerates the metabolism. Since no new stimuli enter the digestive system at night, unless we eat something, the second and final digestion can take place peacefully. So from the food consumed during the day, which has already gone through the first digestion, new energy is generated for the following day during sleep.

Since the entire food intake—from appetite to the sight and smell of food, the chewing and swallowing process, the passage through the esophagus and stomach, to the further processing in the intestine and finally to the excretion—is hormone-controlled. It can also massively influence sleep. The function of the regeneration of the organ systems runs in homeostatic cycles in the sleep-wake regulation. In the waking state, the organs are challenged because performance, movement, transport, digestion, filtering, etc. must be carried out. This keeps the organism active and awake. In return, the sleep breaks are urgently needed for the organism to calibrate, "clean" and regenerate all body systems. If an organ (-system) is exhausted and urgently needs a break, we also feel this during the day with fatigue and exhaustion. For example, if we have drunk too little and the kidneys cannot work adequately, we also feel fatigue and exhaustion during the day. With sufficient fluid intake, this feeling can be alleviated. In the evening, however, we should not drink so much anymore in order to not stimulate the kidney function, which is to be regenerated at night. In the nocturnal final digestion, fluid is removed from the food mush in the large intestine in order to stimulate kidney function again.

The more diverse the intestinal flora is, the better the sleep quality and duration.

Melatonin, Nutrition and Digestion

A basic pacemaker for the sleep-wake rhythm is our "sleep hormone" melatonin. If we stay in bright light, there is only a small amount of melatonin in our circulation and in the darkness our pineal gland in the brain begins to secrete melatonin. Recently it has been discovered that melatonin is also produced in the intestine. The melatonin level in the gastrointestinal tract can exceed the serum concentration of the blood, controlled by the pineal gland, by 10 to 100 times. There it stimulates peristalsis and thus ensures good digestion. However, if the melatonin level is too high, digestion becomes slower and food remains in the intestine for too long. Then the food is still deprived of water and it can lead to constipation. In the winter months, when there is little daylight to inhibit melatonin production, it is therefore particularly important to drink enough and to move. Protein-rich evening meals also have a positive effect, as one gram of protein can bind up to 6 g of water, which is reflected in the smoothness of the food. The regulation of water balance is therefore also an important function of sleep.

Melatonin can only be produced if there are sufficient raw materials available for our sleep hormone to be produced. However, our body cannot produce these raw materials itself, they must be absorbed through food. First, serotonin is produced from tryptophan, vitamin B6, zinc and iron. Serotonin is then converted into melatonin and then secreted into the circulation. All these substances are mainly found in nuts, sprouts and seeds, meat, fish and seafood (Sanlier and Sabuncular 2020).

Food = Nutrition

As the name suggests, food should nourish us. This means that it should contain minerals, vitamins, proteins, fats, carbohydrates and fiber. For a restful sleep it is important to pay attention to when we take which food, how they are composed and how they are prepared. There are a number of studies that have shown a sleep-promoting or sleep-inhibiting effect of various foods.

For a sleep-promoting diet it is not enough to eat in the evening not too late and not too heavy. However, for a start in nutritional therapy with a patient, this can be a first point of attack.

Sleep-promoting foods for dinner:

- Light, warm, high-protein, and vegetarian meals
- Warm milk with honey
- Soothing magnesium-rich spices, such as cinnamon, cloves, and nutmeg
- Bananas
- Amino acid-rich nuts, such as walnuts, almonds, cashews

Sleep-disrupting foods in the evening are, for example:

- Heavy meat and sausage products
- Cold dishes
- Green salads
- Vegetables with a long digestion time, such as broccoli, spinach, leafy vegetables
- Mushrooms (hence the saying: "Mushrooms at night lie heavily in the stomach")
- Raw onions or garlic
- Alcohol
- Caffeine-containing stimulants, such as coffee or green/black tea

Fasting for a Better Sleep

There are also fasting methods and specific diets for which a positive influence on sleep has been proven. For example, the 16:8 fasting method has been shown to be particularly effective in reducing sleep disorders and early waking, as the body is given the opportunity during the longer fasting phase (14–16 h) to digest the food consumed during the day evenly and over a longer period of time. This represents a recovery phase for the body.

This benefits the liver in particular, as it switches to an "autophagy" mode. The term "autophagy" comes from the ancient Greek and means "self-consumption". During this phase, the liver cells actually break down their own components, primarily toxins and also carbohydrates that have not yet been stored, which are to be converted into fats for storage. This small "hunger phase" detoxifies the liver and thus sustainably supports health. Since fewer toxins are "stored" in this way, fewer such substances need to be broken down at night, which leads to a more restful sleep (Binks et al. 2020).

However, the 16:8 fasting method should not omit dinner. A full stomach doesn't like to sleep, but an empty one doesn't either. If the body gets a "hunger signal", it will be alert in order to be able to go in search of food again for evolutionary reasons. Going to bed hungry can cause sleep disorders and early waking in particular. Therefore, it is more advantageous to take a light early evening meal, for example to eat a warm and filling soup at 6 p.m. Breakfast the next morning can then be omitted or taken later in favor of an early lunch. With Information Sheet IS12: Interval fasting for sleep disorders, you can instruct your patients to try interval fasting.

Therapeutic fasting

Other methods of therapeutic fasting also have a healing effect in principle and can thus bring great benefits for health. However, I primarily do not recommend this treatment to sufferers of sleep disorders, as this can initially worsen sleep even further. In addition, it must be borne in mind that the mere thought of giving up meals may already cause stress, and this should be reduced by means of therapy. Therefore, I recommend therapeutic fasting only when the sleep quality has improved significantly. Therapeutic fasting should not be carried out in everyday life, but rather during an inpatient or outpatient fasting cure with medical and therapeutic supervision.

Since hunger, as mentioned, makes one vigilant, an adequate fast is helpful against daytime sleepiness. This is a tightrope walk: On the one hand, a slight hypoglycemia can sharpen the senses, increase concentration and make fatigue less noticeable. On the other hand, severe hypoglycemia leads to exhaustion. If there is not enough fuel available, of course no energy can be provided. Severe hypoglycemia or hyperglycemia should be avoided in general. With simple sugar (industrial white sugar in sweets and ready-made meals), the body gets a quick rise in blood sugar. This should be immediately buffered by the pancreas, which is why a lot of insulin is secreted to process the sugar. On the one hand, this leads to excess fat deposits, on the other hand, one gets into an even stronger hypoglycemia, into a vicious circle.

It is always advisable to plan one's meals well in order to always have enough energy available from the nutrients. Long-chain carbohydrates, as found in whole grain products, or (preferably plant-based) proteins satisfy hunger for a long time and provide good energy without landing on the hips.

In the area of specific nutritional diets, so-called diets, positive effects on sleep could above all be shown for the Mediterranean whole food diet (Campanini et al. 2017):

- Lots of fresh and seasonal fruit and vegetables
- Little meat and sausage, but fatty fish like salmon, herring or sardines
- Healthy oils with simple or multiple saturated fats, like olive oil, flaxseed oil or walnut oil
- Plant-based protein from legumes
- Whole grain products with complex carbohydrates
- Nuts and seeds
- Herbs and spices

Figure 3.22 gives an overview of which foods should preferably be incorporated into the daily diet in the corresponding amount.

Many people find it very difficult to give up habits, even if they know exactly that they are not good for them. Therefore, mere enlightenment about a healthy lifestyle is not enough. In holistic therapy of sleep disorders, it has proven to be helpful to give as concrete instructions for action as possible and in this case meal plans.

On Information sheet IS13: Healthy nutrition for a refreshing sleep, important information about a fundamentally beneficial diet is presented.

With the worksheet WS 20: My diet plan—part 1, you can first sensitize your patients with regard to their eating habits. An excerpt from the worksheet can be found in Fig. 3.23.

With the worksheet WS 21: My diet plan—part 2, you can develop a concrete meal plan together with your patient in the further course of therapy, which should be clearly visible to the patient in his everyday life (e.g. on the fridge). To be-all and end-all of is the practicability:

1. Eating is enjoyment, so it must taste good.
2. The menu must fit into the patient's everyday life.
3. Nutrition must allow exceptions for a good quality of life.

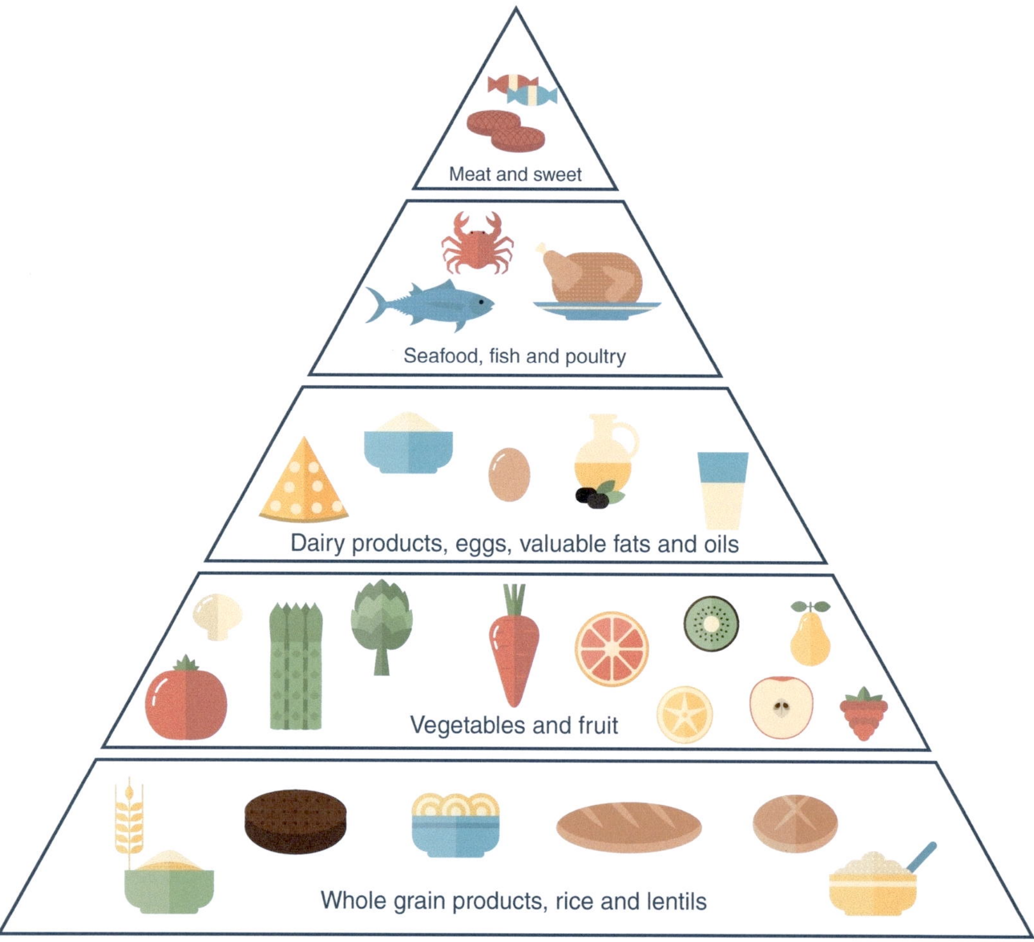

Fig. 3.22 The food pyramid

Try to either reduce the foods that prevent sleep or avoid eating them after 4 pm.

Food	Sleep disturbing?		When can I eat this?
	😊	😟	
	😊	😟	
	😊	😟	

Please observe your dietary changes for four weeks and evaluate afterwards:

- *How are you doing with it?*
- *Do you feel restricted?*
- *Do you feel comfortable in your skin?*
- *Are you more efficient than usual?*
- *Has your weight changed?*

Fig. 3.23 Excerpt from Worksheet WS 20: My nutrition plan—Part 1

To 1 Applying a healing diet is a temporally limited health application. In such a time it may be necessary that the patient has to do without beloved food. However, a change of diet should be permanent. Therefore, it is necessary to integrate favorite dishes and delicacies into everyday life.

To 2 People with sleep disorders usually have an extremely busy day-to-day life. Stress is often the cause of poor sleep. Therefore, it is important not to cause even more stress with the therapeutic interventions. Complicated diet plans and recipes that don't end up filling you up can actually create even more stress. A meal plan doesn't have to be perfect! It just needs to be implementable and balanced. Maybe the food in the cafeteria isn't the healthiest. However, there is a hot meal available every day. Often, there is a choice of different dishes and the patient can choose "the healthiest" one. In larger cities, there are numerous delivery services that have now gone with the trend of healthy eating. These can be a good alternative for a balanced midday meal. Cooking seems very time-consuming for many people. However, it is worth it to start with your patient on a specific attempt, for example, by cooking one extra portion that he can take with him the next day, once a week at first. It is important and necessary to be able to eat in peace. Even very digestible meals can cause indigestion and stomach ache if they are gulped down in a hurry or eaten during a strenuous work lunch. Try to work out as specifically as possible what the patient can eat, when, where and how. Worksheet WS 21: My Nutrition Plan—Part 2 can be a good basis for this and can also be given as homework to some extent.

To 3 In order to ensure that your patient changes his dietary habits permanently, it is important to allow "exceptions" on a regular basis. Clear rules help here to keep enjoyment in moderation without falling back into old patterns right away. For example, there may be one piece of chocolate allowed per day, a little alcohol may be consumed on weekends (not too late at night), and cake may be eaten once a week.

3.7.6   Module: Movement and Sport

Overview (Table 3.33)

Background

Numerous studies have shown that regular physical exercise improves sleep quality significantly. Exercise helps against insomnia and early waking, and also improves circulation and thus oxygen transport in the body. In addition, regular physical activity helps against obesity, which is often present in people with sleep apnea syndrome.

For groups of people who have been physically inactive in the past and who begin regular physical activity to improve sleep quality, however, the first noticeable effects only occur after at least four weeks of regular training (Kredlow et al. 2015). This is very important information for patients, as they expect to sleep better in the night following the increased fatigue during the day. However, patience pays off, as sleep quality, i.e. sleep depth and sleep stability, can be positively and durably influenced by an appropriate exercise program.

> In order to be able to fall asleep in the evening and sleep through the night, we need a relaxed state of wakefulness with sufficient fatigue before going to bed.

This state can be achieved by regular physical activity, which has two sleep-promoting aspects:

- Exercise produces endorphins (hormones of happiness), which make us satisfied.
- Exercise makes us physically tired.

The release of endorphins increases the subjectively perceived satisfaction of people and promotes relaxation processes. In combination with the increased fatigue caused by the physical activity, the satisfaction and relaxation caused by the release of endorphins has a positive effect on the latency to fall asleep, the overall duration of sleep and sleep quality (Miles 2007).

Most people find it very easy to get mentally exhausted today: constant screen work, a lot of thinking, planning, researching and structuring, telephoning and writing messages or making decisions are part of our mental effort during the day. This overload tires us out mentally. However, the primary sedentary activities mean that many people lack movement and thus physical fatigue.

Cortisol and Movement/Sport

For our ancestors, it was vital for survival to react to dangerous situations with flight or fight, that is, to start a stress reaction. The body is on alert during stress and ready to give everything. Today, however, we no longer have to fight in times of stress, and the energy provided is not used, but remains in the body. This is harmful and can lead to serious stress-related illnesses and sleep disorders.

Moderate exercise can break down this energy and thus act as an antagonist to chronic

Table 3.33 Overview Module: Movement and Sport

Indications	In insomnia, sleep-related breathing disorders, circadian sleep-wake disorders, especially in people with sedentary occupations
Contraindications	None, possibly somatic diseases that prohibit movement or sport
Effectiveness	Very well proven
Working principle	Movement and sport favor hormonal and other body processes that aim at homeostasis and thus also favor sleep. Movement and sport exhaust the body, thus contributing to relaxation and contentment
Treatment requirements	Basic knowledge of the use of sport and movement in a therapeutic context
Treatment goal	Holistic health, self-responsible action

stress. 20–30 min of lighter activity, such as walking, hiking or cycling, can reduce tension and thus consume excess cortisol.

The point of the exercise is not to power through and get tired. On the contrary, too much or too hard training actually increases cortisol secretion and the surplus may not be broken down by bedtime.

Procedure

First of all, it is important that your patients understand why it is so important for their health in general and their sleep in particular to exercise regularly. To illustrate and read again at home, you can give your patient the Information sheet IS14: Exercise, Sport & Sleep to take home. As with all other therapy components, it is also important with exercise and sport that these can be integrated into the patient's everyday life as a targeted intervention. Therefore, when choosing the exercise, it is important to consider that the physical activity

- Is fun,
- Can be organized in time and space,
- Corresponds to the patient's basic constitution (age, health status, fitness level, ambition),
- Corresponds to the chronotype,
- Is conducive to the goal.

Do not put your patient under pressure to "finally start exercising". This pressure creates stress and is therefore sleep-inhibiting. In addition, too much pressure can also create reactance on the part of the patient, making it even more difficult for him to start training. Go to work with joy by perhaps first collecting which sports and types of movement would be conceivable. With worksheet WS 22: Sports, your patient can get an overview of the ways in which one can physically exert oneself. For sleep, endurance exercises are particularly beneficial, such as Nordic walking, brisk walks, slightly faster bike rides, etc. To give the patient a guideline as to which heart rate is favorable for the training, I always give the advice:

You should walk fast enough that you can still talk, but not sing anymore. It would also be good if you ran a few minutes faster from time to time, so that you can't talk anymore.

There are people who prefer to train alone. However, for most people, having a training partner for regular overcoming of the inner pig-dog is also favorable. Some people need a varied training plan, others are very satisfied with regularly doing the same sport. In any case, it is important that as many muscles in the body are moved and strengthened as possible.

The most difficult step for everyone is the beginning of a regular exercise program. You help your patient the most when you "nail him down" in the therapy session and agree very specifically when and which sport will be tried in the next few days. Clarify that the patient has all the necessary equipment and the appropriate clothing for it, so that there are no excuses available.

> A first step to getting more movement into everyday life could be small changes in everyday life that only take a few more minutes but have a very positive effect on overall health and, of course, sleep.
>
> - Walk home from work
> - Take public transportation and get off two stops earlier or park the car further away
> - Make plans for a walk, etc.
> - If there are several stops along the way, leave the car at one point and walk the rest
> - And of course the classic: take the stairs instead of the elevator

Discuss different weather options and set clear cut-offs, for example: "Only if the outside temperature is below 5 °C, may the training be postponed." A small tip at this point: You can also do very well with rain. As is well known, there is no bad weather, but only the wrong clothing. In the best case, your patient will notice that it can be very nice to experience nature to the full. Also discuss which place or which route should be used for the training. This is sometimes the hardest decision. If your patient decides to train in a sports club or gym, discuss when he should make an appointment for a trial training. Many people do not find the time to call there. Everything boils down to outsmarting the inner pigdog and making no more excuses possible. For a structured approach, you can use worksheet WS 23: More movement—Part 1 (Fig. 3.24).

After the first training and movement units, it should be discussed in a therapeutic session how the patient feels with the additional movement. It should be discussed which problems have arisen and how they can be remedied if necessary. Everything has a beginning! Therefore, encourage your patient even if he has not been able to implement the new movement plan so far. Then it is important to adjust for as long as it takes to create an implementable plan. For this you can use the worksheet WS 24: My movement plan.

3.8   Manual Procedures

3.8.1   Background

For the sake of completeness, the mention of manual methods must not be missing from a book on holistic treatment of sleep disorders. Although most sleep disorders are of a psychological nature, the body must be included in the therapy. Here too, the various cultures of naturopathy offer numerous very helpful methods. In addition to the traditional relaxation massages for regulating the peripheral nervous system, each school has specific manual therapy methods. The body is a key part of the pathogenesis of sleep disorders and therefore offers wonderful starting points for sustainable therapy. As described in *Sect. 3.6*, body-oriented exercises offer enormous potential to positively influence the overall symptomatology.

It is a myth that psychotherapists are not allowed to touch their patients. Therefore, I would like to encourage my colleagues here to also include body-oriented elements. It is also important here that you as a therapist have solid expertise and only use the therapy methods whose effectiveness has been scientifically proven.

A complete overview of manual therapy measures would exceed the scope of this book. Nevertheless, I would like to introduce three basic variants that you can include in the therapy planning. No doctor or therapist can do everything. Various therapy components, especially manual therapy, can be wonderfully delegated to experts (e.g. physiotherapists, TCM and Ayurvedic physicians).

3.8.2   Hydro- and Thermotherapy

The best-known applications from the field of manual therapy are the hydrotherapeutic approaches of Sebastian Kneipp (Stier-Jarmer et al. 2021). The great advantage of these therapy techniques lies in the low-cost and uncomplicated application in the home environment. As long as there are no serious physical illnesses, especially in the cardiovascular system, they are low in side effects and risks.

Within the framework of hydro- and thermotherapy, both cold and warm stimuli can be set. With some disorders and especially for hardening the immune system, changes between heat and cold are very effective. With a cold stimulus, the vessels contract at the corresponding body site. In response, there is then increased blood flow. The cold stimulus generates the so-called "active" heat and thus promotes increased blood flow. This effect is interesting to note on the opposite side of the body. Through this paradoxical effect, cold stimulus therapy is more sustainable than heat application with passively generated heat. It stimulates the body to regulate itself. With heat applications, there may be more perspiration and thus heat loss leading to cold or hypothermia.

The regulation of the body's own heat balance is an essential part of sleep. In the evening, the body temperature is highest, cooling down at night, reaching its lowest point in the morning.

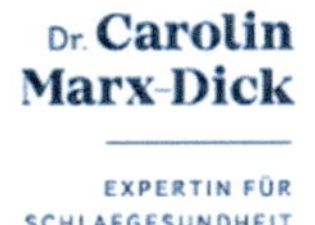

WS23 - Worksheet: More Movement

How can you integrate more exercise into your everyday life?

Please go through your daily routine and see when there would be an opportunity to move more. Please also rate how much you would like to do this.

Exercise doesn't necessarily mean working out. For example, you could walk to work or home, or at least part of the way, enjoy a walk during your lunch break, or even visit a gym in the evening.

	Here I can take my time (MO-FR)	So gladly I do it
morning		😀 😐 ☹
		😀 😐 ☹
morning		😀 😐 ☹
		😀 😐 ☹
at noon		😀 😐 ☹
		😀 😐 ☹
afternoon		😀 😐 ☹
		😀 😐 ☹
evening		😀 😐 ☹
		😀 😐 ☹

In the near future, try out different possible exercise and sports variants. observe and note how you feel about them. Enter your plans in the following table and note the days of the week. You will see that individual activities do not disrupt your schedule too much.

Day and time	Movement type and place	With whom?	How did I do?
			😀 😐 ☹
			😀 😐 ☹
			😀 😐 ☹
			😀 😐 ☹

Fig. 3.24   Worksheet WS 23: More movement

WS23 - Worksheet: More Movement

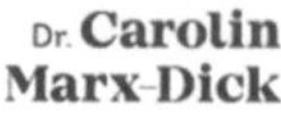

Day and time	Movement type and place	With whom?	How did I do?
			🙂 😐 🙁
			🙂 😐 🙁
			🙂 😐 🙁
			🙂 😐 🙁
			🙂 😐 🙁
			🙂 😐 🙁
			🙂 😐 🙁
			🙂 😐 🙁
			🙂 😐 🙁
			🙂 😐 🙁
			🙂 😐 🙁
			🙂 😐 🙁

There is no such thing as the wrong weather, only the wrong clothing. Try a workout in "unfavorable" weather conditions. A walk in the rain, well wrapped up in Raincoat and rubber boots, can be a real pleasure. The inner pig dog is a strong opponent who will use any excuse not to train. You can only conquer when there is no doubt that you are actually taking the first step.

Therefore, set up a very **specific** training or exercise plan and make sure you have everything you need to do it.

Checklist for my movement:

Clothing/Equipment	Check
The right sports ski boots	☐
The right clothes (preferably weatherproof)	☐
Possible equipment: rackets, sticks, weights	☐
Training partner (it is easier to train in company)	☐
Other:	☐

As soon as you start to question whether you really still want to exercise today, because you are too tired, the day was too exhausting and the weather is not suitable anyway, your inner pig has already won. The answer is always YES!

Don't forget: a short walk is much better than sitting on the sofa.

Fig. 3.24   (continued)

The cooling of the body is a necessity in order to rest and find sleep. If this does not happen, sleep remains superficial. Insomnia and sleep disorders are the result. However, if we support our body in the down-regulation of our body core temperature, falling asleep and sleeping through can be favored. Informationsheet IS15: Leg wraps for sleep disorders contains instructions for a cool leg wrap that has already "worked wonders".

In particularly strong states of excitement, a whole-body wrap can be applied in the same way. After an initially unpleasant cold sensation over the whole body, a pleasant warmth sets in after a few minutes, which at the same time calms the peripheral nervous system. Many people fall asleep unintentionally with this application.

In addition to the calming effect on falling asleep and sleep disorders, such hydro or thermo applications can also be very effective in restless legs syndrome. The corresponding wraps can then also be applied to the arms.

Heat applications promote the circulation of the skin as well as the metabolism and, depending on the body region, the activity of individual organs.

Their areas of application also include painful muscle complaints and tension. Through the heat, a reduction in muscle tension and pain can be achieved.

Heat applications are carried out with warm-hot water (36–40 °C), they last between 3 and 5 min. In part, a conclusion with a short cold application is recommended in order to avoid sweating (risk of hypothermia).

3.8.3 Acupuncture

The term "acupuncture" comes from Latin and is made up of *acus*, needle, and *punctura*, sting. It is probably the best-known healing method of Traditional Chinese Medicine (TCM). By puncturing certain body points that are located on different energy pathways (meridians), the "life energy of the body" (the Qi) is stimulated to circulate. The effect of acupuncture has been scientifically proven for various disorders. A search on the scientific platform "PubMed" yielded more than 37,000 entries. It is effective for pain disorders, respiratory diseases, gastrointestinal disorders and mental illnesses. It has also been shown to be effective for sleep disorders, especially insomnia and REM sleep behavior disorders (e.g. Liou et al. 2021; Li et al. 2021). Due to its balancing effect on the body, acupuncture counteracts nervous unrest and tension, and is therefore helpful against sleep disorders. It also has a positive effect on sleep apnea syndrome (Wang et al. 2020). Acupuncture may only be used by doctors or naturopaths who have undergone intensive training and have as much experience as possible under supervision.

3.8.4 Marmatherapy

Marmatherapy, which originates from India, is a manual therapy of Ayurveda. Simply put, it could be said to be the counterpart to acupuncture, but without needles. By means of a special massage of the sensitive marma points, which in turn are also located on energy channels (nadis), blockages are dissolved. These blockages arise over long periods of time as a result of an unfavorable lifestyle with too much stress, shallow breathing, inertia, poor posture, etc. Ayurveda assumes that, as a result of the blockages, internal organs, the cardiovascular system and our nervous system are constricted and cannot function properly. By dissolving the blockages, the organs and systems are given back their space and thus their full functionality. Scientific research into the effectiveness of marmatherapy is only just beginning. First studies show positive effects on high blood pressure and states of excitement of the peripheral nervous system (e.g. Gautam et al. 2021). Both are possible causes of sleep disorders.

The patients lie on a massage table or take a relaxed sitting position. The marmatherapist massages the blocked points and strokes the clearly noticeable blockages into the nadis. For a positive influence on sleep as well as for the targeted relief of insomnia, Ayurveda has identified and defined a special marma point. It is located on the occipital lobe on the central median line (Oz). Nevertheless, it can make sense to also dissolve other blockage points on the body. For example, there is a concentration of many marma points on the sternum (breastbone). A targeted treatment at these points can have a positive effect on a sleep apnea syndrome, on feelings of tightness and panic, strong heart palpitations or high blood pressure. A targeted treatment of the marma points on the calves or arms can have a very positive effect on a restless legs syndrome. In this way, the physiological-energetic flow is stimulated. Already one treatment can have a noticeable effect on patients. Even though this description of marmatherapy sounds easy to carry out, it requires a detailed multi-day training and a lot of experience to be able to apply this technique safely to the patient.

are supposed to work together are connected by neuronal connections. Nerve connections or missing neuronal connections that lead to pathological patterns (such as post-traumatic stress disorder) are interrupted or built up.

Neurotherapy is used in many areas. It is particularly popular as biofeedback in orthopedics and neuroprosthetics, neurology, psychotherapy, bladder, bowel and digestive disorders. In the subconsciously controlled neuronal networks, the body's own healing powers are activated, as nature intended. For example, in REM sleep, emotional events are processed by rapid eye movements. In the case of mental disorders, especially post-traumatic stress disorder (PTSD), neurotherapy stimulates processing processes in the limbic system. The limbic system is primarily responsible for the processing of emotions.

3.9   Neurotherapy

Neurotherapy brings "dysregulated" networks of the human nervous system back into harmony. It acts directly on the central nervous system and modulates brain rhythms so that the structures of the central and peripheral nervous systems work together again in a synchronous and functional manner (Chapin and Russell-Chapin 2014). The eye movement integration (EMI; Beaulieu 2003) and polyvagal therapy presented here, based on the polyvagal theory (Porges 1995), do not require suggestibility, special sensitivity, concentration or belief in the efficacy of the therapy technique. The mechanism of action is based on functional neuroanatomy: structures that

3.9.1   Therapy Module: Eye Movement Integration (EMI)

Overview (Table 3.34)

Background

Eye Movement Integration (EMI) is a neuro-psychotherapeutic technique originally developed for the treatment of trauma victims. EMI is a method for activating the self-healing of subconscious neural networks. In the case of mental disorders, especially post-traumatic stress disorder (PTSD), neurotherapy focuses on the limbic system or the amygdala of the limbic system. The limbic system is primarily responsible for the processing of emotions, the

Table 3.34 Overview of Module: Eye Movement Integration

Indications	Parasomnias (nightmares, sleepwalking), insomnia with comorbid post-traumatic stress disorder, distressing/traumatic experience of sleep disorder
Contraindications	Psychotic symptoms, suicidality
Effectiveness	From practical experience: very good
Working principle	Strongly aversive or traumatic experiences are processed on a conscious and subconscious level
Treatment requirements	Solid knowledge of Eye Movement Integration, self-experience desirable
Treatment goal	To alleviate and reduce strongly negative dreams or to find insomnia less burdensome

associated impulse control of instinctive behavior and the associated intellectual abilities. The amygdala enables a mammal to quickly recognize and evaluate danger in order to subsequently initiate the corresponding vegetative reactions.

The amygdala only acts as an intermediate storage for the sensory impressions. The emotional information is added later and initially exists in loose fragments. The feelings are "split off" and the neurological speech center shows little activity when talking about the trauma. Therefore, a pure verbal psychotherapy (depth psychology or cognitive behavioral therapy) is usually not sufficient. Scientific studies show that bimodal stimulations (e.g. sound and image) are significantly more successful because they activate more neurons (e.g. Calvert 2001).

Clinical studies on the efficacy of EMI already show a reduction of 48.33% of the self-reported trauma symptoms after only one treatment. After a holistic treatment, 83.30% fewer symptoms are reported (Beaulieu 2003).

EMI was developed by Andreas and Andreas in 1989 and subsequently refined by Danie Beaulieu. The trauma researchers assume that traumatic life events then lead to pathological post-traumatic stress disorders if they are maintained fragmented in short-term memory and the amygdala and not transferred as a complex event to long-term memory. Only with the integration of all involved senses and emotions can the fragments be adapted to a total picture and transferred to long-term memory. Affected persons can integrate acquired competencies, e.g. maturation, into the memory as a resource (Beaulieu 2003).

▶ *EMI promotes the integration of experience fragments through neuronal activation.*

Neuroscientists have discovered a direct connection between eye movements and sensory or emotional memory. In nature, this process can also be found in REM sleep, as eye movements during subconscious, i.e. sleeping, promote emotional regulation.

Through an exchange of information between short-term and long-term memory during deep sleep, current experiences are linked to experiences already anchored in memory. This means that primarily during deep sleep, old memory content is reactivated and combined with new experiences, so that "bad experiences" from earlier times can be compensated for with new, possibly more positive ones. Overall, this can make the experience less bad or move it emotionally further into the background. And on the other hand, negative experiences of the current day can be combined with older experiences, so that, for example, problem-solving strategies can be triggered.

EMI in Insomnia

Many sufferers of insomnia report that staying awake in bed is "hell". Of course, being awake in bed is not threatening. But even in the definition of trauma, it is assumed that the experiences are purely subjectively experienced as threatening. Descriptions of patients with sleep disorders often include the subjectively experienced loss of control over the automatic and natural state of (falling) asleep. In the nocturnal wakefulness phases, there are sometimes strong depressive and even suicidal thoughts. Drifting into dissociative states allows patients to endure this subjectively threatening situation. This means that this part of the disorder is indeed experienced as traumatic and therefore treatment techniques from trauma therapy can be adapted and adapted to the treatment of people with sleep disorders.

EMI in Nightmares

Since many people who suffer from pathological nightmares experience this dream situation as subjectively very aversive, therapy techniques for the treatment of nightmares could be very effective.

EMI is a very technical and less cognitive method that can be carried out after a short introductory preparation phase (3–5 therapy hours). This was followed by 1–3 EMI sessions. Finally, a debriefing takes place. It is therefore well suited for use in a clinically limited time frame.

In 5–8 sessions, massive fears of staying awake or in bed or bad nightmares can be alleviated.

Procedure for Eye-Movement Integration

First, a comprehensive medical history should be taken of the patient's symptoms. The night-time situation must be queried in detail. If the patient experiences lying awake in bed as extremely stressful, there is an indication for the use of EMI. If the patient suffers from nightmares, a detailed exploration of the dream content must first be carried out, as described in *Sect. 3.5 (nightmare therapy).*

Preparing the Patient

In the preparatory sessions, descriptions and personal statements that establish a verbal connection to the problematic or traumatic situation are collected. When selecting these personal statements from the patients, it is important to ensure that they are concrete and simple. They should represent the situation factually and accurately. There is no need, and it is rather disturbing, to delve too deeply into emotional content or even imagination of the stressful situation (as in EMDR [Eye Movement Desensitization and Reprocessing], i.e. desensitization and processing through eye movement).

In addition, the patient's resources should be uncovered in advance, which will be used during the EMI treatment. Typical resources are:

- "I am a "professional" at staying awake."
- "Even if I am awake in bed, I don't have to be afraid/I can relax."
- "It's all just a dream."
- "Nothing can happen to me when I'm asleep."

At the end of the EMI session, these resources are incorporated into the patient's mindset.

Conducting the EMI Session

The therapist sits opposite the patient. Before the session starts, the therapist must scan the patient's field of view, not the field of vision. The therapist should align his own position to this and ensure maximum use of the eye movement field, as shown in Fig. 3.25. The patient should keep his head forward and relaxed.

During the eye movements led by the therapist, the therapist speaks the previously worked-out personal sentences. The patient's eye movement follows the therapist's finger movement. The patient only has the task of listening and following the therapist's movements with his eyes. The respective movements (Fig. 3.25) are carried out several times during a sequence. The therapist pays attention to the patient's "hotspots". These are then displayed when the patient cannot follow an eye movement evenly with his eyes and the eyes "jump". These hotspots are signs that restructuring is taking place in the patient's neural network (Beaulieu 2003). With continued movement, the neural network is "massaged". Often, the hotspots already decrease during the second or third immediate repetition of the eye movement in the sequence. Between the individual movement sequences, the patient and the therapist have the opportunity to communicate. This serves above all to query the patient's condition on all five sensory modalities. After sequence F (in Fig. 3.25), the patient's previously discussed resource is introduced.

At the end of the EMI treatment, the eyes are "decoupled" from the trauma by the patient moving his eyes in spirals (G and H in Fig. 3.25). The eye movements are "anchored" and solidified with the resources.

Post-Processing

After the EMI procedure is completed, there should be room for open questions and comments. However, it is important to let the neural network do its job and not to interrupt the subconscious processes by over-interpretation. EMI can cause side effects. Headaches are often reported, which disappear on their own after

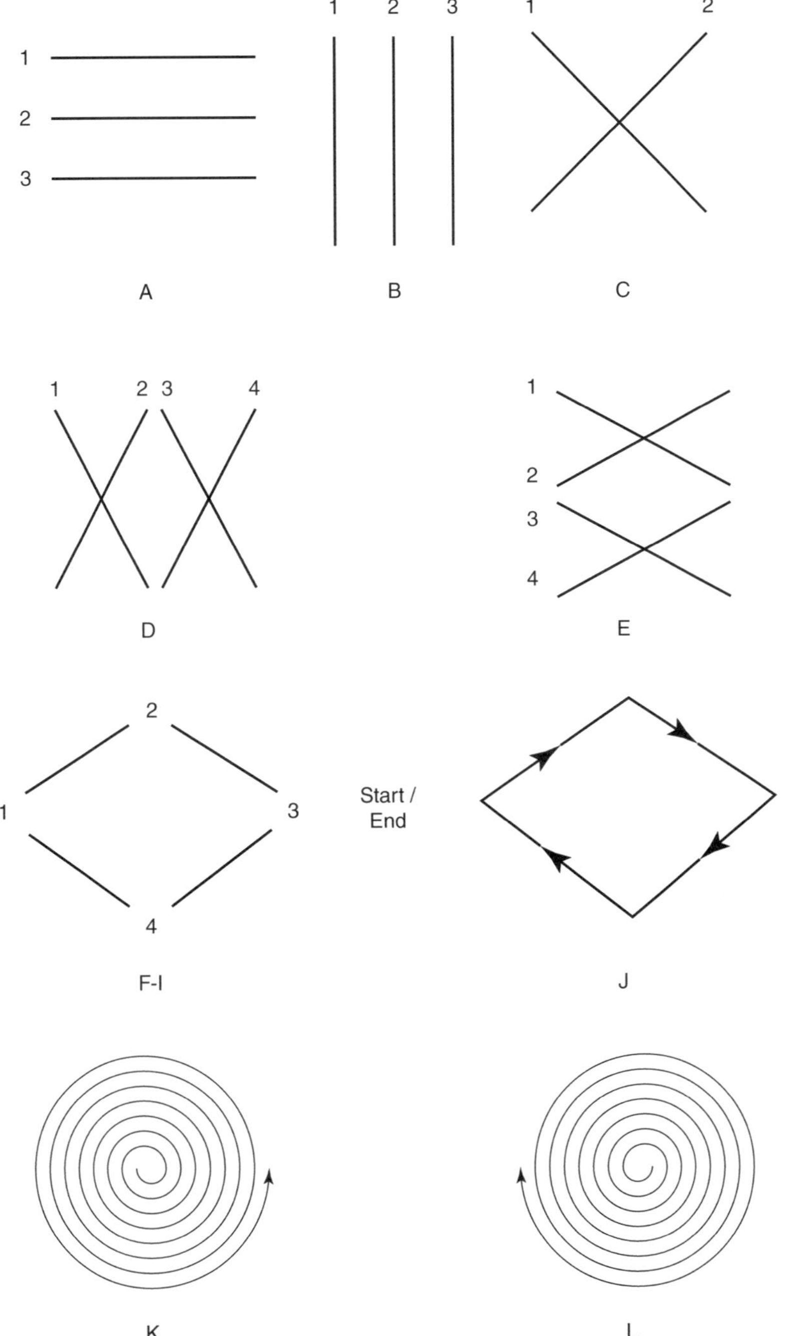

Fig. 3.25 Representation of eye movements during the EMI session

hours or 1–2 days. Many patients also describe a feeling of "standing next to themselves", which also disappears on its own.

In the next regular therapy session, usually a week after the EMI session, the EMI session is discussed. The positive change should be reinforced by the therapist.

▶ *The reading of the description of a therapy with EMI carried out here is by no means sufficient to be able to carry out this technique safely in everyday clinical practice. A multi-day training course for EMI therapists is generally necessary.*

3.9.2 Module: Polyvagal Therapy

Overview (Table 3.35)

Background

Polyvagal therapy is based on the polyvagal theory. The name is made up of "poly", meaning "many", and "vagal" (wander or roam). It describes the functions of the vagus nerve, the 10th cranial nerve. It is the longest of our twelve cranial nerves and is relatively widespread and heavily branched in the periphery. The anatomy makes it clear that the vagus nerve has many functions. It is the cranial nerve that supplies the most organs, tissues and nerve cells. It is divided into head, neck, chest and abdominal parts. In addition, the vagus nerve provides most of the nerve fibers for the parasympathetic reaction.

The anatomy of the vagus nerve is shown in Fig. 3.26. It shows the strong branching in the human body. The dark blue lines represent the individual branches of the vagus nerve. It can be seen very well that the individual strands run from the brain stem over the tongue root, the larynx, over the heart and lungs, liver, kidneys and digestive organs to the intestine. This representation makes it clear how versatile the functions of the vagus nerve are (Table 3.36).

The polyvagal theory was first presented in 1995 by Stephen Porges (Professor of Psychiatry and Biomedicine) (Porges 1995). The combination of evolutionary, neuroscientific and psychological theories shows the many functions of the vagus nerve in stress and emotion regulation as well as in social behavior. This perspective should not be missing in a holistic treatment of sleep disorders.

Excursus: The Polyvagal Theory—Short and Sweet
It has long been assumed that the peripheral nervous system consists of two feedback loops: 1st Stress and 2nd Relaxation, also known as sympathetic and parasympathetic. The sympathetic has the task of making us ready for "fight or flight", thus building up a time-limited stress reaction in a (potentially) dangerous situation. The focus here is on "survival", all currently unnecessary functions, such as digestion, are switched off. In return, the body is perfectly prepared for flight or fight: optical focusing and tunnel vision, increased blood flow to large muscle groups, muscle tension, faster breathing, increased heart rate and blood pressure, etc. The parasympathetic controls the nervous counter-reaction: relaxation. The organism turns to other functions, such as digestion, building up reserves, secretion of various enzymes, etc.

In this sympathetic-parasympathetic model, it was assumed that these functions are innervated antagonistically by a strand of the vagus nerve.

Table 3.35 Overview Module: Polyvagal Therapy

Indications	Chronicization of the fight-flight reflex (fight-flight mode), teeth grinding, massive body tension, hard abdomen, shallow breathing, social withdrawal
Contraindications	Not known
Effectiveness	From practical experience: very good
Working principle	The massive body tension under chronic maintenance of the fight-flight mode is softened
Treatment requirements	Solid knowledge of the polyvagal theory, self-experience desirable
Treatment goal	The chronically tense body relaxes and the patient regains confidence in himself and his body

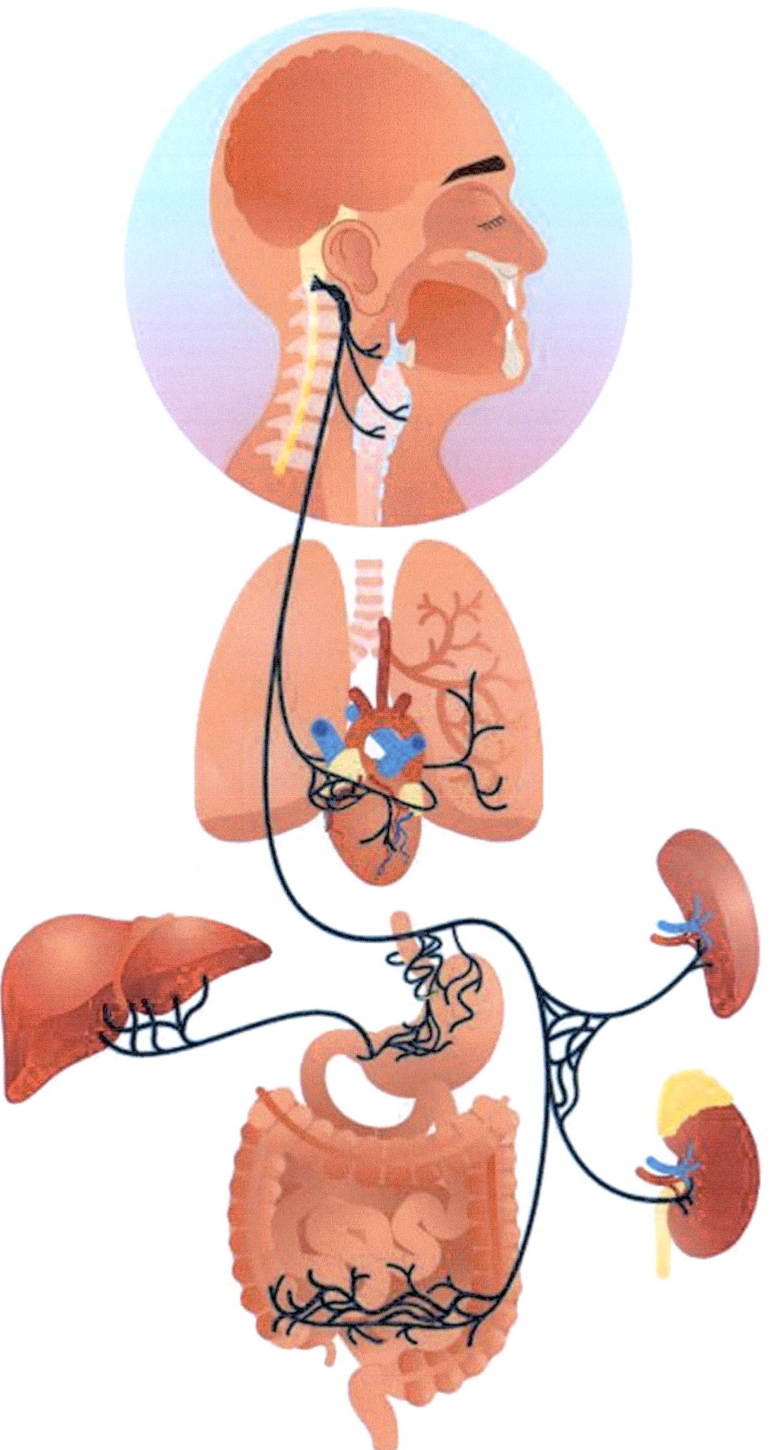

Fig. 3.26 Anatomical structure of the vagus Vagus

Table 3.36 Functions of the vagus nerve

Process	Organs	Function
Information conduction from the periphery (Viscerosensory stimulus conduction)	Cardiovascular system	Detecting blood pressure changes
Motor regulation	Throat, larynx, vocal cords, trachea	Modulation of voice loudness and melody
Vegetative-autonomous control of the smooth muscles and glands of the gastrointestinal tract	Heart, lungs, liver, kidney, adrenal gland, gastrointestinal tract, including digestive glands	Parasympathetic regulation of the heart, lungs and abdominal organs
Sensory information conduction (perception)	Throat, epiglottis, larynx, trachea and esophagus	Taste perception of epiglottis and tongue base; Perception of pressure, touch, vibration, pain and temperature in the throat, trachea and esophagus

However, Porges recognized another function of the parasympathetic. He showed a division of the vagus nerve into a anterior (ventral) and a posterior (dorsal) vagus branch, which arise in adjacent areas of the brain stem. The circulation and respiration, which are necessary for the regulation of the sympathetic and parasympathetic reaction, are influenced by both branches. The anterior (ventral) branch houses more afferent nerve fibers, thus sending information from the periphery to the central nervous system, from where our "gut feeling" comes. The posterior (dorsal) branch houses more efferent nerve fibers and sends signals from the brain to the periphery.

Porges recognized that the vagus nerve allows us to react appropriately to different dangers in all phases of life:

- acute danger to life with little prospect of survival
- dangerous situations in which one should fight or flee
- safe and trusting situations in which one can relax completely

There are thus not only the two antagonistic processes of sympathetic and parasympathetic reaction, but a total of three reaction patterns:

1. Freeze or shutdown in the dorsal branch:
   a. Slowing down, shutting down, freezing
   b. Excites feelings of helplessness, hopelessness, apathy
   c. Initiates withdrawal

2. Fight or Flight in the boundary cord of the sympathetic nerve
   a. Physiological and emotional mobilization of the body in response to danger
   b. Stress reaction
3. Social-Engagement-System (SES) in the ventral branch:
   c. Social engagement and relaxation
   d. Contact and communication
   e. Promotion of rest and relaxation

These cycles interact with each other so that they regulate our physiological and emotional experience. There is a need for a flexible switching of the activity of the different strands as a respective reaction to different demands:

- Greatest life danger/trauma: The dorsal branch is active, body physiology and perception ability sink. The body is thus hardly able to act or react. The exhausted and depressive lethargy and apathy are the result. This reaction is typical for shock states.
- Dangerous situation/stress: The sympathetic trunk is activated, we are ready to show great performance, to "fight" through everyday life and to endure stress.

> • Safety and security: The ventral branch is active and brings the relaxation necessary for sleeping. In addition, the possibility arises to show open social behavior, which is essential for our mental health.

A state to be striven for or a necessary process in the holistic treatment of people is the flexible switching between the activation of the three reaction patterns. Only this allows adequate reactions to the different situations that occur in life: stress/danger, overload and joy/security.

These feedback loops regulate our homeostasis and are the basis for our mental and physical health. A flexible exchange of functions is also very important for sleep: Only if the day is right, can the night be good too. The body and psyche must be able to adapt to the different situations of the day in order to be able to react physiologically and psychologically appropriately. If the range of reaction is limited, the homeostasis cannot be maintained and illness occurs.

Therapeutic Possibilities

In the last two decades, numerous clinical studies have found evidence for the validity of this new approach to the peripheral nervous system. This has led to the development of many multimodal and especially direct therapeutic approaches. They show good efficacy in the treatment of:

- Pain in the jaw-shoulder-neck area
- Migraine
- Anxiety disorders
- ADHD and hyperactivity
- affective (especially bipolar) disorders
- Posttraumatic stress disorder
- Disorders in the autism spectrum

In the course of my treatment practice, it became apparent that people with sleep disorders often experience the nocturnal wakefulness as traumatic and also develop great generalized fears in everyday life. Frequent comorbidities are migraine, great inner restlessness, hyperactivity and of course the affective disorders. In addition, most sufferers suffer from chronically increased muscle tone, especially in the shoulder-jaw-neck area. All of these are typical comorbidities in non-organic sleep disorders. Nocturnal arousals make it more difficult to fall asleep and stay asleep. Therefore, it is logical to use the approaches of the Polyvagal Theory to develop therapeutic techniques for the holistic treatment of sleep disorders.

The Polyvagal Theory can directly stimulate the peripheral nervous system and thus also inhibit its overactivity. The additional advantage of this method is that it can simultaneously affect and thus treat comorbid mental disorders of any kind. Polyvagal therapy is therefore a very economical therapy technique that can also enable patients to quickly relieve their overall symptoms. Since Polyvagal Theory is more of a body therapy, it is particularly suitable for patients who are very "heady" and have difficulty getting involved in cognitive techniques. People of all educational levels and different intelligence, as well as with limited suggestibility, which is required, for example, for imagination techniques and hypnotherapy, also respond very well to Polyvagal Theory.

Therapeutic Means of Polyvagal Theory

The Polyvagal Theory offers various direct points of attack to promote the variability of reaction patterns: eye and tongue muscles, fascia, muscles (especially around the spine and chest), and the gastrointestinal tract. These areas can be loosened and made variable using targeted eye exercises, tongue exercises, breathing and stretching exercises using yoga therapy, massages, breathing exercises, targeted meditation, and appropriate nutrition.

▶ *However, in order to be able to use Polyvagal Theory safely, it is necessary to attend a multi-day training with supervision on this topic.*

Procedure

The following tongue exercise, which only takes a few minutes and can therefore be easily integrated into the treatment routine, offers a first start to the application of Polyvagal Theory. It can also be used diagnostically to give your patients feedback that their flexibility in reacting to stress and relaxation situations in everyday life is limited.

Most sufferers of sleep disorders have a chronic overactivation of the vagus nerve to the sympathetic nervous system. They are permanently ready for action, "alert" and struggle through the stressful everyday life. If there is time for recovery, relaxation and social contacts, many patients are not able to enjoy this time. This is shown, for example, by a tongue that is sticky, hard and sometimes pointed at the front.

Below you will find two exercises to get started with Polyvagal Theory with your patient.

Basic Exercise for Training the Vagus Nerve with the Tongue

Notes and "reading guide": This exercise consists of three parts: an introduction, the actual exercise and a debriefing. It is intended to help the patient better accept difficult-to-change situations in their lives.

Discuss a situation or complex topic with your patient in advance. The exercise will build on this.

We assume that every symptom has a function. So does a sleep disorder. The exercise will also address what function the patient attributes to their sleep disorder or could attribute to it.

It is important to read the instructions slowly and with a calm voice. Take breaks between sentences and give your patient time to find their way in the exercise.

Introduction

[Read the instructions slowly and with a calm voice, give your patient time to sense everything].

Take a comfortable sitting position and relax as much as possible. Take a deep breath and exhale completely. Find your rhythm for relaxed breathing.

Now focus your attention on your tongue and feel exactly where it is in your mouth. For many people, the tongue "sticks" to the palate. Or is your tongue in the back of your mouth? Now focus your awareness on the shape and tension of your tongue. Does the tongue touch the teeth? How hard or loose does it feel? Now focus your attention on your jaw. This is often tense and the teeth are clenched. If possible, loosen the jaw. Make some chewing movements and let the lower jaw circle.

Now feel your mouth space with the tip of your tongue. At the very back is the soft palate. This is difficult for some patients to reach with their tongue. It is not absolutely necessary to touch it with the tip of your tongue. On the way forward you will find your hard palate. Finally, stroke over your gums and come to your incisors. Explore your mouth in this way and stroke with the tip of your tongue from the back, from the soft palate, over the hard palate, over the gums, the incisors and the gums of the lower row of teeth to the back of the tongue. Wander back on the same path from the back of the tongue over the gums and teeth, to the hard palate and finally to the soft palate. Repeat this movement a few times.

[Give your patient 2–3 min to repeat this forward and backward movement several times at his own pace. Ask your patient how he feels and how he felt the sensation.]

How does your tongue feel now? Where is it in your mouth? What is your tongue touching? Is it tight or loose? How does your jaw feel?

Now guide your tongue tip a little to the middle of the hard palate and move to the left side. You feel your gums, teeth and finally your soft palate. Now walk back the same way over the hard palate and then continue with your tongue tip to the gums on your right side, over the teeth to the palate. Now move your tongue from right to left and from left to right. Feel what your tongue perceives.

[Give your patient 2–3 min to repeat this forward and backward movement several times at his own pace. Ask your patient how he feels and how he felt the sensation.]

How does your tongue feel now? Where is it in your mouth? What is your tongue touching? Is it tight or loose? How does your jaw feel?

Now let your tongue be completely loose and let your tongue dance. It should now move in your mouth as it pleases. Let your tongue dance a waltz or do figure eights in your mouth. Your tongue can do what it wants. Also feel free to stick your tongue out.

[Ask your patient how he feels and how he felt the sensation.]

How does your tongue feel now? Where is it in your mouth? What is your tongue touching? Is it tight or loose? How does your jaw feel?

Exercise instructions for reading: The Yes-saying-exercise

Take a comfortable sitting position and relax as much as possible. Take a deep breath and exhale completely. Find your rhythm for relaxed breathing.

Now focus your attention on your tongue and feel exactly where it is in your mouth. For many people, the tongue "sticks" to the palate. Or is your tongue in the back of your mouth? Now focus your attention on the shape and tension of your tongue. Does the tongue touch the teeth? How tight or loose does it feel. Now focus your attention on your jaw. This is often tense and the teeth are clenched. If possible, loosen the jaw. Make some chewing movements and let the lower jaw circle.

What if you accepted your sleep disorder just as it is? Say "yes" to all symptoms and to how you experience them. Your sleep disorder has also come to

help you. It protects you from _________

____

___. *E.g. overload, stress, etc., possibly include topics from therapy. Give your patient 2–3 min to be able to take on this function.]*

Now start moving your head gently back and forth, start nodding. Allow all thoughts that come. Perhaps a part of you wants to shake your head, but please stay with the nodding.

No matter what cognition, inner images, feelings or body sensations come now, everything is welcome. Stay with the nodding.

[After your patient has tuned in to the nodding and has automated it as much as possible]

Now feel your mouth with your tongue tip. The soft palate is located at the very back/top. For some patients it is difficult to reach with the tongue. It is not absolutely necessary to touch it with your tongue tip. On the way forward you will find your hard palate. Finally, stroke over your gums and come to your incisors. Via the upper and lower rows of teeth you reach your lower gums with your tongue tip and finally the base of the tongue. Explore your mouth in this way and stroke with your tongue from the back, from the soft palate, to the front, over the hard palate, over the gums, the incisors and the gums of the lower row of teeth to the base of the tongue. Wander back on the same path from the base of the tongue over the gums and teeth, to the hard palate and finally to the soft palate. Repeat this movement now a few times.

[Give your patient 2–3 min to repeat this forward and backward movement several times at his own pace.]

Find yourself relaxed in the movements and stay with your tongue movement with the head movement. Combine the nodding with the tongue stroking. You can of course include the entire upper body. Start gently rocking back and forth and stay with the nodding and stroke your tongue back and forth. Remember the situation __________________ *[Name the situation the patient has chosen for the exercise]* and stay with the movement.

Post-discussion

This exercise can be maintained for 5–15 min. After the exercise, explore how the patient feels and what he now thinks about this situation. Also ask about possible intermediate states.

If the exercise was successful, the patient has now gained distance from the selected situation, as he has accepted it and said "yes" to it.

3.10   Pharmacotherapy: Opportunities and Risks

The first port of call for sufferers of sleep disorders is usually general practitioners, psychiatrists, neurologists or other medical specialists. Contrary to all recommendations, i.e. also those of the S-3 guideline, pharmacological treatment of the symptoms with hypnotics is still often the first measure offered in the healthcare system. Pharmacological treatment of sleep disorders has the advantage that the symptoms can usually be safely reduced and an effect occurs. However, medications cannot cure the cause of many sleep disorders (insomnia, circadian sleep-wake disorders and parasomnias), but only act on the symptom of wakefulness or the suppression of nocturnal phenomena. The cause remains untouched. In addition, pharmacological treatment cannot be continued indefinitely. After discontinuation of the medication, the symptoms may even worsen, as the psychodynamics are very unfavorable. In this way, the patient is told that they can only sleep with medication. They lose confidence in their own body. Many medications interfere with the healthy sleep process, sleep architecture and the circadian-controlled hormone and neurotransmitter release. Then, despite sufficient sleep duration and depth, they report not to feel rested, psychologically unstable and cognitively impaired.

However, there are certainly situations, life phases, diseases and age structures in which the intake of hypnotics is beneficial and partly also necessary. It must therefore be assessed to what extent a pharmacological treatment is appropriate and useful and whether the expected benefit exceeds the possible risk.

The 6-K-Rule Provides a Guideline for the Assessment
- Clear indication
- Smallest possible dose
- Shortest possible treatment time
- Never stop abruptly
- Consider contraindications
- Combination with non-medicinal methods

In any case, the patient must be fully informed about the mode of action and the risks. It is also important to show the person concerned other treatment options and, if necessary, to refer him or her to the corresponding specialist (psychotherapy, neurology, psychiatry, etc.).

The term hypnotics refers to various drugs that are used as sleeping pills. It is a general term for all active ingredient groups and pharmacological treatment approaches for sleep disorders. The common feature is that they influence sleep, i.e. in most cases they should initiate and maintain it. A large number of drugs are available:

Hypnotics—Substance Groups
- Benzodiazepine hypnotics
- "Z-substances" (substances similar to benzodiazepines, non-benzodiazepine hypnotics, benzodiazepine receptor antagonists)

- Antihistamines
- Melatonin
- Antidepressants
- Antipsychotics (neuroleptics)
- Phytopharmaceuticals (herbal preparations)
- Dietary supplements
- Placebo

A preparation must be selected that catches the patient's current complaints and has as few side effects as possible or has as little negative effect as possible (Hajak and Riemann 2008). Hypnotics usually relieve the suffering and symptoms of sufferers quickly, but do not have a lasting effect on the cause of the non-organic sleep disorder. Medication treatment often has other disadvantages such as tolerance development, dependence risk and hangover effects.

A drug therapy, especially that of the psychologically strongly modulated sleep disorders (insomnia, hypersomnia, circadian sleep-wake disorders, parasomnias), should only be started after exhausting non-pharmacological methods, the failure of behavioral and causal treatment attempts (Benkert and Hippius 2020). A long-term therapy should only be considered in exceptional cases and should be very well weighed (Stuck et al. 2018, p. 111). It should also be combined with non-drug methods in principle.

All hypnotics have in common the influence on the sleep architecture in more or less invasive way. With the manipulation of the sleep architecture, the human body no longer has the opportunity to go through all the nightly processes of regeneration, calibration, and the build-up and breakdown of various structures, cells and tissues optimally. This means that all processes that do not take place during the day because the conscious waking mind lacks the capacity for them can take place neither nor only to a limited extent under hypnotics at night. Therefore, many affected people report insufficient fatigue despite measurable sleep.

There is the possibility to use shorter-acting drugs that are only useful in falling asleep disorder. These preparations shorten the latency to sleep and do not destroy the sleep architecture, so that many processes that take place exclusively or primarily during sleep can still take place.

As with many mental disorders, the HPA axis (hypothalamic-pituitary-adrenal axis) is important in the psychically modulated sleep disorders. Here, the sleep-inhibiting corticotropin-releasing hormone and the sleep-promoting growth hormone-releasing hormone influence each other. Both control the release of the hormone cortisol (for the production of performance and stress resistance) and the growth hormone. Therefore, the hypothesis is still held that too little sleep inhibits children's growth. If the balance of these two releasing hormones is disturbed and thus also the subsequent hormones are out of balance, sleep is permanently impaired. Thus, by restoring the balance pharmacologically, a positive effect can be exerted on sleep.

For the short-term treatment of severe sleep disorders, Hajak and Rüther (Hajak and Rüther 2013) suggest benzodiazepines or non-benzodiazepine hypnotics. Since these have a high risk of dependence with tolerance development, sedative antihistamines and antidepressants are recommended for longer-term treatment. In general, an intermittent administration should be considered, with administration frequencies of 4–6 nights per month.

> ▶ *In general, hypnotics should not be used continuously for more than 4 weeks.*

It should always be started with a low dose and titrated until a safe entry and sufficient maintenance of sleep occur. Different sleep aids should not be combined. In older patients, a lower dose is usually recommended.

The advantages of benzodiazepines and non-benzodiazepines lie mainly in a rapid and safe onset of action. However, the disadvantages of tolerance development and dependence potential are also of weight and must be taken into account. Antidepressants and antipsychotics that have a sleep-inducing effect do not show such a rapid and safe effect, but they also do not cause tolerance development and dependence risk. However, it should be noted that these preparations act intensively on the neurotransmitter balance and, in addition to a sleep-inducing function, also influence the mood and perception of the affected person.

3.10.1 Benzodiazepines

Overview (Table 3.37)

In the past, benzodiazepines were classified as "sleeping pills of first choice" (Parkes 1985). Depending on the active ingredient and dosage, benzodiazepines have a relaxing and finally sleep-inducing effect. In acute stress reactions that require a safe and rapid relaxation of the organism, benzodiazepines are still the drugs of choice. However, they are not suitable for long-term use in the treatment of sleep disorders, as tolerance develops quickly and there is a high risk of dependence.

Background

Benzodiazepine hypnotics provide a stable and seemingly deep sleep with significantly fewer interruptions. They thus prolong the effective sleep time and sleep efficiency. However, they can also reduce the proportion of deep and REM sleep (Borbély et al. 1981) and thus influence or destroy the natural sleep architecture. It is therefore possible that various functions of sleep, such as memory formation and emotion regulation, cannot be fulfilled despite phenotypic sleep. The after-effect can also be felt the night after without prior intake of a benzodiazepine. Occasionally, paradoxical reactions were also observed, i.e. despite taking a benzodiazepine, no sleep occurred and the patients stayed awake all night. It should also be noted that insomnia can intensify significantly after discontinuation of benzodiazepines. Therefore, a careful risk-benefit assessment must be made when using benzodiazepines. Benzodiazepines are rather unsuitable for the treatment of chronic sleep

Table 3.37 Overview: Characteristics of Benzodiazepines

Indications	Approved for short-term treatment of insomnia
Contraindications	In general increased vulnerability to addiction and existing addiction diseases, allergy to an ingredient, sleep apnea syndrome, respiratory and liver insufficiency, glaucoma
Advantages	Faster and safer onset of action, large therapeutic range, anxiolytic and sedative, hardly any fatal overdose possible
Disadvantages	Even in small doses quickly addictive, promotes the rebound effect, change in sleep architecture
Important side effects	Sedative, hangover effects, increased daytime sleepiness, deficits in cognitive performance, prolonged reaction times, possibly anxiety or amnesia, dizziness, slowed reaction, coordination problems, paradoxical reactions in geriatric patients possible, drowsiness, visual disturbances muscle hypotonia, ataxia and nocturnal falls, headaches, appetite loss, abuse and dependence potential, less deep and REM sleep (after discontinuation REM rebound with nightmares)
Working principle	They increase the affinity for GABA at $GABA_A$ receptors, thus the inhibitory effect of GABA in the CNS is increased and deep sleep is promoted
Application recommendations	Short-term and as needed, careful risk-benefit assessment, especially in older patients
Therapeutic goal	Quick and short-term symptom relief

Table 3.38 Overview: Frequently used benzodiazepines (selection)

Preparation	Active ingredient	Equipotent dosage (mg/day)	$t_{1/2}$ (h)
Flunibeta, Fluninoc, Flunitrazepan	Flunitrazepam	0.5–2	17–27
Loretam, Lormetazepam acis, Lormetazepam AL	Lormetazepam	0.5–2	8–14
Eatan N, Mogadan Nitrazepam AL	Nitrazepam	2,5–5	18–30
Norkotral Tema, Planum	Temazepam	10–20	5–13
Halcion	Triazolam	0,125–0,25	1,5–5

$t_{1/2}$ Half-life

disorders. The method of choice for chronic insomnia is psychotherapy.

Ultra-short, short- and long-acting benzodiazepines are distinguished. As a compromise, medium-acting preparations have also been developed. Table 3.38 gives an overview of frequently used preparations.

3.10.2 Barbiturates

Barbiturates were considered the sleep aid of choice for many decades. Today, with a few exceptions, they are no longer approved for use as a sleep aid in Germany and Switzerland. They are used to initiate and maintain anesthesia. In contrast to benzodiazepine hypnotics, barbiturates not only have a sleep-inducing effect, but also a sleep-forcing effect. Paradoxical reactions under barbiturates are therefore not possible.

The reason for the withdrawal as a sleep medication is the difficult to control and high risk of using barbiturates. They have very long half-lives and often require an antidote to regain wakefulness. There is also the danger of paralysis of the respiratory system, which can lead to death. Barbiturates were often abused in suicidal acts. Prominent examples of deaths associated with barbiturates are Marilyn Monroe and Judy Garland.

▶ Today, barbiturates are used in assisted suicide because they make it possible to transition from the waking state to sleep and then to death in a comfortable way.

3.10.3 "Z-Substances" (Non-Benzodiazepines)

Overview (Table 3.39)

GABA = γ-aminobutyric acid, ARAS = ascending reticular activating system

Background

The newer non-benzodiazepines (Table 3.41) have, like benzodiazepines, a safe onset of action. They differ structurally from these, but act on the same receptors. As GABA receptor agonists, they increase the inhibitory effect of GABA in the CNS. The ascending reticular activating system (ARAS) is inhibited and deep sleep is promoted. The newer hypnotics have a much lower potential for dependence, as tolerance develops more slowly than with benzodiazepines. In addition, they have a weaker muscle-relaxing effect, which is why the risk of falling is lower. According to current state of knowledge, they are the drugs of choice for the pharmacological treatment of insomnia. The drug names begin with "Z" (zaleplon, zolpidem and zopiclone), which is why the non-benzodiazepines are also called "Z-substances". The common hypnotics are listed in Table 3.40.

Z-substances are the drugs of choice for treatment accompaniment, with the goal of gradually phasing out this medication. A good treatment result is also achieved if, at the end of therapy, non-benzodiazepines are only taken occasionally in exceptional situations (e.g. driving on vacation, extraordinary psychological stress, etc.) (4–6 doses per month). Z-substances

Table 3.39 Overview: Characteristics of the "Z-Substances" (Non-Benzodiazepines)

Indications	Approved for short-term treatment of insomnia with significant severity if all non-pharmacological procedures did not provide significant relief
Contraindications	Pathological muscle weakness, sleep apnoea syndrome, respiratory insufficiency
Advantages	Faster and more secure onset of action, more specific effect than benzodiazepines, therefore fewer side effects and less influence on sleep architecture, shorter half-life, therefore less hangover effects
Disadvantages	Potential for dependence, influence on sleep architecture, falls possible, retard preparations intensify hangover (e.g. StilnoxCR)
Important side effects	Increased daytime sleepiness, headaches, visual disturbances, amnesia, restlessness, irritability, perceptual disturbances, delusions
Working principle	GABA agonist, increases binding affinity to GABA receptors, the ARAS is inhibited and deep sleep is promoted
Application recommendation	Short-term
Therapeutic goal	Fast and short-term symptom relief

Table 3.40 Overview: Frequently used non-benzodiazepine hypnotics (selection)

Preparation	Active ingredient	Equivalent dosage (mg/day)	$t_{1/2}$ (h)
Stilnox, Bikalm, Zolpidem	Zolpidem	5–10	5–2.5
Espa-dorm, Somnosam, Optidorm, Ximovam, Zopiclodura, Zopiclon	Zopiclon	7.5	2–6
Sonata	Zaleplon	5–20	1–1.5
Luniva (neu zugelassen 04/2021)	Eszopiclon	1–3	5–8

t½ half-life.; Starting dose is initially ½ tablet

also have a non-negligible addiction potential. Depending on the preparation, the duration of use should be limited to two and in exceptional cases to four weeks with daily use. It is important to note that tolerance development is primarily oriented towards the number of times of use and less towards the dose taken. Patients tend to halve, quarter or even smaller divide the sleeping pills and take a small dose several times a night. If, nevertheless, a small crumb of a Z-substance is taken every evening, there is a greater risk of addiction than with one- to two-time administration of half or a whole tablet per week.

▶ In patients over the age of 65, long-term medication under close supervision is conceivable.

3.10.4 Melatonin

Overview (Table 3.41)

Background

Melatonin is a hormone produced in the epiphysis (pineal gland). The production of melatonin is suppressed by light. With fluctuating brightness or darkness of the day-night rhythm, melatonin production and secretion are also subject to periodic changes: during the day, when it is light, the production is suppressed, then there is little or no fatigue. With increasing darkness, melatonin is produced and secreted more and more. During the day, it would be enough to cause fatigue with a small dose of melatonin and even initiate sleep. In the evening, however, the melatonin level rises exponentially. To promote

Table 3.41 Overview: Characteristics of Melatonin

Indications	Primary insomnia (approved), sleep-wake rhythm disorders and jet lag syndrome (*off label*)
Contraindications	Liver and kidney dysfunction; Patients with hereditary galactose intolerance, lactase deficiency or glucose-galactose malabsorption, the use is not recommended in autoimmune diseases
Advantage	No influence on sleep architecture, long-term administration (over 13 weeks) possible, not addictive, also safe in overdoses
Disadvantages	No certain onset of action, not sufficiently potent in severe sleep disorders, patients report hypersensitivity to the preparation
Half-life	40–50 min
Important side effects	Nausea, vomiting, headache, irritability, nervousness, restlessness, dizziness, constipation, drowsiness
Working principle	Synthesis in the epiphysis from serotonin, sleep-inducing, -maintaining, controls the sleep-wake rhythm
Application recommendation	People over 55 years, medium-term, up to 13 weeks in primary insomnia
Dosage	0.5–5 mg before bedtime
Therapeutic goal	Quick and short-term symptom relief
Trade name	Circadin

falling asleep and maintaining sleep, very high doses are necessary at this time to have a noticeable effect. Between 3:00 and 4:00 a.m., melatonin secretion reaches its maximum and then decreases again in the morning and with increasing brightness.

After melatonin could be synthesized for the first time, great hope arose among those affected and carers that it would now be possible to treat insomnia causally. First, the synthetic hormone was introduced and researched on the American market, in 2013 it was also introduced on the German market. As early as 2009, melatonin could be purchased as a prescription drug in Switzerland.

However, the desired effect of improved control and control of the sleep-wake rhythm or a sleep aid for people with insomnia did not occur with the administration of melatonin. Since the melatonin level increases in the natural cycle in the evening with decreasing brightness, very high doses of melatonin must be administered for a noticeable intervention. These are often not tolerable for those affected and they reacted with nausea and vomiting. There are patients who benefit from melatonin administration. Melatonin is known to be helpful, especially in shift work or jet lag syndrome.

The so-called seasonal affective disorder ("winter depression") is also coupled to the melatonin rhythm. In winter it is also dark for many hours during the day. The sun only rises in the late morning and sets in the afternoon. The available light is often not enough to suppress melatonin production. Consequently, more melatonin is produced than in the brighter spring and summer months, and fatigue occurs. In addition, a relative serotonin deficiency results, which can lead to depressive symptomatology. In addition to low spirits and lack of motivation, fatigue is also promoted in those affected. This can be the beginning of a downward spiral into a depressive symptomatology. Here, light therapy or medication can be used.

It has not yet been defined when a melatonin deficiency exists. Nevertheless, melatonin has been used as a medication in Germany since 2013 for people over the age of 55.

▶ *For some years, melatonin preparations in the form of tablets, juices or sprays have been available as dietary supplements in the free trade.*

3.10.5 Antihistamines

Overview (Table 3.42)

Background

Antihistamines are mainly used in the treatment of allergies. They act inhibitory on the body's own histamine complex and suppress reactions such as those typical for intolerance to primarily harmless substances (pollen, nuts, etc.). When used against allergies, they have an unwanted effect that is desired when treating sleep disorders, especially insomnia: They make you tired. They have a sleep-promoting effect through the blockade of histamine H1 receptors.

The research situation on the effectiveness of antihistamines for the treatment of insomnia is not very extensive. A systematic review from 2012 points out that the targeted use of antihistamines has a slight to moderate effect in the treatment of insomnia, which is primarily due to the sedative effect of the substances and their long half-life. At the same time, it must be noted that the body develops tolerance very quickly and the stability of the treatment effect is rather low. There are also frequent side effects, such as drowsiness, dry mouth, restrictions on cognitive and motor skills or blurred vision. Positive for those affected is that these substances are freely available. Medications from the group of antihistamines, which are generally intended for the treatment of insomnia, have a corresponding name that suggests their sleep-promoting function. For mild forms of insomnia with temporary cause (short-term stress, travel, noise, etc.) and for people over 65 years, antihistamines can be an alternative. A purely pharmacotherapeutic treatment of insomnia with antihistamines is not recommended on the basis of the described cost-benefit ratio according to the current state of research.

In Table 3.43 preparations are listed which are offered for the treatment of sleep disorders.

Table 3.42 Overview: Characteristics of antihistamines

Indication	Short-term treatment of insomnia
Contraindications	Acute intoxication, respiratory diseases, various functional disorders in the metabolism/excretion system
Advantage	Faster and safer onset of action
Disadvantages	Faster loss of efficacy, therefore moderate dependence potential, hangover effects with pronounced daytime sleepiness; since not prescription, less control of interaction with other medications, unfavorable side effect profile, especially for older people
Important side effects	Increased daytime sleepiness, gastrointestinal disorders
Mode of action	Mediation of a sleep-inducing effect through the blockade of central H_1 receptors
Application recommendation	Short-term
Therapeutic goal	Safe symptom relief

Table 3.43 Overview: Commonly used antihistamines for sleep disorders (selection)

Preparation	Active ingredient	Equipotent dosage (mg/day)	$t_{1/2}$ (h)
Atosil, Closin, Promethazine	Promethazine	25–50	10–12
Gittalun, Hoggar Night	Doxylamine[a]	25	17–27
Beta-dorm, Dolestan, Emesan, Hevert-Dorm	Diphenhydramine	50	7–12

[a] Not available on prescription; taking is not recommended

3.10.6 Antidepressants—Off-Label as Hypnotics

Overview (Table 3.44)

Background

In recent years, the use of sedative antidepressants in the treatment of chronic sleep disorders has proven to be very effective. Since sleep disorders are often the leading symptom of a depressive disorder or sleep disorders can cause depression, the prescription of an antidepressant with a sleep-inducing effect is a logical measure. When prescribing off-label as a pure hypnotic, the dosage can be set significantly lower than for antidepressant treatment. Modern antidepressants such as SSRIs (selective serotonin reuptake inhibitors) or SNRIs (selective serotonin-norepinephrine reuptake inhibitors) have a narrow range of side effects and are well tolerated by most patients after the first two weeks. Nevertheless, these substances fundamentally interfere with the natural processes of the CNS and influence nerve transmission and hormonal cycles. Antidepressants can significantly influence sleep architecture and thus suppress important processes. Doxepin, for example, suppresses REM sleep. It is therefore well effective against nightmares, but interferes with memory formation and emotional regulation. Some preparations shorten deep sleep, which in turn has effects on the subjectively experienced recovery effect and memory formation. Therefore, despite generally good tolerability, risks and benefits should always be weighed up.

Another positive aspect is the possibility of long-term prescription without dependence risk, although there are no relevant long-term studies. Depending on the cause of the sleep disorder, however, sufferers report that they do not feel any effectiveness with regard to the sleep disorder. Antidepressants therefore do not have such a safe effect of action as Z-substances or benzodiazepines.

Excursus Agomelatin

Agomelatin is a chemical compound structurally related to melatonin from the group of antidepressants. It is considered the first melatonergic antidepressant and has been used for the treatment of major depression in adults since its approval under the trade name Valdoxan in 2009. Agomelatin has a high affinity for melatonin receptors. Current studies have shown that agomelatin has positive effects on the duration of deep sleep, general sleep quality and daytime vigilance, and is also very well tolerated. Therefore, agomelatin preparations may be an alternative to the usual medications for the treatment of insomnia for some patients. However, a safe efficacy cannot be guaranteed here either.

The antidepressants commonly used for sleep disorders are listed in Table 3.45.

Table 3.44 Overview: Characteristics of Antidepressants—Off-Label as Hypnotics

Indications	Sleep disorders (Off-Label; there is no approval for this indication)
Contraindications	Cardiovascular diseases, suicidality, manic episodes, blood cell changes, possibly epilepsy, gastrointestinal bleeding. Cave: central serotonin syndrome
Advantage	In addition to treating the insomnia, therapy can also treat the often comorbid affective symptomatology, longer-term prescription possible, few side effects with good tolerance, fewer hangover effects because of the short half-life when used as a hypnotic
Disadvantages	Partially long half-lives, especially at the beginning of therapy → hangover effects, drive inhibition, effect only after 7–14 days, side effects are possible
Important side effects	Dry mouth, headaches, loss of appetite, influence on sleep architecture, restless legs, other psychovegetative symptoms possible
Mode of action	Sedative effect mediated by antihistaminic and 5-HT$_2$-antagonistic properties, control of the day-night rhythm through the activation of serotonergic or noradrenergic receptors, blockade of adrenergic receptors
Application recommendation	Low dosage, can be prescribed for long-term
Therapeutic goal	Increasing the effective sleep time, stabilizing the sleep or increasing the drive in hypersomnia

Table 3.45 Overview: Antidepressants frequently used for sleep disorders (selection)

Preparation	Active ingredient	Equipotent dosage (mg/day)	$t_{1/2}$ (h)
Saroten, Tryptizol	Amitriptylin (TZA, *off label*)	25–50	8–51
Aponal	Doxepin, suppresses REM sleep (TZA, *off- abel*)	50	17
Remergil, Remeron	Mirtazapin (SNRI)	15–45	20–40
Thombran, Trittico	Trazodon (SSRI)	100	13
Herphonal, Stangyl	Trimipramine (TZA)	100	24
Valdoxan	Agomelatine (Melatonin receptor agonist, SSRI)	25–50	1–2

TZA tricyclic antidepressant, *SNRI* selective serotonin-norepinephrine reuptake inhibitor, *SSRI* selective serotonin reuptake inhibitor

3.10.7 Neuroleptics—Off-Label as Hypnotics

Overview (Table 3.46)

Background

Neuroleptics (or antipsychotics) are used primarily in psychopharmacology to treat psychotic disorders and schizophrenia.

In addition to their use in treating insomnia, the advantage of prescribing antipsychotics lies in the possibility of achieving parasomnias medicinally. Due to their depressing effect on the dopaminergic system, the probability of occurrence of dreams with great emotional stress and emotional outbursts (as in pavor nocturnus, which is associated with sudden great fear) is reduced. Especially the newer, "atypical" neuroleptics such as olanzapine, quetiapine or clozapine have a sedative effect even in very low doses. However, it should be noted that antipsychotics influence sleep architecture and thus can suppress or inhibit important night-time processes. Dreams have the function of memory formation and emotional regulation. If these nocturnal sequences are suppressed, the actual symptomatology may worsen. Treating sleep disorders with neuroleptics appears to be very promising at first glance, as most patients respond well to them and there is an observable effect. However, neuroleptics have a wide range of side effects. In cases of milder symptomatology, a thorough weighing of risks and benefits is particularly important, as the use of antipsychotics is often exaggerated here and there are more favorable treatment options.

In Table 3.47 the neuroleptics commonly used in sleep disorders are listed.

3.10.8 Anxiolytics

Anxiolytics are substances that relieve anxiety. Benzodiazepine anxiolytics are the main representatives, as they have a muscle-relaxing and sedative effect. In the past, such substances were also called tranquilizers, because they have a calming effect on the organism. The main area of application is the therapy of anxiety disorders, in which they should only be used as an accompaniment to psychotherapy.

In the therapy of sleep disorders, anxiolytics are used to promote somatic relaxation. The primary goal is to create a relaxed state of wakefulness that is absolutely necessary to fall asleep. Anxiolytics are specifically prescribed to support the therapy of nightmares. They cause REM sleep suppression and thus prevent intensive and

Table 3.46 Brief overview: Characteristics of neuroleptics—off-label as hypnotics

Indications	Sleep disorders (Melperon and Pipamperon are approved for this indication)
Contraindications	Acute intoxication, epilepsy or brain organic damage, various functional disorders in the metabolism/excretion system
Advantage	Low addiction potential, long-term prescription possible, partly mood-enhancing effect
Disadvantages	Hangover effects, generally depressing effect, reduction in quality of life, no use in older patients
Important side effects	Anticholinergic properties: delirium, arrhythmias, bladder dysfunction, late dyskinesias, increased daytime sleepiness, temporary dysphoria, induction of euphoric mood, increased irritability
Mode of action	Suppression of dopaminergic overactivity in the CNS
Recommendation for use	Short- to medium-term
Therapeutic goal	Safe symptom relief

Table 3.47 Overview: Neuroleptics commonly used in sleep disorders (selection)

Preparation	Active ingredient	Equipotent dosage (mg/day)	$t_{1/2}$ (h)
Zyprexa	Olanzapine	5–40	23–43
Seroquel, Quentiax	Quetiapine	200–800	6–11
Leponex, Elcrit	Clozapine	25–600	8–16
Dipiperon	Pipamperone	20–80	17–22
Dominal	Protipendyl	40–80	2–3
Melperon generics	Melperon	50–400	4–6

extensive dreaming. This can only be done to a limited extent, as dreams play an important role in memory formation and emotion regulation. If REM sleep is suppressed permanently, those affected are emotionally unstable, irritable and have significant memory deficits. Dreams have an important function, their suppression is not exclusively beneficial. Therefore, nightmares should be treated specifically.

In addition, there are other groups of active substances in the field of anxiolytics that can be prescribed for non-organic sleep disorders, such as pregabalin, buspirone, opipramol or various phytopharmaceuticals, whose effect is based on a relaxation effect through muscle relaxation.

▶ A very positive property of anxiolytics is the positive influence on pain.

3.10.9 Cannabinoids (Tetrahydrocannabinol, THC)

Overview (Table 3.48)

Background

CBD is the abbreviation for cannabidiol, an extract of the hemp plant. So far, more than 100 cannabinoids have been extracted, each with very different properties. CBD and THC are among the best known cannabinoids. Tetrahydrocannabinol (THC) and cannabidiol (CBD) are phytocannabinoids, which are mainly obtained from the hemp plant (cannabis plant). Cannabinoids have a high affinity for cannabinoid receptors within the so-called endogenous cannabinoid system. This system is responsible for the diverse effects of cannabinoids in our body, although the exact

Table 3.48 Overview: Characteristics of Cannabinoids

Indications	Sleep disorders
Contraindications	Acute intoxication, epilepsy or brain organic damage, various functional disorders in the metabolism/excretion system
Advantage	Long-term prescription possible, partly mood-enhancing effect
Disadvantages	Hangover effects, generally depressing effect
Important side effects	Anticholinergic properties: delirium, arrhythmias, bladder dysfunction, late dyskinesias, increased daytime sleepiness, temporary dysphoria, induction of euphoric mood, increased irritability
Mode of action	Inhibition or activation of the endogenous cannabinoid system (part of the nervous system)
Application recommendation	Controversial
Therapeutic goal	Safe symptom relief, but controversial

mechanisms of action of THC and CBD have not yet been sufficiently investigated. It is important to distinguish THC and CBD fundamentally from each other, because their mode of action is very different in the human organism.

Tetrahydrocannabinol (THC) is a psychoactive substance that occurs in its highest concentration in the resinous flowers of the female hemp plant and produces an intoxicating effect in the human body. Therefore, THC is attributed psychoactive effects, such as changes in affect, perception and consciousness. Contrary to many opinions, THC can lead to psychological dependence and cause lasting psychological and especially neurovegetative deficits as well as withdrawal symptoms.

Cannabidiol (CBD) is a non-psychoactive cannabinoid that occurs mainly in the female hemp plant and, in contrast to THC, does not produce an intoxicating effect in the human body. CBD is said to have an antispasmodic, anti-inflammatory, anti-anxiety, antipsychotic and anti-nausea effect.

Nevertheless, THC has very positive effects on various symptoms and diseases, provided it is used conscientiously, in the right dosage form and dose. In Germany, the cannabis-containing prescription drugs "Sativex" for the treatment of multiple sclerosis and epilepsy and "Canemes" for the treatment of chemotherapy-induced nausea, vomiting and appetite loss are approved. In addition, medical cannabis in the form of dried cannabis

flowers (marijuana) has been a prescription drug in Germany since 2017 and can be prescribed by any doctor. Corresponding indications are chronic pain, chronic inflammatory bowel diseases, epilepsy, Tourette syndrome, tremor or—in cancer or AIDS patients—nausea, vomiting and appetite loss.

In the fight against sleep disorders, there is a rather heterogeneous effect, which is why the use of THC as a medication must be well weighed and currently takes place as an off-label medication. In human history, reports of the soporific benefits of the cannabis plant can be found dating back more than 5000 years. In Western societies, the majority of consumers say they consume cannabis also because of the subjectively strong soporific effect. Current systematic reviews conclude that THC and CBD as medical cannabis can have positive effects on sleep latency and subjective sleep quality in patients with sleep disorders (Bhagavan et al. 2020; Gates et al. 2014). The sedative effect of the substances seems to be responsible for the reported effects. At low doses, positive effects on REM and non-REM sleep, subjective sleep quality and sleep latency could be demonstrated for THC. At higher doses, even opposite effects were observed (Garcia and Salloum 2015). In general, it was shown that the soporific effect of THC is only temporary. With longer use, there is often a habituation and a decrease in the positive effects. If the regular use of THC is interrupted, withdrawal symptoms often occur, which are accompanied by a decrease in sleep quality, increased daytime sleepiness and an increase in sleep latency (Babson et al. 2017). For the prescription-only cannabis preparations approved in Germany, convincing studies are still lacking today, and the general evidence base is very thin in this context (Bhagavan et al. 2020).

Cannabidiol (CBD), on the other hand, can be used to a large extent without any concerns, but is just as heterogeneous in terms of efficacy in sleep disorders, dosage recommendations and times of intake. It is sold in Germany as a non-prescription dietary supplement and is mostly very cost-intensive. Studies report positive effects on total sleep duration and a subjectively overall improved sleep for medium to high doses of CBD (Babson et al. 2017).

From experience, it is rather a small group of patients for whom CBD shows a solid effect. Since CBD oils are freely available for sale as dietary supplements, you will find recommendations for dosage and administration under the heading Phytopharmaka.

3.10.10 Orexin Receptor Antagonists

Overview (Table 3.49)

Background

Orexin receptor antagonists are a popular subject of current research into pharmacotherapy for sleep disorders. The neurotransmitter orexin (also called hypocretin) was discovered in 1998. It is produced in the hypothalamus and plays a key role in regulating sleep-wake cycles in the central nervous system by stabilizing wakefulness. Orexin regulates both REM and non-REM sleep. Orexin deficiency leads to fatigue and can even cause narcolepsy.

Orexin receptor antagonists block the orexin receptors and thus have a sedative effect. Studies have shown that the use of the orexin receptor antagonist "suvorexant", which has been approved for use in the United States since 2014, has positive effects on the subjective sleep duration, especially on REM and non-REM sleep of patients with insomnia (Patel et al. 2015; Holst et al. 2019). In addition, a shorter latency to sleep was reported (Michelson et al. 2014). In recent reviews, "suvorexant" is explicitly recommended for the treatment of sleep onset and sleep maintenance disorders (Atkin et al. 2018; Krystal et al. 2019). In previous studies, no dependence syndromes have been found. However, a hangover effect is observed due to the longer half-life. Applications for the approval of orexin receptor antagonists for use in Europe have been submitted.

Orexin receptor antagonists must not be used in narcolepsy because orexin is detectable in cerebrospinal fluid in smaller amounts and contributes to the already pronounced daytime sleepiness. In addition, it increases suicidal thoughts. Orexin is also involved in metabolic

Table 3.49 Brief overview: Characteristics of orexin receptor antagonists

Indication	Insomnia, especially difficulty falling asleep
Contraindications	Narcolepsy, diabetes mellitus, anorexia, obesity, possibly with comorbidities: depression, anxiety disorders, psychosis
Advantage	Faster and more secure onset of action
Disadvantages	Moderate dependence potential, hangover effects with pronounced daytime sleepiness, unfavorable side effect profile, interactions with comorbidities (especially depression, anxiety disorders, psychosis), ability to drive and operate machinery impaired
Important side effects	Headache, drowsiness, dizziness, abnormal thinking and dreams, diarrhea, dry mouth, sleep paralysis, hallucinations, tachycardia, psychomotor hyperactivity
Mode of action	Central nervous system depressant (CNS), blockade of orexin receptors, thus promoting fatigue and sleep
Application recommendation	Rather short-term, but controversial
Therapeutic goal	Safe symptom relief

Table 3.50 Orexin receptor antagonist approved for sleep disorders

Preparation	Active ingredient	Equipotent dosage (mg/day)	$t_{1/2}$ (h)
Belsomra	Suvorexant[*]	10–20 mg	8–13
Quvivig[**]	Daridorexant	25–50 mg	approx. 8

[*] approved in USA
[**] approved in Germany

diseases such as diabetes mellitus, anorexia or obesity (Hungs and Mignot 2001). There have also been links found with alcohol dependence.

Depending on the preparation, the recommended doses are between 10 and 50 mg. At least 8 h of sleep should be planned, as the half-life of this orexin receptor antagonist is between 8 and 13 h (Table 3.50).

3.11 Phytotherapeutics

Phytotherapeutics are over-the-counter preparations based on plants. The treatment with medicinal plants is one of the most commonly used complementary treatments for sleep disorders. Products with valerian, hops, lavender, balm and passion flower are particularly popular. Although some studies have already been able to document positive effects of these substances on the sleep latency and the sleep duration of patients with sleep disorders, there is still no sufficient proof of efficacy (Cravotto et al. 2010; Fernández-San-Martín et al. 2010; Colalto 2018). Nevertheless, the use of phytotherapeutics is worth a try, as some patients respond very positively to it, the side effect profile is narrow and no dependency diseases can occur.

Valerian and hops can help those affected above all against difficulty in falling asleep. However, they are less successful in the case of sleep through disorder. Lavender and melissa are less effective, but can calm down during the day, so that the overall stress level and the accompanying hormone levels remain lower. Often, various extracts of medicinal plants are combined, especially with passion flower.

In order to achieve an efficacy of the phytopharmaceuticals, it is important to take a potent dose regularly and over a long period of time. The extracts available in drugstores and pharmacies promise a fast effect. In contrast to potent chemical drugs, the extracted active ingredients of the capsules, tablets or drops of the medicinal plants do not act immediately, so patience is required here. Sometimes the noticeable effect only occurs after weeks.

In addition to the extracted active ingredients, it is possible to take the medicinal plants in the form of teas, tinctures, medicated oils or juices. Since these contain not only the concentrated active ingredients, but also the secondary plant active ingredients, they act more regulative than exclusively sleep-inducing. It is advisable to consume the natural preparations several times a day. The feared effect by many patients, then to be more tired during the day, does not occur due to the regulative effect of the natural preparations.

Another advantage of consuming the entire medicinal plant in tea or other natural preparations is that the natural smell and taste of the phytopharmaceutical are retained. The peripheral nervous system is addressed directly by the stimulation of the olfactory and gustatory buds, which is why these preparations sometimes work better and faster than concentrated extracts contained in capsules, which only contain the basic active ingredient of the medicinal plant. These have to be metabolized by digestion first before the active ingredient arrives where it is needed. Part of the active ingredient has already been filtered out, which is why in this case significantly higher doses have to be taken.

Phytopharmacology has attracted the interest of research in recent years, and so numerous studies have been carried out on the effectiveness of many preparations. Since the research situation is still very thin, the data situation is still inconsistent. However, some preparations showed good potency in these studies, so that clear recommendations can be made.

3.11.1 European Medicinal Plants

Background

Valerian is sleep-inducing, which is scientifically proven. In order to achieve a noticeable effect here, proven. In order to achieve a noticeable effect here, it must be consumed regularly over a longer period of time. In the dosage form as an extract in drops, powder, pressing or in tea, the unpleasant bitter taste already has a calming effect on the nervous system on the tongue and can be incorporated into an evening ritual in this way. Therefore, I recommend my patients to forego the more pleasant intake of the concentrate preparations in capsules and to consume the mostly unpleasant smelling and tasting unprocessed valerian roots in the appropriate form. When used in combination with other calming and sleep-inducing herbs such as hops, melissa or passionflower, the effectiveness is increased. Clinical studies showed few side effects, so that these preparations can be taken safely and for a long time and should be effective for them. In Table 3.51 you will find a list of common phytopharmaceuticals for the treatment of sleep disorders.

3.11.2 Ayurvedic Medicinal Plants

Background
Not only the European herb garden has effective medicinal plants to offer, but other forms of naturopathy also have potent phytopharmaceuticals. In the over 5000 year old medicine of Ayurveda, a good benefit has been observed in many medicinal plants. In fact, the Ashvanganda, also known as the sleep berry, winter cherry or Indian ginseng, is shown to be soporific. In clinical studies, it has a similar efficacy to modern antidepressants, as it acts on the HPA axis. Studies show a regulatory influence on cortisol levels (Cheah et al. 2021).

In Table 3.52 you will find a list of Ayurvedic phytopharmaceuticals for the treatment of sleep disorders.

3.11.3 Herbal Medicines from Traditional Chinese Medicine (TCM)

Background
TCM views health and illness differently than Western medicine. As such, the diagnostics and description of syndromes used to describe and treat sleep disorders are also unique. Starting with the diagnostics, TCM describes various syndromes that can cause sleep disorders, such as an imbalance between Yin and Yang, a Liver

Table 3.51 Overview: European medicinal plants for sleep disorders (selection)

Heilpflanze	Wirkweise	Darreichungsform	Einnahme
Baldrian	Sleep-inducing, relaxing (acts, similar to benzodiazepines and Z-substances on GABA receptors).	l Root as tea, drops, powder, dragée, capsule combination preparation	3 times daily
Hops	Soothing, relaxing	Hops cones as tea, lozenge Combination preparation	3 times daily
Lemon Melissa	Soothing, antispasmodic, digestive, antiviral	Flowers as tea, drops, lozenges, and capsules Combination preparation	3 times daily
Passionflower	Soothing, anxiety-reducing	Herb, popular combination preparation	2- to 4-times daily
Lavender	Soothing and actually sleep-inducing	Flowers as tea, drops, dragées, and capsules, bath additive, lavender pillow	Depending on dosage form, as tea 3-times daily
Mugwort	Relaxing, temperature-regulating (also said to have an antidepressant effect)	Tea	2- to 3-times daily
St. John's wort	The antidepressant effect can have a positive effect on sleep Attention: Consider interactions	Flowers as tea, drops, dragées, and capsules	Depending on the dosage form, 1 to 3 times daily

Table 3.52 Overview: Ayurvedic medicinal plants for sleep disorders (selection)

Medicinal plant	Mode of Action	Dosage form	Intake
Ashvanganda *(Withania somnifera)*	Balancing, calming sleep inducing	Roots as powder, pressed or capsule	2 to 3 times daily 2-6 g, approx. 90 min before going to bed
Brahmi (Bellyflower)	More against fatigue during the day Solves inner tension, neuroprotective, promotion of cognitive performance	Dried herb, fresh herb juice especially effective	2 times daily, 1–2 g
Jatamansi	Soothing, relaxing and thus promotes sleep, does not make primarily tired	Dried herb, as a combination preparation with valerian and Brahmi	2 to 3 times daily, 1–3 g
Tulasi (broad-leaved basil)	Stress-regulating	Dried herb in tea, capsules, tablets, often as a combination preparation Fresh herb juice especially effective	2- to 3-times daily, 1–3 g

Table 3.53 Overview: Herbal medicines from traditional Chinese medicine for sleep disorders (selection)

Medicinal plant	Mode of Action	Dosage form	Intake
Shenqi Wuweizi	Sleep inducing, extended effective sleep time	Tablets, decoction	Different
Zaoren Anshen	Calms the mind, cools the "false" heat of the liver and heart, eliminates irritability	Capsules, decoction	Different
Yangxin Anshen Therapy (TYAT)	Improvement of sleep quality (total sleep time, sleep efficiency, sleep latency, wake time after falling asleep)	Pressing, capsules, decoction	Different
Paeoniae Radix-containing (Chinese Peony)	Promotes circulation, relaxing and antispasmodic, promotes thermal regulation, therefore good against RLS and also insomnia (especially for women in menopause)	Root and seed as tablets, capsules, decoction	Different

Yin deficiency, Liver Fire, or a raging Heart. According to these syndromes, various herbs and manual methods, especially acupuncture, are used. Phytopharmaceuticals include herbs and mushrooms. Minerals and animal products are also often used as medications in combination preparations. Numerous studies have been published in recent years. Some substances, according to these studies, show similar effect strengths to benzodiazepines and Z-substances.

In Table 3.53 you will find a list of phytopharmaceuticals for the treatment of sleep disorders from TCM.

(Ni et al. 2015)

> ▶ *In addition to phytopharmacology, naturopathy has a number of mental and manual therapies that are very helpful against sleep disorders.*

3.12 Dietary Supplements

3.12.1 Background

The market is currently flooded with dietary supplements that promise to quickly lead to a restful sleep. Promises are made of grandiose proportions, such as "falling asleep within 5 minutes", never having trouble sleeping again and never being tired during the day. Attractive names of the products reinforce their supposed effectiveness. I believe such healing promises are not ethically defensible.

Nevertheless, there are serious products that are difficult to identify in the jungle of the large and fast-moving offer. Dietary supplements are usually harmless and can be used for a long period of time if prescribed dosage and tolerability are observed. However, despite this, health problems or damage can still occur with overdose and incorrect use. Blood tests and close cooperation with the patient's treating GP are therefore advisable.

Deficiencies of various vitamins, minerals and (essential) amino acids that are contained in dietary supplements can actually lead to health problems and also sleep disorders. If there is not enough "raw material" to produce serotonin or melatonin, the body cannot produce the corresponding neurotransmitters and hormones that are necessary for regulating the sleep-wake cycle. Serotonin is produced from tryptophan, vitamin B6, zinc and iron. In the pineal gland of the brain, serotonin is finally converted into melatonin. If one of these starting materials is missing, this complex conversion process is inhibited. Melatonin can cross the blood-brain barrier. Therefore, direct intake of melatonin via food or as a dietary supplement (e.g. as a spray that is sprayed directly onto the tongue) can be helpful if there is a melatonin deficiency.

Vitamin D supplements can also improve sleep quality according to a recent study (Majid et al. 2017). The vitamin can be produced by our body itself. However, sufficient sunlight is necessary for this. In winter, many people suffer from a vitamin D deficiency, so substitution is also sensible in this case. However, caution is advised in the event of an overdose, which can cause calcification of the vessels, among other things.

On closer inspection of the ingredients of dietary supplements for better sleep, it becomes apparent that these preparations contain concentrated extracts of phytopharmaceuticals and substances that are necessary for the synthesization of serotonin and melatonin. Since most of these combination preparations are very expensive, I recommend that my patients weigh up carefully whether this investment is really worthwhile or whether a corresponding change in diet with targeted intake of phytopharmaceuticals, vitamins and minerals would be more sustainable and helpful.

Most of these preparations are combination preparations that are additionally enriched with vitamins, minerals and amino acids. It should be noted that some of the ingredients cannot cross the blood-brain barrier, such as serotonin. Therefore, some of the promised effects cannot be achieved on this basis alone. Popular ingredients can be found in Table 3.54. Dosage, duration and time of intake are very different. Detailed instructions for the producer's recommendations can be found on the package inserts and product descriptions.

3.12.2 Cannabidiol (CBD)

Background

Cannabidiol (CBD) is an extract of the cannabis plant. Unlike other cannabis products, CBD is not psychoactive and therefore largely unproblematic to use. In Germany, as already seen, it is sold as a non-prescription dietary supplement and is very cost-intensive. The state of research on efficacy in sleep disorders is inconsistent despite many research efforts. Some studies report increased total sleep duration and subjectively improved sleep quality for medium to high doses of CBD (Babson et al. 2017). With difficulty falling asleep and staying asleep, CBD oil can have a calming effect and in most cases does not lead to hangover effects the next day.

► CBD can also have a positive effect on the often occurring comorbidities such as anxiety disorders, depression and burn-out as well as pain disorders due to its anti-inflammatory effect.

For the symptoms and diseases listed in Table 3.55, CBD can have positive effects.

The effects have not been conclusively scientifically confirmed. However, many people report the described positive effects on the mentioned symptoms and diseases.

Table 3.54 Overview: Dietary supplements for sleep disorders (selection)

Ingredient	Description and mode of action
Baldrian extract	Sleep-inducing, relaxing
Hop extract	Soothing, relaxing
Melissa extract	Soothing, antispasmodic, digestive, antiviral
Passionflower extract	Soothing, anxiolytic
Lavender extract	Soothing and actually sleep-inducing
Melatonin	Sleep-inducing
L-Tryptophan	As a precursor of serotonin and melatonin: mood-enhancing, antidepressant, sleep-inducing
Serotonin	Mood-enhancing, antidepressant, as a precursor of melatonin sleep-inducing
5-HTP (5-Hydroxytryptophan)	As an intermediate product for the production of serotonin mood-enhancing
Vitamin B	Important component of melatonin production
Vitamin D	Improves sleep quality, often under-supplied in winter months
Magnesium	Muscle relaxant
Selenium	Controls hormone production of the thyroid, imbalance can cause restlessness, sleep and wakefulness problems, can affect the production of melatonin
Gamma-Aminobutyric Acid (GABA)	Inhibits entire nervous system, inhibits nerve conduction and thus shuts down the senses, stress, tension and anxiety relief
Iron	Important component of melatonin production

Table 3.55 Overview: Indication for the use of CBD

Diseases and comorbidities	Description and mechanism of action
Sleep disorder	Stress reduction through calming effect, relaxing
Anxiety disorders and depression	Anxiety-reducing, calming, relaxing
Pain disorders	Pain-relieving, antispasmodic, relaxing
Nausea (resulting from fatigue)	Reduction of nausea

Application and Intake of CBD Oil

CBD is administered orally by dripping a drop of oil under the tongue. CBD is also available as globules. In this case, the corresponding amount of beads is placed on or under the tongue. In this way, the active ingredient is quickly transported to the peripheral nervous system and can take effect there. CBD is also available in capsules, the active ingredients of which enter the circulation via digestion. Here, the desired effect therefore only starts later. Since the product is also metabolized, only higher doses are potent here. It is important to choose high-quality products with a corresponding potency and to slowly introduce the dosage. If well tolerated, the dose can then be gradually increased until the desired effect is noticeable. CBD preparations can be taken in combination with other phytopharmaceuticals or dietary supplements. There are also combination preparations with different ingredients specifically for the treatment of sleep disorders, such as lavender, valerian or passion flower extract.

► Unfortunately, CBD oils can also not work miracles. Experience has shown that it is rather a small group of patients for whom CBD shows a solid effect.

3.13 Placebo

There is a drug that can help against all symptoms and diseases. The ingredients are very different. Sugar beets, salt water and gel capsules are very popular. The dosage form can also range from tablets, capsules, drops, infusions to "irradiation" and "operations". However, all of them are equally ineffective according to the current state of scientific knowledge and cannot take specific action on the respective symptomatology. This "miracle drug" is called placebo. The targeted placebo research began as early as the 1950s and has produced thousands of high-quality studies to date. This knowledge is indispensable for doctors and people with sleep disorders when making the responsible decision to prescribe or take a hypnotic.

For a long time, the question was asked what the basic effect of placebos is. The answer is, from today's point of view, quite different: The conviction that a medication or treatment will help against suffering creates trust. The previously known mechanism of action of the placebo is in the relaxation effect in the affected persons and thus a reduction of the chronically elevated cortisol level. The importance of cortisol regulation for sleep has already been described in detail in *Sect. 1.5.3*.

In order to investigate the placebo effect in the pharmacological treatment of sleep disorders more closely, numerous pure placebo studies have been carried out in the past in patients with insomnia. Comparison groups with hypnotics were included in these studies in order to specifically investigate the actual placebo effect. A meta-analysis of these studies showed that in

patients with insomnia who received a placebo over a period of two weeks, the subjective sleep latency decreased significantly and the subjective total sleep time increased significantly. The objectively measured polysomnographic data only reflected this feeling to a limited extent and not significantly (McCall et al. 2003). However, it is important to note that the subjective quality of life of the affected persons improved significantly. This is our task in the treatment of sleep disorders.

Another meta-analysis showed that potent hypnotics did not perform significantly better than placebos. Compared to the placebo, Z-medications caused only slight improvements in subjective and polysomnographic sleep latency, but only at higher doses (Huedo-Medina et al. 2012).

Even with the use of sleep-inducing antidepressants, a similar picture emerged. With a short-term use of doxepin and trazodone, there was only a slight improvement in sleep quality compared to the placebo. Again, side effects were reported in some studies. Despite frequent use in clinical practice, no basic efficacy could be demonstrated for amitriptyline (Everitt et al. 2018).

In the meta-analysis by Winkler and Rief (2015), a moderate efficacy was already shown in the placebo control groups in both subjective statements and objective measurements across all substance classes, with a symptom improvement of approximately 60% of symptoms. These meta-analyses and systematic reviews show that even potent hypnotics do not create a significant improvement in sleep duration and quality compared to placebo. However, the side effects of hypnotics often limit the quality of life of those affected to a very large extent (e.g. Rösner et al. 2018; Kong et al. 2018). Due to publication bias, one must read the studies very carefully. Many studies show significant improvements in sleep in the pre-post test, but often only slightly better results of hypnotics compared to placebo control group.

Of course, there are numerous studies and large meta-analyses that clearly demonstrate the superiority of hypnotics over placebo (Nowell et al. 1997). However, the overall situation is unclear, which is why a responsible weighing of risks and benefits should be carried out in the treatment with hypnotics. The placebo effect can also be considered as a treatment option.

3.14 Relapse Prevention and Follow-Up

3.14.1 Relapse Prevention

Relapse prevention should be integrated and dealt with alongside therapy after acute treatment in various sessions. For this purpose, it is necessary to summarize again and again and make it clear to the patient which are the personal early warning signs for a possible relapse and which strategies help. It is favorable to set up two hierarchies for this:

- First of all, the person concerned must be able to recognize first symptoms of sleep disorders and also be aware of how their development will continue or which symptoms will follow. This results in the realization of when it is time to take countermeasures.
- Secondly, the strategies helpful for the person concerned should be listed. Here, a subdivision, which strategies are effective but low-threshold, can be useful. These help in everyday life and the person concerned can prepare for them from the therapy experience, with what probability and in what time frame they will work. The other category is that of the actual emergency strategies.

▶ It is important that the awareness for problematic symptoms is sharpened and the strategies are mastered safely.

The imagination of the therapist and the patient is the only limit: A "emergency kit" could be packed for bad nights, which could contain a CD with relaxation stories, herbal tea, etc., or a note could be attached to the computer screen, which reminds to take regular breaks. Even a card in the wallet, which points out to do something good regularly, is one possibility. Such memotechniques should be individually adapted and helpful, and it makes sense to test such methods already in the follow-up phase.

3.14.2 Aftercare

Aftercare immediately follows the actual treatment of the symptoms. In this phase, the learned skills and abilities should be consolidated and anchored in everyday life in particular. Only a few new contents are offered. In the sessions, the current state of affairs and the implementation of the effective strategies are discussed. There is a fine-tuning of the methods in everyday life. To do this, the sessions should be held at increasingly longer intervals so that the support of the therapist does not suddenly disappear, but fades out. This phase should and may extend over several months.

▶ Sleep is a sensitive stress and mood seismograph.

For people who suffer from or have suffered from sleep disorders, sleep is particularly susceptible to disturbance. Therefore, even after apparently successful therapy, fluctuations can still occur. These should be supported as much as possible. It is important to prepare the patients for these fluctuations so that they do not find it catastrophic if sleep suddenly gets worse again. This possibility always exists, especially if the life circumstances of the affected persons change and the learned structures no longer work.

Determining the end of therapy is often not easy for patients with sleep disorders. Many patients have the expectation of regaining a "normal" sleep after therapy. The definition of "normal" sleep includes a wide range of (im)possibilities. Therefore, it is important to lead the patients to realistic goals at the beginning and during the therapy. This mainly affects the duration of sleep and nocturnal awakening. Psychoeducation is the method of choice here.

After the therapy, so-called booster sessions are recommended, at which the therapist and patient meet again a few months after the end of therapy to discuss the current situation and possibly refresh topics that have been forgotten. The booster sessions can also be implemented very well in a group setting, as the patients can benefit and learn from each other directly.

References

Atkin T, Comai S, Gobbi G (2018) Drugs for insomnia beyond benzodiazepines: pharmacology, clinical applications, and discovery. *Pharmacol Rev* 70:197–245

Babson KA, Sottile J, Morabito D (2017) Cannabis, cannabinoids, and sleep: a review of the literature. Curr Psychiatry Rep 19:23

Badura B, Ducki A, Schröder H, Klose J, Meyer M (2020) Fehlzeiten-Report 2020: gerechtigkeit und Gesundheit. Springer, Berlin

Bankar M, Chaudhari S, Chaudhari K (2013) Impact of long term Yoga practice on sleep and quality of life in the elderly. J Ayurveda Integr Med 4:28–32

Beaulieu D (2003) Eye movement integration therapy. The comprehensive clinical guide. Crownhouse Publishing, Williston

Benkert O, Hippius H (2020) Kompendium der Psychiatrischen Pharmakotherapie, 10th edn. Springer, Berlin Heidelberg New York

Bhagavan C, Kung S, Doppen M et al (2020) Cannabinoids in the treatment of insomnia disorder: a systematic review and meta-analysis. *CNS Drugs* 34:1217–1228

Binks H, Vincent GE, Gupta C, Irwin C, Khalesi S (2020) Effects of diet on sleep: a narrative review. Nutrients 124:936

Black DS, O'Reilly GA, Olmstead R, Breen CE, Irwin MR (2015) Mindfulness meditation and improvement in sleep quality and daytime impairment among older adults with sleep disturbances. JAMA Intern Med 1754:494–501

Borbély AA, Baumann F, Brandeis D et al (1981) Sleep deprivation; effect on sleep stages and EEG power density in man. Electroencelphalogr Clin Neurophysiol 51:483–493

Braid J (1844–1845) Magic, mesmerism, hypnotism etc., historically and physiologically considered. Medical Times XI:203–204, 224–227, 270–273, 296–299, 399–400, 439–341

Calvert GA (2001) Crossmodal processing in the human brain: insights from functional neuroimaging studies. Cereb Cortex 111110–1123:1047–3211

Campanini MZ, Guallar-Castillón P, Rodríguez-Artalejo F, Lopez-Garcia E (2017) Mediterranean diet and changes in sleep duration and indicators of sleep quality in older adults. Sleep 403:1–9

Chapin TJ, Russell-Chapin LA (2014) Neurotherapy and neurofeedback: Brain-based treatment for psychological and behavioral problems. Routledge/Taylor & Francis Group, New York

Cheah KL, Norhayati MN, Husniati Yaacob L, Abdul RR (2021) Effect of Ashwagandha *Withania somnifera.* extract on sleep: a systematic review and meta-analysis. PLoS One 169:e0257843

Colalto C (2018) What phytotherapy needs: Evidence-based guidelines for better clinical practice. Phytother Res 32:413–425

Cravotto G, Boffa L, Genzini L, Garella D (2010) Phytotherapeutics: An evaluation of the potential of 1000 plants. J Clin Pharm Ther 35:11–48

Crönlein T (2013) Schlafstörungen: ein Gruppentherapieprogramm für den stationären Bereich. Hogrefe, Göttingen

Dobos G, Paul A (2019) Mind-Body-Medizin: integrative Konzepte zur Ressourcenstärkung und Lebensstilveränderung. Urban & Fischer, München

Ellis A (1979) Handbook of rational-emotive therapy dt. Urban & Schwarzenberg, München

Erickson MH (1954) Special techniques of brief hypnotherapy. J Clin Exp Hypnosis 2:109–129

Everitt H, Baldwin DS, Stuart B, Lipinska G, Mayers A, Malizia AL, Manson CCF, Wilson S (2018) Antidepressants for insomnia in adults. Cochrane Database Syst Rev – Interv (5):CD010753

Farré N, Torres M, Gozal D, Farré R (2018) Sleep and circadian alterations and the gut microbiome: associations or causality? Curr Sleep Med Rep 41:50–57

Fernández-San-Martín MI, Masa-Font R, Palacios-Soler L, Sancho-Gómez P, Calbó-Caldentey C, Flores-Mateo G (2010) Effectiveness of valerian on insomnia: A meta-analysis of randomized placebo-controlled trials. Sleep Med 11:505–511

Garcia AN, Salloum IM (2015) Polysomnographic sleep disturbances in nicotine, caffeine, alcohol, cocaine, opioid, and cannabis use: a focused review. Am J Addict 24:590–598

Gates PJ, Albertella L, Copeland J (2014) The effects of cannabinoid administration on sleep: a systematic review of human studies. Sleep Med Rev 186:477–487

Gautam AS, Verma P, Pathak AK (2021) Blood pressure normalizing effect of Talahridaya marma therapy: a case report. J Ayurveda Integr Med 123:553–555

Geuter U (2006) Geschichte der Körperpsychotherapie. In: Marlock G, Weiss H (eds) Handbuch der Körperpsychotherapie. Schattauer, Stuttgart

Geuter U (2009) Emotionsregulation und Emotionserkundung in der Körperpsychotherapie. In: Thielen M (ed) Körper-Gefühl-Denken. Körperpsychotherapie und Selbstregulation Giessen: psychosozial. pp 69–94

Geuter U (2019) Wirksames Handeln in der Körperpsychotherapie – ergebnisse der Forschung.

In: Praxis Körperpsychotherapie. Psychotherapie: Praxis. Springer, Berlin

Hajak G, Riemann D (2008) Diagnose und Therapie von Schlafstörungen. Der Neurologe & Psychiater 7:21–30

Hajak G, Rüther E (2013) Insomnie – schlaflosigkeit-Ursachen, Symptomatik und Therapie. Springer, Berlin

Hariprasad VR, Sivakumar PT, Koparde V et al (2013) Effects of yoga intervention on sleep and quality-of-life in elderly: a randomized controlled trial. Indian J Psychiatry 55(suppl 3):S364–S368

Hayes SC, Strosahl KD, Wilson KG (1999) Acceptance and commitment therapy: an experiential approach to behavior change. Guilford, New York

Holingue C, Mueller NT, Tanaka T, Differding MK, Chia CW, Wu MN, Spira AP (2020) Self-reported sleep and gut microbiome composition and diversity: associations in well-functioning older adults. *Sleep* *43*(Suppl_1):A53–A53

Holst SC, Werth E, Landolt HP (2019) Pharmakotherapie von Schlaf-Wach-Störungen. Praxis 108:131–138

Huedo-Medina TB, Kirsch I, Middlemass J, Klonizakis M, Siriwardena AN (2012) Effectiveness of non-benzodiazepine hypnotics in treatment of adult insomnia: meta-analysis of data submitted to the Food and Drug Administration. BMJ

Hungs M, Mignot E (2001) Hypocretin/orexin, sleep and narcolepsy. BioEssays 235:397–408

Jacobson E (2002) Entspannung als Therapie. Progressive Relaxation in Theorie und Praxis. Klett-Cotta, Stuttgart

Kabat-Zinn J, Massion AO, Kristeller J, Peterson LG, Fletcher KE, Pbert L, Lenderking WR, Santorelli SF (1992) Effectiveness of a meditation-based stress reduction program in the treatment of anxiety disorders. Am J Psychiatry 1497:936–943

Kanfer HK, Reinecker H, Schmelzer D (2000) Selbstmanagement-Therapie, 3rd edn. Springer, Berlin Heidelberg New York

Khalsa SS (2004) Treatment of chronic insomnia with yoga: A preliminary study with sleep-wake diaries. Appl Psychophysiol Biofeedback 29(4):269–278

Kong D, Run L, Song L, Zheng J, Zhang J, Chen W (2018) Altered Long- and Short-Range Functional Connectivity Density in Healthy Subjects After Sleep Deprivations. Frontiers in Neurology (9)

Krakow B, Zadra A (2006) Clinical management of chronic nightmares: imagery rehearsal therapy. Behav Sleep Med 41:45–70

Kredlow MA, Capozzoli MC, Hearon BA, Calkins AW, Otto MW (2015) The effects of physical activity on sleep: a meta-analytic review. J Behav Med 383:427–449

Li J, Casanova JL, Puel A (2018) Mucocutaneous IL-17 immunity in mice and humans: host defense vs. excessive inflammation. Mucosal Immunol 11, 581–589

Li M, Yang X, Jiang L, Yang D (2021) Acupuncture for rapid eye movement sleep behavior disorder in Parkinson's disease: a case report. Acupunct Med 40(2):203–204. https://doi.org/10.1177/09645284211041125

Linehan MM (1987) Dialectical behavior therapy: a cognitive behavioral approach to parasuicide. J Personal Disord 14:328–333

Liou KT, Garland SN, Li QS, Sadeghi K, Green J, Autuori I, Orlow I, Mao JJ (2021) Effects of acupuncture versus cognitive behavioral therapy on brain-derived neurotrophic factor in cancer survivors with insomnia: an exploratory analysis. Acupunct Med 396:637–645

Liu B, Lin W, Chen S, Xiang T, Yang YY, Xie L (2019) Gut microbiota as a subjective measurement for auxiliary diagnosis of insomnia disorder. Front Microbiol 10:1770

Lorenz N, Heim E, Roetger A, Birrer E, Maercker A (2019) Randomized controlled trial to test the efficacy of an unguided online intervention with automated feedback for the treatment of insomnia. University of Zurich, Zurich Open Repository and Archive, Main Library

Majid MS, Ahmad HS, Bizhan H, Hosein HZM, Mohammad A (2017) The effect of vitamin D supplement on the score and quality of sleep in 20–50 year-old people with sleep disorders compared with control group. Nutr Neurosci 217:511–519

Man, H, Chen B, Wang Q, Fu S, Xie G, Wang J, Zhao C, Gai Z, Zhang C, Heng X, Huo S (2020) Correlations of Gut Microbiome, Serum Metabolome and Immune Factors in Insomnia. [https://doi.org/10.21203/rs.3.rs-35596/v1] (PREPRINT (Version 1) available at Research Square)

Maurer-Groeli Y, Hausmann D, Massenbach K (2005) Maßnahmen zur Überprüfung der Wirksamkeit der Körperzentrierten Psychotherapie IKP. Schweiz Arch Neurol Psychiatr 156:257–265

McCall WV, D'Agostino R Jr, Dunn A (2003) A meta-analysis of sleep changes associated with placebo in hypnotic clinical trials. Sleep Med 41:57–62

Meibert P, Michalak J, Heidenreich T (2006) Achtsamkeitsbasierte Stressreduktion – mindfulness-Based Stress Reduction MBSR. nach Kabat-Zinn. In: Heidenreich T, Michalak J (eds) Achtsamkeit und Akzeptanz in der Psychotherapie, 2nd edn. DGVT, Tübingen

Michelson D, Snyder E, Paradis E et al (2014) Safety and efficacy of suvorexant during 1-year treatment of insomnia with subsequent abrupt treatment discontinuation: a phase 3 randomised, double-blind, placebo-controlled trial. Lancet Neurol 135:461–471

Miles L (2007) Physical activity and health. Nutr Bull 32:314–363

Müller T, Paterok B (2010) Schlaftraining: ein Therapiemanual zur Behandlung von Schlafstörungen, 2nd edn. Hogrefe, Göttingen

Mustian K, Sprod L, Janelsins M et al (2013) Multicenter, randomized controlled trial of yoga for sleep quality among cancer survivors. J Clin Oncol 31:3233–3241

Nagendra RP, Maruthai N, Kutty B (2012) Meditation and its regulatory role on sleep. Front Neurol 3:54. mini review article

Neuendorf R, Wahbeh H, Chamine I, Yu J, Hutchison K, Oken BS (2015a) The effects of mind-body interventions on sleep quality: a systematic review. Evidence-Based Complementary and Alternative Medicine, Article ID 902708, 17 pages, 2015

Neuendorf R et al (2015b) The effects of mind-body interventions on sleep quality: a systematic review. Evid Based Complement Alternat Med, 902708

Ni X, Shergis JL, Guo X, Zhang AL, Li Y, Lu C, Xue CC (2015) Updated clinical evidence of Chinese herbal medicine for insomnia: a systematic review and meta-analysis of randomized controlled trials. Sleep Med 16(12):1462–1148

Nowell PD, Mazumdar S, Buysse DJ, Dew MA, Reynolds CF, Kupfer DJ (1997) Benzodiazepines and zolpidem for chronic insomnia: a meta-analysis of treatment efficacy. JAMA 27824:2170–2177

Pace-Schott EF, Bottary RM, Kim SY, Rosencrans PL, Vijayakumar S, Orr SP, Lasko NB, Goetter EM, Baker AW, Bianchi MT, Gannon K, Hoeppner SS, Hofmann SG, Simon NM (2018) Effects of post-exposure naps on exposure therapy for social anxiety. Psychiatry Res 270:523–530

Parkes JD (1985) Sleep and its disorders. Sounders, Philadelphia

Patel KV, Aspesi AV, Evoy KE (2015) Suvorexant: a dual orexin receptor antagonist for the treatment of sleep onset and sleep maintenance insomnia. Ann Pharmacother 49:477–483

Porges SW (1995) Orienting in a defensive world: mammalian modifications of our evolutionary heritage: a polyvagal theory. Psychophysiology 32:301–318

Röhricht F, Papadopoulos N, Priebe S (2013) An exploratory randomized controlled trial of body psychotherapy for patients with chronic depression. J Affect Disord 151:85–91

Rösner S, Englbrecht C, Wehrle R, Hajak G, Soyka M (2018) Eszopiclone for insomnia. Cochrane Database Syst Rev 10(10):CD010703

Rusch HL, Rosario M, Levison LM, Olivera A, Livingston WS, Wu T, Gill JM (2019) The effect of mindfulness meditation on sleep quality: a systematic review and meta-analysis of randomized controlled trials. Ann N Y Acad Sci 14451:5–16

Sanavio E (1988) Pre-sleep cognitive instructions and treatment of onset-insomnia. Behav Res Ther 26:451–459

Sander C, Hensch T, Wittekind DA, Böttger D, Hegerl U (2015) Assessment of wakefulness and brain arousal regulation in psychiatric research. Neuropsychobiology 72(3–4):195–205

Sanlier N, Sabuncular G (2020) Relationship between nutrition and sleep quality, focusing on the melatonin biosynthesis. Sleep Biol Rhythms 18(2):89–99

Schulte W, Tölle R (1971) Psychiatrie. Springer, Berlin, Heidelberg New York

Segal ZV, Williams JMG, Teasdale JD (2002) Mindfulness-based cognitive therapy for depression: a new approach to preventing relapse. Guilford, New York

Smith RP, Easson C, Lyle SM, Kapoor R, Donnelly CP, Davidson EJ, Parikh E, Lopez JV, Tartar JL (2019) Gut microbiome diversity is associated with sleep physiology in humans. PLoS One 14(10):e0222394

Spielman AJ, Saskin P, Thorpy MJ (1987) Treatment of chronic insomnia by restriction of time in bed. Sleep 101:45–56

Steinberg H, Hegerl U (2014) Johann Christian August Heinroth on sleep deprivation as a therapeutic option for depressive disorders. Sleep Med 821:43–51

Stier-Jarmer M, Throner V, Kirschneck M, Frisch D, Schuh A (2021) Effekte der Kneipp-Therapie: Ein systematischer Review der aktuellen wissenschaftlichen Erkenntnisse 2000–2019. Complement Med Res 282:146–159

St-Onge MP, Zuraikat FM (2019) Reciprocal roles of sleep and diet in cardiovascular health: a review of recent evidence and a potential mechanism. Curr Atheroscler Rep 213:11

Stuck BA, Maurer JT, Schlarb AA, Schredl M, Weeß HG (2018) Praxis der Schlafmedizin – diagnostik, Differenzialdiagnostik und Therapie bei Erwachsenen und Kindern, 3rd edn. Springer, Berlin Heidelberg New York

Thimmapuram J, Yommer D, Tudor L, Dumitrescu C, Davos R (2020) Heartfulness meditation improves sleep in chronic insomnia. J Commun Hospital Int Med Perspect 10:1

Wang L, Xu J, Zhan Y, Pei Y (2020) Acupuncture for Obstructive Sleep Apnea OSA. In adults: a systematic review and meta-analysis. BioMed Res Int, Article ID 6972327

Wang YY, Chang HY, Lin CY (2014) Systematic review of yoga for depression and quality of sleep in the elderly. Hu Li Za Zhi J Nursing 61(1):85–92

Winkler A, Rief W (2015) Effect of placebo conditions on polysomnographic parameters in primary insomnia: a meta-analysis. Sleep 38(6):925–931

Yano JM, Yu K, Donaldson GP, Shastri GG, Ann P, Ma L, Nagler CR, Ismagilov RF, Mazmanian SK, Hsiao EY (2015) Indigenous bacteria from the gut microbiota regulate host serotonin biosynthesis. Cell 161(2):264–276. https://doi.org/10.1016/j.cell.2015.02.047

Young C (2006) One hundred and fifty years on: the history, significance and scope of body psychotherapy today. Body, Movement Dance Psychother 1(1):17–28

Case reports

Case report: Mrs. and Mr. M.-Sex ban in bed as an intervention for falling asleep disorders

Medical history of Mrs. M.

At the initial consultation, Mrs. M. reported suffering from insomnia for several years. She goes to bed at 9 pm, but is not really tired then. Since she sometimes needs up to 2 h to fall asleep, she prefers to go to bed early enough to have enough sleep time. The alarm clock rings at 6 am, the patient's need for sleep is about 7.5 h, so she always hopes to be asleep by 10:30 pm at the latest. Her husband comes to bed at about 10:30 pm. He is a very nice and considerate person and does not try to disturb her. However, she often wakes up after a short nap exactly then. The man then cuddles up to her, which puts her under additional pressure and prevents her from falling asleep.

Medical history of Mr. M.

Mr. M. reported suffering from insomnia for several months. His wife has had it for several years, so he has been familiar with the associated suffering for a long time. Because of his wife's long-standing sleep disorder, he has got into the habit of being very considerate in the evening. He actually goes to bed according to "his time". He is often very tired by 10 pm. However, he wants to give his wife the opportunity to sleep deeply before he goes to bed so that he does not disturb her. Sometimes he gets a real energy boost at 10:15 pm, he can't think about sleeping before midnight. Since he also has to get up at 6 am, he feels insufficiently rested in the morning. He needs at least 7 h of sleep to be reasonably rested. Since he is not really tired at 10:30 pm, but still goes to bed, he cuddles up to his wife to make use of the time spent awake "sensibly". Smiling, he added that this usually leads to sex, which of course pleases him (relaxes and shortens the process of falling asleep).

Biographical history

The 56- and 58-year-old married couple have been married for 26 years and have a good marriage. They live in a house with a garden. They have a solid group of friends with whom they spend holidays, celebrations and outings. It was the "great love" for both of them, and they are grateful for this "gift". Of course, there have been ups and downs over the years. They were not always in agreement on the upbringing of their son (22 years old) and their daughter (26 years old). After the "turnaround", financial problems burdened the relationship. However, they always pulled themselves together and grew closer with each crisis. The sex life is satisfactory for both and takes place regularly every 1–2 weeks. Both were satisfied with their respective workplaces. She is a nursery teacher with heart and soul. He is a carpenter and still loves this profession. There have been no financial difficulties for years. They share many hobbies, such as cycling, hiking and travel.

C. Marx-Dick, *The Holistic Treatment of Sleep Disorders*, https://doi.org/10.1007/978-3-662-67176-4

Somatic anamnesis

At the time of admission, Mrs. M. reported that she had suffered from massive hormonal problems between the ages of 30 and 40. The cycle had been completely mixed up, which had led to sexual disinterest and pain in part. Mr. M. reported that he had broken both legs in a work accident about 4 years ago. However, the fractures had healed completely. Currently there are no physical complaints.

Diagnostics
Psychopathological finding

A very well-groomed, fashionably dressed, much younger-looking couple appear for the admission interview. They appear exhausted, helpless, open and motivated in the first contact. Both were oriented in all qualities, attentive and concentrated.

Mnestic appeared undisturbed. From the clinical impression and linguistic expression, an intelligence above the average was shown. There was no indication of past or present psychotic experiences.

Both showed slight signs of impaired attention and memory. Concentration problems were clearly evident in Mrs. M. The formal thought process was unbroken. There were content-related thought complexes regarding the sleep disorders and loss of own health. There was no current suicidality that could be credibly denied by both and there was also no past suicidality. The affect was variable, only slightly depressed. The drive was not reduced in both. There were no fears or compulsions.

Behavioral analysis of Mrs. M. Micro level according to SORKC (-schema)

Situation:	evening in bed not falling asleep and lying awake, "spasmodic attempt", to fall asleep
Organism variables:	increased muscle tone, fond of harmony, want good relationship

Reaction:	lying awake
Cognition:	"I absolutely have to fall asleep before him. If I'm still awake then, he wants sex. I'm just not in the mood today. But I don't want to reject him either. I find it terrible when he's sad."
Emotion:	restless, worried, anxious
Physiologically:	tense, tired, restless
Motor:	cannot sleep
Consequences:	exhausted during the day, rising tension (physical and emotional)
Contingency:	almost every night unless she feels like sex

Higher-order Condition Analysis

Predisposition: internal image of a good marriage with regular sex, does not want to reject husband

Triggering Conditions: massive stress situation, because she does not want to reject her husband

Sustaining Conditions: does not want sex every night, but also does not want to reject husband, tries to "cramp" to fall asleep in front of him, in order not to have to reject him

Behavioral Deficits: clear communication about the topic of sexuality with the husband

Behavioral Excesses: none

Resources: couple relationship, friends, intelligence, motivation, reflection

Behavioral Analysis Mr. M. Micro Level according to SORKC (-scheme)

Situation:	in bed at night, cuddle up to wife, "explore" to what extent the wife is still awake and possibly has a desire for sex, does not fall asleep, stay awake

Organism Variables:	increased muscle tone, harmony-loving, "normal" sexual desire
Reaction:	"Feel out" to what extent the woman has a desire for sex, stay awake
Cognition:	"I don't want to disturb her if she's already asleep. But if she's not asleep yet, I could see if she might be in the mood for sex."
Emotion:	empathic, considerate, loving, hopeful and worried, anxious
Physiologically:	tense, restless, slightly excited
Motoric:	cuddles up
Consequences:	exhausted during the day, increasing tension (physical and emotional)
Contingency:	every night

Higher-order Condition Analysis

Predisposition: very respectful image of women in general and his wife in particular, considerate and loving

Triggering Conditions: massive stress situation due to the sleep disorder of the wife, wants to give her space and time to sleep

Sustaining Conditions: sleep disorder of the woman, nevertheless sexual desire for the woman, tension due to the "exploration", whether sex will take place

Behavioral Deficits: clear communication about the topic of sexuality with the wife

Behavioral Excesses: none

Resources: couple relationship, friends, intelligence, motivation, reflection

Diagnoses

Both: F 51.0 Non-organic insomnia

Therapy

Therapeutic goals

The following therapeutic goals were formulated together with the patient:

1. Relief of sleep disorder, to be rested and fit during the day
2. Promotion of communication between both partners, especially on the subject of sexuality and needs
3. Maintaining a good couple relationship with regular sexual contacts

Prognosis

Both have a high motivation to change, are punctual and work actively in therapy, so a good therapeutic success is to be expected.

Course of therapy

At the beginning of therapy, the establishment of a complementary relationship and relieving conversations took place. The patients were open and could well engage in the therapeutic relationship offer. With accompanying behavior analyses and mood and sleep protocols, a disorder model was worked out against the biographical background. After a more detailed analysis and everyday diaries, the situation in bed in the evening appeared as a key stress factor.

In the foreground of the therapy was the alleviation of the sleep disorders of both. Their symptomatology was also analyzed in detail using sleep diaries. Accompanying psychoeducational modules were integrated into the architecture of sleep and the associated error expectations and sleep hygiene, etc. In this way, conditions that lead to the patient not being able to fall asleep could be found and a significant countermeasure could be offered.

Therapeutic Intervention

Homework: No sex in bed!

Communication training for the direct communication of needs, fears, anxieties and tension.

Mode of action

Due to different sexual needs, there was an evening "exploration" of the possibilities, misunderstandings and enormous tension in the evening and especially in the bedtime situation in bed. Although well-intentioned consideration, but lacking direct communication led to both partners rather orienting themselves to the needs of the other, rather than openly communicating their own needs and well-being. Due to the communication training, both partners dared to speak about their feelings and thoughts, and it could be communicated more clearly to what extent there is a desire for sexuality.

With the therapeutic instruction not to have sex in bed anymore, the evening "exploration" took place before going to bed. Both partners experienced a fulfilling and also new form of sexuality in other places. From then on, the bed was only for tired reading and sleeping.

Case report: Mr. J.—Systematic nutrition therapy for bipolar and sleep disorder as an alternative to medication therapy

Medical history

The 63-year-old Mr. J. reported at the first consultation that he has been suffering from massive sleep and sleep problems for several weeks (insomnia). His mood is strongly dependent on sleep. He knows light phases of sleep disorders from the past. However, it is currently particularly pronounced.

Until the age of 57, the patient was in good health, but then a series of diseases followed.

At the age of 57, Mr. J. was diagnosed with early-stage colon cancer. The treatment was purely surgical, and he did not require any follow-up treatment. Mr. J. had been doing well since then and had not experienced any fears or concerns about it.

At the age of 59, the patient was diagnosed with heart failure. During the operation, 2 heart valves were replaced. The recovery process was surprisingly fast, and sleep and mood remained stable. Again, the patient did not worry about any health limitations.

Finally, at the age of 60, he suffered a complicated fracture of the neck of the femur. This "completely threw him off track". At that time, he consciously experienced his first depressive phase with pronounced sleep disorders. This was treated with antidepressant psychotherapy.

In retrospect, it turned out that this first depressive phase turned into a manic phase in which he exercised excessively, skied excessively and riskily, and was extremely socially active. The need for sleep was greatly reduced during this phase.

In the following course, light depressive phases alternated with hypomanic episodes up to manic episodes. Depending on the quality of the mood, there were short-term sleep disorders, which, however, subsided on their own with the change of phase. The depressive symptomatology was not so pronounced overall that it caused great suffering, and Mr. J. found explanations for the depressed mood in everyday life.

At the age of 63, the patient developed pronounced symptoms of insomnia. This prompted Mr. J. to come to my special practice for non-organic sleep disorders. After a thorough diagnostic phase, insomnia and a mild depressive episode were diagnosed at this time. The mood was depressed at the time of admission and the drive appeared to be reduced.

A cognitive behavioral therapy of insomnia was carried out, which will be described in more detail in the following. During the treatment period, (hypo-)manic episodes alternated with depressive phases. At first, the manic episodes were only weakly pronounced, but with increasing intensity, so that at first no direct indication of a bipolar disorder was given, and only became noticeable in the further course of treatment.

Since the patient did not show any insight into his illness during the manic episodes, it took another 3 years in the course of treatment until the correct diagnosis "bipolar disorder" and "insomnia" was made. It was made during a moderate depressive episode with enormous suffering in the patient. Psychosomatic symptoms, which mainly affected the gastrointestinal tract, accompanied the patient throughout the time.

At the time of diagnosis, there was enormous suffering, so that Mr. J. agreed to inpatient treatment and was admitted to a special clinic for bipolar disorder. Insomnia should also be treated. During the inpatient stay, various medication treatment strategies were tried with Mr. J. The patient suffered from severe gastrointestinal side effects as well as from feelings of emotional flatness, which the patient experienced as very burdensome. He refused further medication treatment. Mr. J. was finally discharged to continue outpatient therapy in a hypomanic phase without medication. First, an extensive cognitive behavioral therapy with psychoeducation, mindfulness, day structuring and targeted therapy of the fluctuating sleep disorders took place. Light improvements occurred, but the patient slipped into moderate depressive episodes in about 3-month cycles, alternating with hypomanic and manic phases. Sleep disorders also occurred phase-wise more or less.

Biographical anamnesis

The 63-year-old patient lives alone, is currently not in a relationship and has 3 adult children with whom he has a good relationship. The patient reported a stable social network with good friends and colleagues. He works as a civil servant and therefore has no financial or existential worries. So far, he has enjoyed his work and has been constantly recognized with appropriate promotions. The patient reported a very active sporting life (especially walking, inline skating and cycling). At that time he had deliberately searched for a partner via online portals and had regular meetings.

Somatic anamnesis

At the time of admission, the patient stated that he had no somatic complaints. He did not take any medication that he fundamentally rejected and only took in an emergency.

Diagnostics
Psychopathological finding

A very well-groomed man who looks much younger appears for the admission interview. In the first contact he looks exhausted, helpless, lost, unsure, but open and motivated. He was oriented in all qualities, attentive and concentrated.

Mnestic appeared undisturbed. From the clinical impression and the expressive power of speech, an intelligence above average was shown. There was no indication of past or present psychotic experiences.

He showed mild signs of attention, memory and concentration impairment. Formal thought process was intact. There were content-related thought complexes regarding the sleep disorders, anxiety about the future, loss of own health. A current suicidality could credibly be denied and also did not exist in the past. The affect was depressed, sad and hopeless. The drive was slightly reduced. There were fears about the future. There were no other fears. Compulsions existed in partly excessive sports.

Behavioral analysis *Micro level according to SORKC (-schema)*

Situation: waking up at night and not being able to fall asleep again, lying awake, brooding

Organism variables: low self-esteem, parents wanted children to be "brave"

Reaction:

Cognition:	"I can't fall asleep again, I have to get up early tomorrow, how can I get through the day?"
Emotion:	worried, anxious, angry, irritable, restless, depressed, sad
Physiological:	exhausted, tense, tired, restless
Motor:	wakes up several times a night
Consequences:	tired during the day, not sufficiently tired at night, increasing tension (physical and emotional)
Contingency:	every night, unless the patient is on vacation or staying with friends

Higher-order condition analysis Predisposition: unclear, frequent diseases

Triggering conditions: severe stress situation with diseases, work, loneliness

Sustaining conditions: Fear of a relapse of the disease, avoidance, work load, loneliness

Behavioral deficits: Relaxation, active leisure time, social interaction, sexuality

Behavioral excesses: Sport

Resources: Sport, friends, intelligence, motivation, reflection

Diagnoses: F 51.0 Non-organic insomnia

F 32.0 mild depressive episode

Therapy goals

The following therapy goals were formulated together with the patient:

1. Relief of sleep disorder, to be rested and fit during the day
2. Reduction of depressive symptoms, stabilization at a good level
3. Reduction of tension and restlessness
4. Build a relationship with a partner with trust
5. Become more self-confident and feel comfortable in social relationships

Prognosis

Mr. J. has a high motivation to change, is punctual and actively participates in therapy, so a good therapeutic success is to be expected.

Course of therapy

At the beginning of therapy, the establishment of a complementary relationship and relieving conversations took place. The patient was open and could well engage in the therapeutic relationship offer. With accompanying behavior analyses and mood and sleep protocols, a disorder model was worked out against the biographical background. After a more detailed analysis and everyday diaries, living alone and the demanding and time-consuming work appeared as stress factors.

The focus of the therapy was the alleviation of sleep disorders. The symptomatology was also analyzed in detail using sleep diaries. Psychoeducational modules were integrated as accompaniment, on the architecture of sleep and the associated error expectations, healthy nutrition, daily planning and sleep hygiene, etc. In this way, conditions that lead to the fact that the patient cannot fall asleep could be found and corresponding individual countermeasures could be offered. These included mini-interventions with mindfulness and relaxation breaks during work, a balance of active and recovery breaks in leisure time, and an emotional competence training to perceive one's own feelings and their meaning. To reduce the always accompanying tension and restlessness, physiological and psychological relaxation was offered by progressive muscle relaxation, applied relaxation (according to Öst) or autogenic training, which the patient could not implement in everyday life.

An instruction is given to enjoy, positively activate and entertain social contacts. New positive learning experiences should be made by allowing feelings and small personal weaknesses. Supportive calming and behavior-regulating self-instructions were developed. In the course of treatment, continuous feedback was given on problematic behavior. Mr. J. took part in the individual sessions reliably and motivated. This led to a complete improvement of sleep quality and performance at times.

In the further course of therapy, it became apparent that Mr. J. fluctuated noticeably in his condition from time to time, so that the progress made by the patient was also unstable. At the end of 2017, Mr. J. was in a depressive phase and his disorders met the criteria for non-organic insomnia. This changed over the New Year.

At the beginning of 2018, the patient showed more symptoms of a manic episode: he made various plans for holidays (e.g. Chicago, the Caribbean; while he is living in Germany) and also travelled three times in the first half of 2018. Mr. J. was clearly in a euphoric mood, which lasted until about May 2018, and was overall significantly more active (e.g. sports, appointments, etc.).

He himself described the time as a "roller coaster". Therapy appointments took place at intervals of about 6 weeks during this phase.

At the beginning of June, Mr. J. then changed into a moderate depressive episode. He reported inner restlessness, extreme lack of motivation and lack of joie de vivre. He felt exhausted and "crushed". A clear social withdrawal was observed. Antidepressant strategies (self-care and behavioural activation: e.g. walks, mindfulness) were discussed first.

From 04.09.2018 to 16.10.2018, he was treated for this severe depressive episode in a psychiatric hospital. In the clinic, Mr. J. was initially treated with a phase prophylactic agent. The side effects in the form of gastrointestinal complaints, mild nausea and dizziness caused the patient a lot of problems, so that the medication was changed and now an antidepressant (SSRI) was used. Here too, side effects were observed, which the patient could not tolerate. However, the antidepressant showed an antidepressant effect after only 7 days of use, which put Mr. J. into a manic phase again. The treatment was satisfactory for the patient, the mood stabilized at an expansive level, and Mr. J. felt capable.

After his stay in the clinic, he described life as a "drug" that he could not get enough of. He had no time for work at all. The suspicion of a bipolar disorder was confirmed.

In order to confirm the diagnosis and to treat the patient psychiatrically in accordance with the guidelines, Mr. J. was referred to a psychiatrist. However, he was also reluctant to diagnose and initially prescribed an antidepressant. Mr. J. refused to take it because he didn't feel depressed.

In the autumn, the patient's mood changed again in the depressive direction. Now the patient also came to the insight that he was suffering from a bipolar disorder. Since the patient refused a medication therapy despite psychiatric co-treatment, an alternative treatment strategy had to be developed. First, a consistent disorder model was also developed for the bipolar disorder. At this point I would like to mention that Mr. J. learned 2 years later by chance that his sister and probably his mother also suffer from a bipolar disorder. Psychoeducation on bipolar disorders and development of (early warning) symptoms that announce new phases took place. The skills to establish a balanced daily routine are increasingly being expanded. Mr. J. worked very well in therapy and let himself be open to his disorder. He showed himself to be very committed to a consistent daily rhythm and was very aware of his feelings. He continued to see the psychiatrist regularly, but continued to refuse medication due to fears of side effects.

In addition, Mr. J. had joined a self-help group that he wanted to visit regularly.

Systematic nutrition therapy

As another non-pharmacological therapeutic agent, nutrition therapy was now used, which had an effect on the patient's symptoms in several ways:

Change of diet, with the aim of promoting a greater variety in the microbiome. Since Mr. J. suffered from digestive problems, especially diarrhea (up to 15 times in 24 h), with his phases fluctuating, it was reasonable to assume that the patient's microbiome was also out of balance. Together with the patient, a balanced diet was developed:

- with fermented products such as yogurt or sauerkraut, in order to increase the probiotics,
- whole grain products to promote digestion and to build up the prebiotics in the large intestine,
- reduction in the consumption of yeast and sourdough products, alcohol and cold drinks,
- conversion to mainly warm food according to the ayurvedic diet with steamed fruit and vegetables as well as many gently prepared legumes and sufficient fluid in the form of unsweetened tea.

With the gradual introduction of the new diet, Mr. J. was first pulled out of his depressive episode. He had long experienced pleasure in eating, serenity, enjoyment, and mindfulness. In the further course it turned out that also the manic episodes were milder and only occurred as light hypomania.

In addition to the actual nutrient enrichment, the change in diet also offered another advantage in the structuring of the day. Mr. J. found interest in the topic of healthy nutrition, educated himself increasingly independently and learned to cook. He increasingly went to farm shops and weekly markets to shop and experienced a different quality of social contacts as well as self-care and self-worth in this way. Shopping and cooking offered a new and fixed daily structure that provided balance for both the depressive and the manic mood.

Sleep-promoting foods with warming spices, tryptophan- and melatonin-rich nuts and seeds as well as predominantly vegetarian and protein-rich dishes were specifically included in the menu. In doing so, sleep-inhibiting foods were largely omitted, such as meat and sausage products, raw leafy vegetables or carbohydrate-rich foods in the evening.

The patient was examined using the external rating scales of the Hamilton Depression Scale (HAMD) and the Young Mania Rating Scale (YMRS) to measure affectivity. The Regensburg Insomnia Scale (RIS) was used to collect sleep data. It can be seen that both the depressive and the manic symptoms were significantly reduced after only a few weeks of therapy. The depressive symptoms went from an initial 22 points over a period of 16 months to 2 points. The manic episodes also decreased significantly, from an initial 34 points to 3 points in the further course of therapy. The symptoms of insomnia also decreased significantly over the various measurement points, from an initial 38 points (severe insomnia) to 6 points (unremarkable sleep pattern). Through the targeted nutritional therapy, the patient's mood and sleep could be stabilized at a good level. Mr. J. has now been stable for 16 months, without manic or depressive episodes, and his sleep is successful.

Mode of action

Bipolar disorders are among the most severe psychiatric disorders and are characterized by a very high level of suffering and severe impairments in everyday life. Sleep disorders are a very common accompaniment. However, they not only change psychological and neurological parameters, but also cause physiological dysfunctions such as oxidative stress and chronic inflammation.

Thanks to the increasing research interest in the gut-brain axis, a great deal of informative data has been gathered in recent years on bipolar disorder and sleep disorders. It is assumed that the gut microbiota has a strong influence on the central nervous system via interactions with the immune system, the neuroendocrine system, and the vagus nerve. For example, microbial metabolism is significantly involved in the production of a large number of important neurotransmitters, cytokines, and intermediates such as serotonin, dopamine, and adrenaline. New findings of this kind have changed our understanding of mental illness in particular and created new treatment options.

Medication is the treatment of choice for bipolar disorder. Sleep disorders are also often treated with medication. Unfortunately, there are many patients who do not respond well to treatment with psychopharmaceuticals, there is an increased risk of dependence, and it is associated with unpleasant side effects. Therefore, more non-medicinal therapies are urgently needed.

The groundbreaking results of microbiome research should not be overlooked. The microbiome offers great therapeutic potential because it does not have a fixed structure, but rather represents a dynamic ecological composition of various microorganisms. It consists essentially of a large number of bacteria, but also of fungi, viruses, and eukaryotes. These "good" parasites recognize bad intruders and are designed to make them harmless and integrate them into a health-promoting homeostatic process. The standardized studies show that a greater diversity of gut microbiota is associated with better physical and mental health. Therefore, mental disorders such as bipolar disorder and sleep disorders are also associated with reduced microbial diversity. This aspect can be directly addressed and therapeutically used with a targeted nutrition therapy.

Another important structure of the "gut brain" is our 10th cranial nerve, the vagus nerve. It consists of 3 branches, is very complexly branched in the body, and has 3 essential functions: 1. Balance and social affiliation, 2. Innervation of the flight and fight response, and 3. Stiffening in the face of danger. Particularly fascinating is the fact that 80% of its nerve fibers are afferent and only about 20% are efferent. This means that information from the periphery and the digestive tract is primarily directed to the brain and thus to the structures of emotion regulation, such as the limbic system.

It regulates the psychological balance and can be balanced by targeted nutrition in addition to psychological and manual methods.

The case presented here shows that the microbiome can be a good target for non-pharmacological therapies in people with bipolar disorder and sleep disorders. Further studies with representative samples, methodologically applied nutrition plans and the detailed investigation of the microbiome are of course necessary at this point. Further positive aspects of nutritional therapy such as day structuring, genus training, self-efficacy training and other aspects must be systematically observed. A targeted nutritional therapy can be a great opportunity for patients with bipolar and sleep disorders who cannot tolerate medication.

Case Report Mr. A.—Dependence on Hypnotics and Depression

Anamnesis
Acutely reported symptoms
The patient reports that he has been suffering from massive sleep and wakefulness disorders since he retired about 10 years ago. He would then get up again and again and find wakefulness very stressful. If there was no other way, he would take up to 2 sleeping pills, as one tablet often had no effect. In the morning he would not get out of bed. This would intensify his depressive symptoms. On the days after the bad nights he would be very irritable, he would not want to see anyone and could not muster up to anything. The depression has existed since the "Wende" ("the fall of the wall") in 1989 and has so far been treated exclusively with medication. The patient fears that he will soon be unable to sleep at all, as the sleeping pills are having less and less effect. He also fears that he will sink deeper and deeper into depression uncontrollably. On days when he has slept well, he feels "top fit", he is in a good mood and can do everything.

Biographical anamnesis Mr. A. was born in 1947 and remained an only child. There is no contact with the biological father. Mr. A. never knew him. The mother was 19 years old at the time of the patient's birth and died in 2011. When the mother married his stepfather in 1959, Mr. A. no longer got along with the mother. He spent most of his childhood with his grandparents. This was his great luck, as the grandmother was a strict but loving woman. There was never a good relationship with the stepfather.

Mr. A. remembers his kindergarten years as very beautiful time. He was also well integrated into school and had no problems meeting the requirements. There he made his regular graduation and then started an apprenticeship as a mechanic. Until shortly after the reunification, he worked as a maintenance mechanic for a housing company. He enjoyed this work very much because he could work independently and received a lot of appreciation for his work. Afterwards he carried out various property manager and janitorial tasks. The last job was very stressful for him. He felt at the mercy of his boss's whim. Therefore, Mr. A. was very happy when he could retire.

Mr. A. got married at the age of 20 and had a very beautiful and stable relationship. The couple is very active, often on the road by bike and do most things together. With the entry into retirement, the relationship had to be re-formed, which relatively succeeded. There is a common 42-year-old son and already a granddaughter.

Social anamnesis Since the reunification, Mr. A. has again and again had unsatisfactory and alarming experiences at his workplaces. He has not felt any control over various situations and has been afraid of losing his job. Again and again he has got younger superiors, and they have prevented his own promotion. Mr. A. always wanted to be fair and therefore often spoke up for colleagues. But nobody thanked him for it.

Somatic anamnesis No physical complaints known.

Medication anamnesis The depressive disorder caused by the increasing loss of control and the disrespect of his performance has so far been treated exclusively with medication: Mr. A. receives quetiapine (0-0-1) and lithium (1-0-2).

This medication suggests a bipolar disorder, which can neither be confirmed by the anamnesis nor by the reported and observed symptomatology. Mr. A. reports that he has never heard of this diagnosis and was also not informed about his medication. In addition, he has not been able to notice any effect of the medication on his depressive symptoms. In combination with a depressive episode, he is again and again irritable, but does not know any euphoric phases.

If necessary, Mr. A. should take nitrazepam. The nitrazepam doses have increased greatly, and often one tablet per night is not enough anymore. So a tolerance development is already recognizable.

Diagnostics
Psychopathological finding

Mr. A. is awake, oriented in all qualities and attentive. Concentration and memory appear clearly restricted. There is no recognizable mnestic disorder. The clinical impression and the linguistic expression suggest an average intelligence. There are no indications of previous or current psychotic experiences. The thinking is formally ordered, but content-wise restricted to the depression and the sleep disorder. The affect appears clearly depressed, anxious, sad, but not suicidal. The drive is clearly reduced and the patient overall looks less motivated. Mr. A. reports of constant future and illness fears. There are no other fears. No compulsions can be seen. The patient reports of pronounced sleep disorders.

The patient does not smoke and only drinks alcohol occasionally (1–2 beers). He takes benzodiazepines almost daily. The patient looks unsure and answers questions very extensively. He describes his problems comprehensively. The patient is very reliable and sympathetic. In the previous sessions, the patient seemed idea-less, but open and interested in the solution of his problem.

Behavioral analysis Micro level (according to SORKC scheme)

- Situation: in the evening before going to bed, unrest, tension, brooding
- Organism variables: increased muscle tone, patient has already slept badly as a child
- Reaction:
  - Cognition: "I can't calm down again. What if I can't fall asleep again? My depression will get worse again. I don't want to become addicted."
  - Emotion: anxious, powerless
  - Physiological characteristics: exhausted, tense
  - Motor characteristics: restless and fidgety
- Consequences: benzodiazepine intake, patient sleeps longer in the morning
  - Short-term: patient can relax and fall asleep or make up for lost sleep in the morning
  - Long-term: risk of addiction, lack of daytime structure, patient lies in bed for too long, maintains depressive symptoms
  - Contingency: almost daily, otherwise severe sleep disorders

Higher-order condition analysis

- Predisposition: patient has always slept badly, did not experience security in childhood, more frequent loss of control
- Triggering conditions: change in the world of work after the Wende, start of depression at the same time
- Sustaining conditions: no establishment of a daily routine, experience of efficacy of benzodiazepine
- Behavioral deficit: sleep phase delay until late morning
- Behavioral excesses: patient sleeps long in the morning, takes up to 2 sleeping pills
- Resources: Reflective ability, motivation, support from wife

Diagnoses

- F 51.0 Non-organic insomnia
- F 33.1 Recurrent depressive episode, currently of moderate severity
- F 13.88 Other mental and behavioral disorders
- F 13.1 Mental and behavioral disorders due to sedatives and hypnotics, harmful use

Therapy

Therapeutic goals

The following therapeutic goals are worked out and formulated together with the patient:

- Relief of sleep disorder, quick falling asleep
- Abstinence from hypnotics
- Introduction of a daily routine with self-caring design
- Reduction of anxious and depressive symptoms, stabilization at a good level
- Reduction of tension and restlessness
- Learning to feel pleasure and to participate in life again

Prognosis

Mr. A. has a high motivation to change, is punctual and works actively in therapy, so a good therapeutic success is to be expected.

Therapy plan

At the beginning of therapy, the establishment of a complementary relationship and relieving conversations take place. Repeated behavior analyses and mood, benzodiazepine consumption and sleep protocols serve as the basis for the development of a convincing disorder model (including the functionality of the symptoms in the current relationship) also against the biographical background. In this way, it should be diagnostically clarified to what extent a bipolar disorder actually exists, which would require the current medication.

In the foreground of the therapy are the alleviation of sleep disorders and the abstinence from benzodiazepines. The problems with falling asleep should first be analyzed in detail using sleep and behavior protocols.

Psychoeducational modules on sleep hygiene, sleep architecture and the associated error expectations are integrated as accompaniments. Conditions that lead to the fact that the patient cannot fall asleep are to be analyzed in detail and corresponding individual countermeasures are to be offered (movement, healthy nutrition, daily structure, stress reduction, massages, etc.). To reduce the always accompanying tension and restlessness, physiological and psychological relaxation is learned by means of progressive muscle relaxation, applied relaxation (according to Öst) or autogenic training, the implementation of which takes place in exercise units in everyday life.

In general, an increase in interpersonal control conviction is to be achieved by expanding one's own scope of behavior. Likewise, an increase in feelings of self-competence is to be achieved by allowing for clearer boundary setting, which can be used as structuring aids. This should support and consolidate the abstinence from benzodiazepines. Instructions are given on how to enjoy, positively activate and maintain social contacts.

The purpose of conducting role-playing games with role reversal is twofold: first, for diagnostic purposes, and second, to improve social skills, in particular the ability to assert oneself and set boundaries. The goal is to make new positive learning experiences by allowing small personal weaknesses. Calming and behaviour-regulating self-instructions are to be developed to support this. Furthermore, the aim is to achieve a reduction in self-doubt and perfectionism as well as to reduce guilt feelings through cognitive restructuring (according to Beck). In particular, the techniques of de-catastrophising and reality testing are of particular importance here.

Continuous feedback on updated problem behaviour in therapy is a regular part. Throughout the therapy process, the focus should be on autonomy and taking responsibility. In the final sessions, an outlook for the future and the development of relapse prevention is given, also in the light of the already experienced depressive episode.

The patient wants to learn to accept his disorder and to change his catastrophic image of sleep disorders. He wants to increase his self-confidence and, in particular, to modify the cognitions that cause his depressive experience and persistent fears. He wants to learn to distance himself from negative thoughts and to check them from an observing perspective. For this, the patient's self-awareness is to be trained.

45 individual sessions were requested in weekly single frequency, taking into account the duration and severity of the disorder.

Course of therapy

Despite the patient's great scepticism towards psychologists, the complementary relationship has been established well. First, a thorough diagnostics is carried out with regard to the bipolar disorder. For this purpose, standardized diagnosis manuals are used and a comprehensive clinical impression is gained in conversations. There is still no indication of a bipolar disorder. Rather, it turns out that the patient had received lithium on the recommendation of a acquaintance and had asked his psychiatrist for it. She had prescribed it without asking any further questions.

Mr A. is well accessible with psychoeducation. Biorhythm and sleep architecture are explained to him in detail. This causes a great motivation to discontinue the benzodiazepines. Other therapy components are: therapeutic use of light, self-care (euthymic) therapy, mindfulness, stimulus control and sleep hygiene. In addition, biographical work is done and the patient is validated by means of relieving conversations.

After consulting with the psychiatrist, lithium and quetiapine are tapered off. Mr. A. reports feeling less sleepy during the day. He raves about a new quality of life. He thought the symptoms of lethargy and drowsiness were age-related. Now he can "reboot" once again.

During the course of therapy, the patient documents his benzodiazepine use in a controlled manner and with his own motivation. Depending on his mood during the day, Mr. A. increasingly foregoes the medication until he only uses it in case of exciting events (Christmas, visit, vacation). A self-reinforcement sets in through the documentation of success. For each night without benzodiazepine, Mr. A. enters a red dot in the calendar. With ongoing therapy, he only needs a half dose of nitrazepam once a month. This means that not only the frequency of use could be reduced very significantly, but also a lower dose is effective when needed.

Patient report Mr. K.—shift work and sleep disorders

Anamnesis
Acutely reported symptoms

Mr. K. reports working as a nursing assistant in shift work. In principle, he enjoys the work very much, but he finds the different working hours very stressful. In principle, he would rather work in the early shift, because he is always awake early anyway. However, on the evenings before, he is so excited for fear of oversleeping the next morning that he cannot fall asleep at all. In the morning, the patient is surprisingly fit, he can concentrate well and is productive. In the afternoon, however, a deep exhaustion sets in and Mr. K. can hardly stay awake. He tries to avoid a midday nap, but sometimes this is not possible. In the evening, the patient is "exhausted to collapse" at 9:00 pm. Depending on the shift schedule, this state is extremely stressful.

In addition, the patient has been afraid of prolonged loneliness for a long time, as he has not been able to maintain a lasting relationship with a woman despite his constant efforts. He wants to overcome this during the course of therapy and be able to enter and shape relationships without fear. He can already name his low self-esteem and lack of experience in dealing with emotional closeness and feelings as important causes of his disorder.

Mr. K.'s sleep disorders are characterized by early awakening, difficulty staying asleep and falling asleep again. When he is awake, he often thinks about conflicts and problems from the past and present and worries that he will not be fit enough for work the next day and will therefore stand out negatively to his employer. He often looks at the clock to read the remaining time and then tries to fall asleep again. During the night he feels depressed, lonely, physically and emotionally tense and quickly irritable. During the day he is exhausted, less concentrated and receptive, his thoughts revolve mainly around negative topics and the worry that he will not sleep properly again the next night.

Biographical anamnesis Mr. K., 34 years old, is the second child of his parents. His mother (+27), an engineer during her lifetime, was a temperamental, sociable and unstable woman who fell into alcoholism during his childhood. This experience has been very formative for the patient to this day. His father (+30), a retired mechanical engineer, was a quiet, balanced, Craftsman who tried to bring normality into the family's life. The patient has an 4-year-older sister, whom he describes as ambitious, reliable and self-sacrificing, and with whom he had no good relationship during childhood and adolescence. Later, however, she became his closest relative. The relationship with the father has remained good over the years.

Mr. K. has no significant memories of his kindergarten years. The family did a lot, but the shared activities stopped when the mother's alcoholism started. When the mother was unable to get up for 1–3 weeks after an alcohol binge, her maternal grandmother came to take care of her. During his school years, the patient sometimes experienced bullying, and he never felt quite belonging. The patient completed high school and then trained as a plant fitter and worked in this profession for a year. Then he had to do his civilian service and found pleasure in nursing. He then completed the training to become a nurse and has been working in this profession since then. In 2006, his mother died.

Social anamnesis He is currently working as a nurse full time and is mostly satisfied, but he sometimes feels a time pressure. Mr. K. is currently single and longs for a happy partnership. He has not had a long-term, deep relationship so far and feels great insecurity and fear in this aspect of life. His long-term single life is one of his main burdens, as well as the lack of opportunity to live out his sexuality. For 12 years he has been suffering from early awakening, sleep disturbance and poor sleep recovery on most days of the week. Before starting therapy, these symptoms had become so acute that the patient has only been sleeping 2–4 h a night since then.

In the first conversations, shift work as a nursing home and the family background could be identified as the main current problems and the cause of the sleep disorder.

Somatic anamnesis Back and neck tension, no other physical findings.

Medication history The patient started therapy because of his increasingly burdensome sleep disorder and physical tension. In his desperation, he had the doctor prescribe a medication to relieve the sleep disorder and the physical tension in the back and neck area, which did not work.

Diagnostics
Psychopathological finding
A well-groomed and sportily dressed man appears for the admission interview. Mr. K. appears shy and reserved in the first contact, but also exhausted, helpless, lost and insecure. When asked, the patient is open and motivated. The mnestic appears undisturbed. There are clear signs of attention and concentration impairment. The formal thought process appears undisturbed, is contentually limited to single life, future fear, sleep disorders and the loss of health. A current or retrospective suicidality could be credibly denied. The patient reports that he currently consumes alcohol more often (almost daily), nicotine and caffeine daily.

Behavioral analysis Micro level (according to SORKC scheme):

- Situation: Patient is awake at night, but has to get up in the morning
- Organism variables: low self-esteem, possibly a predisposition for dependency disorders
- Reaction:
  - Cognition: "I can't make it again, I'll be completely exhausted tomorrow, I'm alone, I'm not lovable, I can't make it, I'm helpless."
  - Emotion: worried, anxious, angry, irritable, restless, depressed
  - Physiological characteristics: exhausted, tense, tired, restless
  - Motor characteristics: patient stays awake in bed, saves himself during the day
- Consequences: patient is exhausted during the day, increasing tension (physical and emotional)
- Contingency: almost daily, otherwise strong sleep disorders

Superordinate Condition Analysis

- Predisposition: alcoholism and death of the mother, lack of confrontation experience
- Triggering conditions: loneliness, shift work, occupational uncertainty due to reorientation in the meantime
- Sustaining conditions: loneliness, shift work
- Behavioral deficits: relaxation, active leisure time, social interaction, sexuality
- Behavioral excesses: patient lies in bed and broods, makes worried thoughts
- Resources: family, reflection

Diagnoses

- F 51.2 Non-organic disorder of sleep-wake rhythm
- F 41.2 Anxiety and depressive disorder, mixed
- In particular F10.1 Harmful use of alcohol

Prognosis

- Mr. K. has a high motivation to change, is punctual and works actively in therapy, so a good therapy success is to be expected. Mr. K. is very active in sports, which can be used as a resource. In addition, he has good discipline and eats healthy.

Therapy
Therapeutic Goals
The following therapeutic goals were worked out and formulated together with the patient:

- Find a sleep-wake rhythm that allows for rest and regeneration
- Restrict harmful alcohol consumption
- Stabilize mood at a good level
- Open up to a deep, long-term relationship

Therapy Plan At the beginning of psychotherapy, the patient receives comprehensive psychoeducation on the topics of sleep, sleep hygiene, depressive experience, and anxiety. Sleep-inhibiting factors in the patient's life are to be identified and modified. The patient should be familiarized with relaxation methods in order to relax and reduce stress. With these measures, on the one hand, the patient's ability to perceive stress and tension situations is to be further promoted, on the other hand, he should be given his own methods of tension regulation in everyday life.

Further resources for relaxation during the day and also at work are to be found, in particular as an alternative to alcohol consumption.

In order to improve his communication skills, the patient's ability to express himself and to confront him should be increased, for example, by means of role-playing with subsequent video feedback. This can also be operationalized with regard to the fear of negative external impact. The training in dealing with one's own thoughts and emotions should also contribute to strengthening the patient's self-confidence and self-esteem.

In order to build effective techniques for maintaining one's own boundaries and promoting self-accentuated behavior, a self-confidence training (according to Ullrich and Ullrich de Muynck) is to be used in connection with in-vivo tasks with initially high levels of automatic self-reinforcement.

With cognitive therapy methods, work is to be done on correcting the patient's personal level of demand and facilitating the acceptance of offers of help.

Cognitive therapy methods are used to modify the dysfunctional perception and evaluation patterns in social situations, to test the reality of existing social fears, to soften existing self-esteem beliefs, and to reduce excessive personal performance claims.

Based on a thought diary, the registration and correction of misinterpretations (dysfunctional overestimation of the importance of thoughts and overestimation of the consequences of the fear caused by the thoughts) is to be carried out by cognitive therapy.

The patient is to be guided to explore the content of the intrusive automatic thoughts. Dependent schema content or dysfunctional self-concept components are to be modified by means of cognitive procedures (according to Beck).

With the help of behavior and consumption diaries, the actual alcohol consumption is to be uncovered and documented. Depending on the need, control and abstinence strategies are offered.

In view of the severity of the disorder, 25 individual sessions at a weekly frequency and 5 probationary hours were requested.

Course of therapy First, a stable therapeutic relationship is established with the patient, in which the therapist acts as part of a model for a continuous, safe and appreciative interaction with each other. The patient can well engage in this relationship, appears to be reliable and punctual and, despite professional obligations, keeps the agreed appointments.

During the relationship building, an individual biopsychosocial disorder model is worked out together. This includes acquired behavioral patterns, especially with regard to the poor sleep—both in quality and in quantity—and the living conditions of Mr. K., the loneliness. In addition, the relationship between cognition, emotion and behavior in different situations is analyzed using diaries.

In addition, psychoeducational elements are offered to the patient, as he has false ideas about sleep. He thinks you have to sleep through and need at least 8 h of sleep in a 24-hour cycle. The patient is explained the sleep architecture in detail and it is explained how substances, especially alcohol, influence sleep. This makes sense to him, which is why he now only drinks wine for enjoyment and not as a sleeping aid. The consumption decreases from half a bottle daily to half a bottle weekly. Since the patient usually smoked when drinking wine, the nicotine consumption decreases parallel to this.

The bed phases are analyzed and discussed intensively. Various rhythms are tried out. Since Mr. K. works in shift work, the same rest phases cannot always be granted. In the end, Mr. K. is proposed a biphasic sleep, in which he, in addition to a main sleep phase at night, builds in another rest phase during the day shift. Depending on the shift, this takes place in the late morning or early afternoon. This allows the patient to stay up until about 10:00/11:00 pm and then sleep uninterruptedly until 4:00 or 5:00 am. Overall, Mr. K. feels much better and fitter. After a night shift, a biphasic sleep is also favorable. So Mr. K. sleeps shortly after the night shift for about 4 h and then for another 1–2 h before the night shift starts again.

In addition to the targeted therapy of sleep disorders, a social and emotional competence training is carried out with Mr. K. In this, the unstable childhood of Mr. K. is addressed, in which he was allowed to experience little security and stability. This can be identified as the main cause of the sleep disorder. Mr. K. "had to" be alert as a child, as his mother collapsed not very often, but regularly.

Therapeutic modules used: psychoeducation, sleep restriction, shift work, paradoxical intervention, psychohygiene, sleep hygiene, mindfulness, influence of thinking, social rhythm therapy, alcohol and drugs, therapeutic use of light.

A flirting training was carried out to achieve the other therapy goals.

Case report Mrs. G.—insomnia and chronic depression

Anamnesis
Acutely reported symptoms

A very well-groomed and fashionable 64-years old woman appears for the first contact. She had requested the appointment on the recommendation of her neurologist. From other sides the patient had received little support and help.

For about 30 years Mrs. G. has been suffering from depressions and very burdensome sleep disorders. These are characterized by early awakening, difficulty sleeping and difficulty falling asleep again. Especially in the winter months this symptomatology increases and Mrs. G. loses hope and becomes "life-weary" every year.

Her psychiatrist has always prescribed her medication to relieve inner unrest, depressive symptomatology and also sleep disorders. However, these have shown less and less effect over time. Both the sleep disorders and the depressions have so far been treated exclusively with medication.

Biographical anamnesis The patient was born as a desired child of her parents in the post-war period. The mother (+30), sales outlet manager in her lifetime, was a very thrifty, old-fashioned, prudish and otherworldly woman with whom she had no good relationship. There were hardly any good, open conversations with her possible.

In school, the patient was shy and reserved and rather an outsider, but she was not bullied. Sexuality was not discussed in the family, out of fear of becoming pregnant, she avoided sexual contacts until the age of 20. She suspects that her first partner left her because of her problematic attitude towards sexuality.

She has a close, trusting relationship with her long-term partner and husband (+4), which has been occasionally disharmonious and stressful. Their common daughter (35 years old) was a desired child and a sensitive late developer. She has a good, close bond with her.

Psychological anamnesis About 30 years ago, the patient began to suffer from a depressive mood and a sleep disorder. The event that exacerbated the disorder was the change in 1989. This caused great insecurity in her. In addition, stress with her partner, an unfulfilled desire for a second child and the death of her parents came. Worrying about the welfare of the daughter also occupied a large part of her time.

20 years ago she started a therapy because of the depression, which was interrupted. In 2002 she took part in a 6-week psychosomatic rehabilitation measure, which did her very well.

Because of the intensification of her sleep disorder, the patient had herself examined in a sleep laboratory in June 2015. There she slept better, but also had no deep sleep. At present she suffers from difficulties in falling asleep, sleeping through and falling asleep again on most days of the week, as well as from premature awakening. Her sleep is not restful and phases of particularly burdensome nightmares are characterized. Often she is not really tired. If Mrs. G. is awake at night, she broods and thinks about topics and problems from everyday life and the past. Occasionally she uses autogenic training to become calm and fall asleep again, but without success. Irregular bedtimes, working hours or unfavorable sleeping conditions can so far be ruled out as causes.

During the day, the patient feels depressed, sad, apathetic, without motivation and only forces herself to go through her everyday life. In the first conversations, the family background (both of the original family and of her own) can already be identified as the main cause of current problems and of the sleep disorder in particular. Mrs. G. has not yet found a way to deal with the stress and the dissatisfaction with her marriage and the concern for the development of her daughter, for example. The patient also expresses that she is still struggling with the death of her parents, because, for example, no clarifying conversations about the relationships in the family and in particular about the depressiveness of the mother have ever been held. When she is awake at night and during the day, she suffers from the circling of thoughts around the mentioned topics. During the day she is exhausted, unfocused, less receptive and depressed.

At the moment the patient does not have enough self-confidence and skills in coping with her depressive symptoms, fears and conflicts from a therapeutic point of view. Several attempts to solve the problems independently with selected methods failed.

Somatic anamnesis Loss of appetite, stomach pain, herniated discs.

Mrs. G. suffered a disc herniation about 5 years ago, which was treated with physiotherapy. She still has back pain from time to time. However, since she is no longer working, she can then rest and the pain is tolerable. At that time she decided against an operation, which she is very happy about today. When she was young, she often had circulatory problems. These have decreased with age. There are no other physical complaints.

Medication history The patient has been accompanied by a depression for as long as the sleep disorder, which has only been treated medically so far. Currently she is taking the anti-depressant Escitalopram (SSRI), which does not show any effect.

In addition, she takes the medication Zolpidem twice a week. In a good night she then sleeps for about 6 h, but usually only 3–4 h.
Diagnostics

Psychopathological finding

For the admission interview comes a well-groomed, age-appropriate looking woman. In the first contact she appears exhausted, helpless, lost, unsure and yet open, sympathetic and motivated. In contact behavior, the patient appears adequate. The patient is awake and clear in consciousness, oriented to all qualities. The mnestic appears un disturbed. Perception and concentration are slightly restricted. The thinking is orderly, no indication of content-related thinking disorders. In the affect, the patient is fully modulated, she gives a depressed mood with strong brooding tendency. In terms of content, she describes thought complexes regarding the single daughter, her fear of the future, the sleep disorders and the loss of health. No information is given on perceptual disorders, nor on ego disorders. Psychomotorics are unspectacular, abstraction ability intact. There are social fears but no panic attacks. The patient reports of compulsive actions in the form of slightly pronounced control compulsions. Otherwise, there are no compulsions and obsessive thoughts. There are circadian peculiarities and pronounced sleep disorders. Motivation and drive are clearly restricted, leading to social withdrawal with suffering. There are pronounced appetite disorders with libido and appetite loss. There are no indications of foreign or self-endangerment. Current suicidality can be credibly denied, as well as the consumption of illegal substances. Mrs. G. drinks a glass of sparkling wine or cocktail on certain occasions or on vacation, but she has never smoked nicotine. She drinks coffee every day, but only in the morning.

Behavioral analysis Micro level (according to SORKC schema)

- Situation: The patient cannot fall asleep at night, lies awake, gets up too early in the morning, has to be alone in the apartment.
- Organism variables: The patient falls out of the "norm", has a lot of imagination, is dreamy and has great trust in people, she is criticized by her parents and society for this → low self-esteem
- Reaction:
  - Cognition: "I can't fall asleep again. I can't sleep again. Everything goes wrong. I'm afraid to be alone. I feel so helpless. I

have no desire for anything, nothing gives me pleasure. What is the meaning?"

- Emotion: depressed, worried, anxious, restless
- Physiological: exhausted, tense, tired, restless
- Behavior: The patient lies awake in bed, takes it easy during the day, withdraws from confrontational situations
- Consequences: The patient is exhausted during the day, not sufficiently tired at night, increasing tension (physical and emotional)
- Contingency: almost daily, otherwise severe sleep disorders

Superordinate Condition Analysis

- Predisposition: Depression, lack of lived emotionality and closeness with parents, death of parents, lack of confrontation experience
- Triggering Conditions: Turning point, death of parents, unfulfilled desire for children, disharmony in marriage, worry about daughter
- Sustaining Conditions: Lack of confrontation ability, no appropriate access to and dealing with thoughts and feelings
- Behavioral Deficits: Relaxation, active leisure time, social interaction, sexuality
- Behavioral Excesses: Patient lies awake in bed and broods, makes worried thoughts, watches TV
- Resources: Family, reflection, great motivation

Diagnoses

- F 51.0 Non-organic insomnia
- F 34.1 Dysthymia

Therapy
Therapeutic Goals
The following therapeutic goals were worked out and formulated together with the patient:

- Relief of sleep disorder, to no longer have the burdensome brooding phases and to be rested and fit during the day
- Reduction of the anxious and, above all, depressive symptomatology and stabilization at a good level
- Reduction of tension and restlessness
- Building of socially competent contacts to friends, the daughter and the husband, in order to be able to express and possibly assert one's own needs
- Becoming more self-confident and feeling comfortable in social relationships
- Becoming more productive during the day
- Learning to feel joy and to participate in life again

Prognosis
Mrs. G. has a high motivation to change, is punctual and works actively in therapy, so a good therapy success is to be expected.

Therapy plan At the beginning of therapy, the establishment of a complementary relationship and relieving conversations take place. Repeated behavioral analyses and mood and sleep protocols serve as the basis for developing a convincing disorder model (including the functionality of the symptoms in the current relationship), also against the biographical background. The focus of therapy is the alleviation of depression and sleep disorders as well as the reduction of anxiety problems. The sleep problems should first be analyzed in detail using sleep and behavior protocols. Psychoeducational modules on sleep hygiene, sleep architecture and associated error expectations are integrated as accompaniments. Conditions that lead to the patient not being able to fall asleep are analyzed in detail and corresponding individual countermeasures are offered (movement, healthy nutrition, daily structure, stress reduction, massages, etc.).

In order to reduce the always accompanying tension and restlessness, physiological and psychological relaxation is learned through progressive muscle relaxation, applied relaxation (according to Öst) or autogenic training, the implementation of which takes place in everyday exercise units. In general, an increase in interpersonal control conviction is sought by expanding one's own range of behavior. Likewise, an increase in feelings of self-competence should be achieved by allowing for clearer boundary setting (e.g. towards the husband and daughter), which can be used as structuring aids. Instructions are given for enjoyment, positive activation and social contact. The performance of role-plays with role reversal serves both diagnostic purposes and, on the other hand, is intended to improve social skills, in particular self-assertion towards family members. New positive learning experiences should be made when allowing for personal weaknesses. In addition, calming and behavior-regulating self-instructions are to be worked out. Furthermore, it is the goal to reduce self-doubt and reduce guilt feelings through cognitive restructuring (according to Beck). In particular, the techniques of de-catastrophization and reality testing are of particular importance here. In order to reduce social fears, confrontational methods/*risk taking* are to be used on a continuous basis. This is done by means of a worry confrontation (exposure in sensu), which is worked out and carried out together with the patient. Afterwards, confrontations take place in vivo, with previously avoided situations being visited and reassurance behavior being set.

Continuous feedback on updated problem behavior is a fixed component in therapy. Throughout the therapy process, focus should be on autonomy and assumption of responsibility. In the final hours, a look to the future and the development of relapse prevention take place.

In view of the severity of the disorder, 45 individual sessions are requested at a weekly frequency and 5 probationary hours.

Course of therapy In the first phase of therapy, almost exclusively relieving conversations take place at first. A complementary relationship is established. The patient has repeatedly heard and felt throughout her life that she must adapt and not be as she is. The patient is right here, exactly as she is. She does not fall out of the norm. Characteristics that were usually referred to as weaknesses can be worked out as strengths in therapy. First, old dreams, wishes and needs are brought to the surface and it is discussed what has been achieved and what has not. The patient is very bitter: "I've already missed everything. If only I … ". At this point, the first cognitive restructuring begins. Many things that appear to be missed can now be made up for in retirement. Things that were actually missed (e.g. a second child) can now finally be mourned and thus also processed. Mrs. G. orients herself anew and, for the first time in 30 years, does not need antidepressants over the winter months. There is a new orientation, a loosening of dysfunctional patterns and schemas. A significant reduction in depressive symptomatology can be achieved and confidence, hope and activity can be built up.

During the first phase of therapy, the clearly pronounced sleep symptomatology is already triggered, but it is not yet in the focus of therapy. Through the alleviation of the depressive symptomatology, the evening and night phases of brooding can be reduced and, to some extent, filled with beautiful thoughts and plans. This has the consequence that Mrs. G. no longer has any fear of going to bed and lying awake there. This in turn promotes relaxation. The parallel increase in activity (purchase of a small dog) increases the evening sleep pressure and the latency to sleep is shortened from an average of 120 min to 20 min. However, the pronounced sleep disorders continue.

When analysing sleep habits, it turns out that Mrs. G. has a significantly extended bedtime. She usually goes to bed at 10 p.m. and often does not get up until 10 a.m. due to the depressive morning low. The bedtime is therefore 12 h. About a bedtime restriction from 24:00 to 7:00, the sleep pressure can be further increased and the efficiency of the bedtime increased. Since Mrs. G. suffers from nocturnal bladder pressure, a urologist is consulted for advice, but he can not find an organic reason for the increased nocturnal urination. The bladder pressure therefore has a psychological cause. Therefore, the patient is trained to endure the bladder pressure and fall asleep again. At the end of therapy, the effective sleep time is 6–7 h.

In addition, the following therapy components are used: therapeutic use of light, psychoeducation, cognitive work, healthy nutrition, mindfulness and pleasure therapy. Mrs. G. tries to achieve more relaxation through fantasy journeys. This succeeds her above all when listening to music. Since Mrs. G. has lived socially rather withdrawn, the establishment of social contacts is supportive. Mrs. G. enjoys a lot of fun with friends. With the help of social competence training and role-playing, emancipation from the husband is possible. She can then formulate and, if necessary, also demand needs more clearly. She spends less time with her husband and also drives away with friends or starts activities.

There are regular fears that the symptoms could return or worsen. As part of relapse prevention, Mrs. G. can be given a "emergency kit" with useful exercises and behaviors in the event of a further deterioration of the symptoms. Overall, Mrs. G. feels much better.